The Great Psychotherapy Debate

The second edition of *The Great Psychotherapy Debate* has been updated and revised to expand the presentation of the Contextual Model, which is derived from a scientific understanding of how humans heal in a social context and explains findings from a vast array of psychotherapy studies. This model provides a compelling alternative to traditional research on psychotherapy, which tends to focus on identifying the most effective treatment for particular disorders through emphasizing the specific ingredients of treatment. The new edition also includes a history of healing practices, medicine, and psychotherapy; an examination of therapist effects; and a thorough review of the research on common factors such as the alliance, expectations, and empathy.

Bruce E. Wampold, PhD, ABPP, is the Patricia L. Wolleat Professor of Counseling Psychology at the University of Wisconsin–Madison and director of the Research Institute at Modum Bad Psychiatric Center in Vikersund, Norway.

Zac E. Imel, PhD, is an assistant professor with the counseling psychology program in the department of educational psychology and an adjunct assistant professor in the Department of Psychiatry at the University of Utah.

The Great Psychotherapy Debate

The Evidence for What Makes
Psychotherapy Work

Second Edition

Bruce E. Wampold and
Zac E. Imel

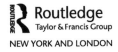

Routledge
Taylor & Francis Group

NEW YORK AND LONDON

Second edition published 2015
by Routledge
711 Third Avenue, New York, NY 10017

and by Routledge
27 Church Road, Hove, East Sussex BN3 2FA

Routledge is an imprint of the Taylor & Francis Group, an informa business
© 2015 Bruce E. Wampold and Zac E. Imel

First edition published by Routledge 2001

Library of Congress Cataloging-in-Publication Data

Wampold, Bruce E., 1948–
   The great psychotherapy debate : the evidence for what makes
psychotherapy work / by Bruce E. Wampold and Zac E. Imel. —
Second edition.
      pages cm
   Includes bibliographical references and index.
   1. Psychotherapy—Philosophy.   2. Psychotherapy—Evaluation.
I. Imel, Zac E.   II. Title.
   RC437.5.W35 2015
   616.89'14—dc23
   2014032867

ISBN: 978-0-8058-5708-5 (hbk)
ISBN: 978-0-8058-5709-2 (pbk)
ISBN: 978-0-203-58201-5 (ebk)

Typeset in Baskerville
by Apex CoVantage, LLC

To all of my collaborators, personal and professional, many of whom have made sacrifices so that this revision could be completed. BEW

To KT, Jiajia, and Lulu. ZEI

Contents

Preface

When one publishes a book with the word *debate* in the title, one must be prepared for rebuttals. In science, rebuttals are best presented as evidence. In the 13 years since the first edition, there have been many arguments about what makes psychotherapy work, best characterized by a debate between proponents of evidence-based treatments and proponents of common factors. This debate often mischaracterizes one side or the other, with more than a few instances when rhetorical accusations have predominated, rather than evidence.

Rhetoric does not keep me up at night but evidence surely does. And since the first edition, there have been many reasons for sleepless nights. As Zac and I discuss in this volume, psychotherapy evidence has proliferated since the first edition. The number of psychotherapy clinical trials and meta-analyses of these trials has increased exponentially. There is more evidence now for the effectiveness of psychotherapy than ever before. Would that evidence trend toward showing the scientific folly of the Contextual Model that I proposed in 2001? If so, then the Contextual Model would fall on the scrap heap of perfectly rational, but empirically unsupported, theories, including chemical theories of fermentation (spontaneous generation), light propagation through aether, and a static universe (Einstein's Universe). Yet, the research conducted in the last decade and a half has not produced evidence that seriously threatens the Contextual Model—indeed, the evidence for the Contextual Model is an order of magnitude stronger than it was in 2001.

In the preface to the first edition I spoke about the meaning of psychotherapy for me personally and dedicated the book in part to my therapist. Sadly, some have used this intimate story to say that my work is biased and should not be trusted. So, let me be clear about this—as is true of all humans, I do indeed have biases. However, one hallmark of science is that we intentionally put our biases aside and attend rationally to evidence. Moreover, the scientific endeavor is a correcting system in that evidence in the end will prevail and theories will be abandoned, despite their ability to attract adherents, should the evidence be sufficiently compelling. As with all theories, the current iteration of the Contextual Model will be modified as anomalies are detected—in the coming decades, evidence will likely emerge that both clarifies and complicates components of the model. In this process, my allegiance is to the evidence and there is no disgrace in having one's theory ultimately to be found in the same dustbin as Einstein's Static Universe.

This edition of *The Great Psychotherapy Debate* differs from the first edition in several ways. Of course, the research corpus is updated and the various chapters reflect the latest evidence. The first chapter now presents a brief history of medicine and psychotherapy to put the current debate into proper perspective. In 2001, the Contextual Model I proposed was just emerging from the work of Jerome Frank. During the last decade, the model has expanded based on social science research—the expanded model is presented in Chapter 2. As in the previous edition, there is a chapter (Chapter 3) that presents what evidence is to be considered and then discusses the conjectures of the Medical Model and the Contextual Model. As in the first edition, there are chapters that examine the evidence for absolute efficacy (Chapter 4), relative efficacy (Chapter 5), and therapists' effects (Chapter 6). In the first edition, evidence related to general effects was limited to a discussion of the therapeutic alliance. We have expanded this section to also include how placebos induce powerful expectations, as well as several other therapeutic factors hypothesized to be powerful in the Contextual Model (Chapter 7). Chapter 8 reviews the literature on the importance of specific ingredients. Chapter 9 makes conclusions related to theory, practice, and policy.

Books have authors. But authorship reflects an amalgamation of influences. To a large extent, my work was spawned from discussions with students and collaborations with colleagues around the world. Zac Imel, from his first days as my doctoral advisee over a decade ago, has challenged me to think deeply about the issues discussed in this edition and expand my methodological expertise. He would bring articles and books to me: "You have to read this!" and "We have to learn new methods to understand this issue," his restless mind collecting and synthesizing information from a variety of spheres. This edition has continued our intellectual collaboration, mutually stimulating and rewarding.

BEW, Madison, Wisconsin, April 1, 2014

Quite unintentionally, my psychology training began in small groups that were a part of church youth camps in the Red Rock Canyons of Oklahoma. I observed the work of talented group leaders who worked to replace emptiness and shame with acceptance and support. While many of my peers were taken with spiritual explanations for these experiences, in me they awoke an appreciation for open and emotionally charged relationships and provided an enduring template that continues to guide my relationships and inform my clinical work.

The intervention we discuss in this book is still mostly a human conversation—perhaps the ultimate in low technology. Something in the core of human connection and interaction has the power to heal. Ironically, the unavoidable complexity of unstructured, emotional dialogue poses an immense challenge to scientists who wish to know why it is that conversations with certain characteristics lead to improvements in psychological well-being, decreases in distress, and recovery from profoundly disabling mental health problems—while other conversations do not.

As we complete this second attempt to summarize the existing evidence for a general model of psychotherapy as outlined by the Contextual Model, we are confronted with interesting times for psychotherapy as a science and profession. Patients prefer psychotherapy as a first-line treatment for many problems, but psychotherapy continues to decrease as an overall percentage of mental health care. There is more evidence for the effectiveness of what therapists do and how they do it than ever before, but much remains unknown. Technology has revolutionized almost every aspect of human life, transforming science, medicine, entertainment, journalism, and social interaction. However, our current gold standard for evaluating the process of change in psychotherapy—human behavioral coding of patient–provider interactions—is based on 70-year old technology first used by Carl Rogers and his students. Simultaneously, computer scientists and electrical engineers have developed techniques that can model the words in all published books and automatically recognize speech from acoustic signal. The American Psychological Association released a general statement on the effectiveness of psychotherapy, but many contend that advocating for the effectiveness of psychotherapy generally is like talking about the effectiveness of "drugs." Instead, they argue we have scores of specific, evidenced-based treatments with demonstrated effectiveness. The Veterans Health Administration launched one of the largest psychotherapy quality improvement initiatives in history by disseminating specific psychotherapies into mental health specialty clinics, but regular monitoring of patient outcomes or provider behavior is mostly absent in community settings.

I am the son and grandson of accountants, engineers, and teachers, and thus it is not surprising that my rebellion into the practice of psychotherapy led back to an immersion in numbers and the academy. I first read The *Great Psychotherapy Debate* after graduating from a small liberal arts college where I thrived in the intellectual space between scientifically oriented psychology and a pluralistic religious studies department with professors who often shared lunch (and maybe a polite argument or two). In psychotherapy, I was frustrated by what I saw as a glut of "true believers" and the persistence of theoretical camps that seemed independent of the evidence. Thus, I was quickly taken by the parsimony of the common factors approach outlined in the book and Bruce's devotion to data and the scientific method. Upon arrival in Madison in 2003, I quickly began what I have come to recognize as an unusually close and productive collaboration, working and thinking about how to make sense of the beautiful mess that is psychotherapy data. Bruce encouraged my natural skepticism and curiosity, and Monday morning espressos were a time to poke holes in our own theories (as well as those of others, of course). I like to think my contributions to this volume began during those meetings.

ZEI, Salt Lake City, Utah, April 2014

Chapter I

History of Medicine, Methods, and Psychotherapy

Progress and Omissions

Examining only the current state of affairs in any field reveals recent trends but can obscure other critical issues. And often it is what is left behind in our efforts to attain progress that reveals much about the field. Psychotherapy, shaped by context, actors, and allied fields (particularly medicine), is no exception. The pursuit of progress—or maybe better said, the inevitable process of progress—comes with a cost. It may well be that what is cast off as archaic is actually the essence, and what is retained is a façade. On the other hand, innovation and progress can be achieved, and nostalgically clinging to the past can be damaging. In this book, a critical examination of the progress in psychotherapy is undertaken with attention to the hidden, forgotten, and ignored factors, as well as to the current practices, policies, and research.

A romantic notion is that progress is a result of knowledge—evidence driving innovation and practice. However, the modern view is that events are the result of human action, and human action is influenced by a myriad of factors, of which evidence is only one. But then, even the notion of evidence is problematic, as evidence is the interpretation of a pattern of data—interpretation is a human cognitive task subject to biases, power, methods, and constraints. The social sciences are particularly vulnerable to these vectors as precision is not great, replication is infrequent, and the subject matter is imbedded in cultural, political, and fiscal contexts. In most instances, psychotherapy exists within a health delivery system that exerts further pressure to progress along a narrow corridor. So constrained, psychotherapy exists as it is, but its future is to be determined, primarily by the actors whose influence is most boldly exerted. This book's thesis, which is outside the canonical view yet built upon the very evidence collected within that canon, provides an alternative course for the future. The course, which was abandoned some time ago and is updated here under the name "The Contextual Model," may, if we can be so bold, be the one that has more potential to benefit patients than the course presently being pursued.

Before the evidence can be presented for a contextual view of psychotherapy, there are certain consequences from history that need to be fully understood. How did we get here? And what was omitted to make certain progressions? Several intertwined stories need to be examined: the stories of medicine, research methods (particularly clinical trials), and psychotherapy. Of course, each of these histories could fill a volume on their own (indeed, there are several volumes on each), but abbreviated versions are sufficient to take notice of important elements.

Medicine

Medicine is the dominant healing practice in Western cultures. It is the application of scientific knowledge to cure disease, alleviate physical suffering, and prolong life. However, modern medicine is a recent invention and one that evolved from a tradition of healing practices, most of which medicine would rather not claim as antecedents.

The Origins of Medicine as a Healing Practice

Healing practices appear in the earliest humans and characterize, in an important way, the essential nature of humanness:

> According to Sir William Osler (1932), the desire to take medicine is one feature that distinguishes hominids from their fellow creatures.... Although nothing is known about the earliest medications or about the first physician, historians date the earliest portrait of a physician to Cro-Magnon times, 20,000 B.C. (Haggard, 1934; Bromberg, 1954). This horned tailed, hirsute, and animal-like apparition had great psychological effect, and it is likely that the treatment used was simply a vehicle for the psychological or placebo effect and was without any intrinsic merit (Model, 1955).
>
> (Shapiro & Shapiro, 1997b, p. 3)

Indeed, it is impossible to identify historically a civilization in which medicines, rituals, and healers were not central features of the culture (Shapiro & Shapiro, 1997b; Wilson, 1978). As societies evolved, the human mind was predisposed to generate explanations of physical, mental, and somatic phenomena (Gardner, 1998)—the particular explanations differed by culture and have evolved over time—but the art of using the explanations to create and apply treatments—that is, the practice of healing—has spanned both culture and time. Indeed, the nature of the healing practice is a large component of the description of any culture, as healing and other cultural practices are so intertwined. The Pythagoreans suggested that the body was composed of four humors (viz., blood, phlegm, yellow bile, and black bile), and personalities were manifestations of various mixtures of humors; illness resulted when the humors, which were thought to be affected by diet, weather, and climate, were unbalanced (Morris, 1997; Shapiro & Shapiro, 1997b; Wampold, 2001a). The Apache shaman, elaborately dressed in animal skins and masks and whose power derived from special status among the spirits or from possession of a sacred object, administered rituals involving dance, drums, rattles, prayers, and chants and to replace evils spirits with protective ones (Morris, 1997). Traditional Chinese medical practices, described in *The I Ching* (Book of Changes) and the *Huang Ti Nei Ching Su Wen* (The Yellow Emperor's Classic of Internal Medicine), postulated five elements: water, fire, wood, metal, and earth and combinations of the yin and yang; diseases were treated with five tastes, five types of grain, and five flavors (e.g., pungent food was used to prevent disintegration of the liver and sour food to drain the liver), supplemented by acupuncture, which has persisted as a Chinese treatment for more than 2,500 years (Shapiro & Shapiro, 1997b). Each with a medical explanation for its effect, the pharmacopoeias of European medicine of the seventeenth century contained such substances as Vigo's plaster (viper's flesh with live worms and frogs), fox lungs, moss from the skulls of victims of violent death, Gascoigne's powder (bezoar, amber, pearls, crab's eyes and claws, and coral), human urine, various sexual organs, excreta (from many different sources), human placenta, saliva from fasting individuals, and wood lice (Shapiro & Shapiro, 1997b).

There is no attempt to romanticize ancient or indigenous medical practices, as it is clear that many such healing practices were ineffective and some dangerous (Shapiro & Shapiro, 1997a,b). Hippocrates prescribed a diet that excluded vegetables and fruits, resulting in vitamin deficiencies. Acupuncture, due to unsterilized needles, caused homologous serum jaundice, a deadly disease that was prevalent in China for centuries and killed many. Dehydrating procedures, such as bloodletting, vomiting, enemas, and leeches "killed more patients than any other treatment in the history of medicine" (Shapiro & Shapiro, 1997a, p. 18). Indeed, George Washington was no doubt killed by his physician, who treated his abscessed tonsil with a variety of procedures that exacerbated the natural dehydration of fever. Nevertheless, effective or ineffective, cultures developed explanations for illness and developed treatments—each explanation and the associated treatment were consistent with the beliefs and practices of the culture and in many ways were defining features of the society.

Although the origins of Western scientific medicine can be traced to the ancient Greeks, the preponderance of the treatments in Europe and the United States remained ineffective, by modern standards of medicine, until at least the nineteenth century. The introduction of the twined concepts of materialism and specificity, arising in the Renaissance era, along with the concept of the *placebo*, allowed modern medicine to ride the crest of the wave created by science and the scientific method.

Materialism, Specificity, and the Placebo as Critical Concepts of Modern Medicine: The Contributions of René Descartes, Benjamin Franklin, and Louis Pasteur

Materialism, as a general philosophical term, considers matter as the sole basis of reality and thus attempts to explain phenomena as the consequence of the interaction of various types of matter. Applied to medicine, materialism implies that any bodily state, including most importantly illness, has a physical substrate. *Specificity*, which is a corollary of materialism, refers to the manner in which treatments render their effects. A treatment is said to be a specific treatment if the components of the treatment address illness by altering those physiochemical aspects of the body that were responsible for the illness. Generally, specificity in medicine relies on demonstrable alterations of the physiochemical process responsible for the disease and either a removal of the disease (i.e., cure) or a reduction in the severity of the disorder above what could be obtained through effects created by the mind by such factors as hope, expectation, and conditioning. Although materialism, as a philosophy, has been around since the ancient Greeks, establishing specificity in medicine depended on the development of the sciences of anatomy and physiology to explain the causes of disease and on the development of research design and statistical methods to appropriately test the effects of treatments.

Before Benjamin Franklin and Louis Pasteur could make their contributions to modern medicine, a philosophical issue needed to be resolved. For most of human history, there was no distinction between physical and mental disorders; indeed the sciences of anatomy and physiology were not sufficient to claim that physical disorders resided in the body and mental disorders in the mind. The imbalances in the Pythagorean humors were sufficient to explain physical and mental disorders and there was no corroboration or refutation of the conjecture relative to these disorders possible. (Of course, the idea of refutation of hypotheses empirically was not yet developed, so it wasn't simply a lack of knowledge of anatomy and physiology.) If medicine were to find the material bases of disorders, it would be in the arena of physical disorders and the distinction between physical and mental disorders was consequently necessary. It was René Descartes, in the early seventeenth century, who made the distinction between mind and body, although it was not his purpose to be at the service of the development of medicine, as he was interested in the mind in an ontological sense. Nevertheless, the distinction placed anatomy and physiology, which were now subject to observation, on an empirical track; the mind remained in the metaphysical realm and, in a manner of speaking, became the province of psychology. Of course, as a note, there is much interest in the past few decades on the interaction of mind and body, and advances in the neurosciences are eliminating, according to some perspectives, the notion of the mind as distinct from the body—rather the mind is what the brain does (Miller, 1996).

As science and the scientific method were evolving in Europe in the Cartesian context, it became apparent that most of the substances in the pharmacopoeias were not effective. Indeed, only a very few seemed to be effective for particular diseases (e.g., foxglove for congestive heart conditions and cinchona bark for malaria) (Shapiro & Shapiro, 1997b). In 1785 the term *placebo* entered the medical lexicon and was applied to treatments that were known to be ineffective physiochemically but satisfied the patient's desire to be treated (Shapiro & Shapiro, 1997b). The term, according to Walach (2003), originated from the Latin psalm verse, "Placebo Domino in regione vivorum" ("I shall *please* the Lord in the land of the living"), which was sung in the Middle Ages as a prayer at the deathbed. Because others were often paid to do the singing, the term placebo became associated with a "nearly fraudulent replacement of the real" (Walach, 2003, p. 178). As will become apparent in subsequent discussions, placebo and the effects that are derived from them are deeply imbedded in several controversies in medicine and in psychotherapy; from the perspective of this volume, an understanding of the placebo effect is critical to an understanding of psychotherapy. Nevertheless, the term placebo, from its origin, has retained a tainted connotation—administration of a substance simply to please the patient became repugnant and claims that a "placebo" was curative would risk being labeled a charlatan, as Franz Anton Mesmer was soon to find out.

Contemporaneous to the development of the notion of the placebo, the Parisian physician Mesmer had a lucrative medical practice. It was populated with the elite of Paris but was also controversial. In his dissertation, Mesmer (1766/1980) claimed that some illnesses were caused by the blockage of the normal flow of an invisible universal fluid, which he called *animal magnetism*. The physician could restore health by removing the blocks, and after further "research," Mesmer found that he could "magnetize" objects with animal magnetism and these could be used to cure his clients (Buranelli, 1975; Gallo & Finger, 2000; Gauld, 1992; Pattie, 1994). The success of this treatment was well documented and led to its immense popularity in the late eighteenth century.

Mesmer, already caught up in several controversies, came under intense scrutiny. Medicine, wanting to disavow practices that were unscientific, found Mesmer's cures uncomfortable. Responding to these forces, King Louis XVI of France established in 1784 a Royal Commission, chaired by Benjamin Franklin, to investigate mesmerism (Gould, 1991). Some of the experiments designed by the commission involved patients being split into two groups, with one group coming into contact with "magnetized" objects and the other group coming into contact with what they believed were "magnetized" objects (i.e., according to modern terminology, a placebo). Care was taken to ensure that the patients did not know whether they were receiving a magnetized object or not, creating one of the first, if the not the first, rigorous blinding in a study (here, a single blind). This design enabled the Royal Commission to demonstrate, as there were no differences in the cures produced by the two groups, that Mesmer's cures did not occur through treatment-specific ingredients.

The noted natural historian Stephen Jay Gould (1989) heralded the testing and discrediting of Mesmer as one of the earliest and exemplary demonstrations of the use of the scientific method to expose pseudoscience and charlatanism. However, imbedded in the Mesmer story are two points that should not be lost in this progressive story. First, Mesmer's treatments were effective, as noted by the Royal Commission—benefits to patients were observable. Second, Mesmer's theories of illness and treatment were grounded in the best science available, namely the theories proposed by Sir Isaac Newton, who only a century earlier had crossed the threshold from a fascination with the occult to the origins of mechanics and the advancement of mathematics (Gleick, 2003). Thus Mesmer was discredited not based on treatment effectiveness or theoretical cogency but on the observation that the proposed mechanism of illness remediation was questionable. This is a standard that mental health treatments, pharmacological as well as psychological, will have, as we will see, a difficult time satisfying. Of course, Mesmer's exposure as a charlatan was a conspicuous event that furthered medicine as a profession.

The third seminal person in the development of modern medicine was Louis Pasteur, the father of germ theory (actually, paternity questions could be raised by Robert Koch, who has a legitimate claim of fatherhood). Pasteur exhibited the optimal blend of theory and experiment to, as the philosopher Ernest Renan noted, "interrogate nature" until certain proofs of conjectures were accomplished. The unifying theme, if one could characterize discoveries across a vast array of areas as a theme, of his work is that Pasteur was able to make inferences about the existence and characteristics of entities too small to be observed directly. The story of how he made fermentation *alive* provides an important anecdote about the inevitable interactions between epistemological and ontological contributions (Latour, 1999).

In the 1850s, chemistry, having thrown off the vestiges of alchemy and finding itself the preeminent field of science, sought chemical explanations for most natural phenomena, including biological processes. The canonical view at the time was that fermentation was the decay of sugars into alcohol by a catalytic but unobserved "disintegrating disturbance," which could be transferred from one batch of fermenting solution to another. Unfortunately for alcohol producers, the process was unreliable and the chemical explanation provided had little pragmatic value. Based on his prior work in crystallography of organic substances, keen observation, and systematic experimentation, Pasteur hypothesized that living microorganisms were responsible for fermentation, rather than being created spontaneously as a result of the process. This discovery led to other conclusions, including the conjecture that disease was caused by microorganisms, which constituted the origins of the germ theory of disease. The pairing of theory and experimentation resulted in medical practices with demonstrable benefits—vaccines using compromised organisms, sterilization of medical environments, and sterilization of foods by heat (i.e., "pasteurization").

Two aspects of the Pasteur story are critical, one quite obvious in retrospect and the other illustrative of more subtle implications for the philosophy of science. Materialism applied to medicine requires physical explanations for illness—the germ theory was exactly "what the doctor ordered." Not only could disease be cured or prevented, but the underlying mechanism could be explicated in a demonstrable manner. To be sure, there was no lack of hypothesized mechanisms prior to Pasteur. It was his beautifully constructed and in the end inconvertible demonstration of how microorganisms caused disease and the developments that followed as a result that changed the status of the explanations.

From today's perspective, the ontological nature of disease was clearly advanced as a result of Pasteur's work on fermentation and the idea of spontaneous generation seems absurd (see Latour, 1999), which brings us to the second point relative to Pasteur. In 1864 the epistemological battle was just beginning to be fought. At the time chemical decomposition was accepted as *the* explanation for fermentation; the microbes observed were due to spontaneous generation as a result rather than the cause of fermentation. Proponents of a microorganismic explanation for fermentation, and there were some, were considered lunatics, in the way we now think of Mesmer. The organisms were *there*, in retrospect, and *not there*, in a contemporaneous way. In the 1860s, the disintegrating disturbance that catalyzed fermentation and the microbes that caused fermentation both were unobservable. Pasteur not only ingeniously designed the experiments so that the organisms could make themselves known and constructed the theory to provide the cogency of the experimental results, but he rhetorically, in papers and presentations, convinced the scientific world of the merit of his explanation—the latter as difficult as the former. In a sense, Pasteur and the microorganisms conspired together; neither one alone could have spawned the germ explanation of disease (Latour, 1999).

What constitutes knowledge in a given field depends, in part, on the people who conduct the research, create the theories, and influence the scientific community, particularly in the social sciences. Knowledge at any given time, as we will argue in this volume, is tenuous—the nature of psychotherapy makes itself known in response to our inquiries, but the nature of those inquiries shapes what we accept as knowledge. We, as researchers, clinicians, and policymakers, influence what is said to be knowledge. Descartes, Franklin, and Pasteur played critical roles in developing, along with others in this the critical period of the nineteenth century, the components that were necessary to form the model of modern medicine.

The Medical Model

The Medical Model, undergirded by materialism and specificity and existing within anatomy, physiology, microbiology, and other biological sciences, is, for our purposes, composed of five components.

Illness or Disease

The first component is an illness or disease. The patient reports to the physician with signs and symptoms, which, along with the history, examination, and laboratory tests, leads to a determination first whether the patient's condition is abnormal (i.e., deviates from what is considered normal human biological functioning) and second, if abnormality exists, a diagnosis. Some interventions are designed to prevent illness (e.g., vaccines); such preventative interventions generally conform to the Medical Model as well.

Biological Explanation

The second component, emanating from the materialistic stance of medicine, is that there is a biological explanation for the illness or disorder. For instance, influenza is caused by a virus, which invades cells in the nose, throat, and lungs of humans, where it replicates and mutates. Of course, the explanation progressively becomes more sophisticated as science illuminates the process. Not infrequently, an explanation will turn out to be false and will be supplanted with a better alternative, as was the progression of the explanation of peptic ulcers from excess acid due to stress or spicy diet to the presence of the bacterium *H. pylori*. Of course, the materialistic stance of medicine dictates that the explanation be biological—something related to the anatomy or physiology of the body.

Mechanism of Change

The third component of the Medical Model is that the basis for treatment be established at the level of the biological system causing the disease and a conjecture about how changing an aspect of the system will eliminate the disease or mitigate the severity or duration of the illness. When the cause of peptic ulcers was thought to be acids produced by the stomach due to stress or diet, the mechanism of change involved neutralizing acids and changing diets, whereas if an *H. pylori* infection were verified, the mechanism of change would involve reducing the population of the bacteria with antibiotics.

Therapeutic Procedures

The presence of an explanation and the mechanism of change lead logically to the design of a treatment, containing therapeutic procedures, which might involve administration of a substance (i.e., a drug) or implementation of a procedure (e.g., surgery). The explanation of excess acid due to stress (the explanation) and the goal to reduce acid (mechanism of change) would suggest the administration of a substance known to neutralize acid (i.e., an alkaline substance, such as an antacid containing calcium carbonate). If an infection of *H. pylori* is verified, then the therapeutic ingredient would be an antibiotic. Medical treatments generally require that the therapeutic procedures be consistent with the explanation for the illness, disease, or disorder and the mechanism of change.

Specificity

Mesmer's treatments based on animal magnetism conformed to the first four components of the Medical Model: patients presented with signs and symptoms of illness, there was a biological explanation for the disorder, a hypothesized mechanism of change existed, and a particular therapeutic procedure was followed. Mesmer's treatment, however, failed the specificity test. Specificity in the context of medicine, as already discussed, implies that the components of the treatment are remedial through alterations of physiochemical aspects of the body that were responsible for the illness. Antibiotics for peptic ulcers are specific to the degree to which they work by killing the bacteria rather than through other means, including but not limited to hope, expectation, or conditioning. Mesmer's cures were not specific because animal magnetism was shown not to be responsible for the benefits of his treatments.

In medicine, specificity is established in two primary ways. First, the treatment can be shown to be more effective than a placebo treatment, thus ruling out incidental causes related to the context of the treatment. For example, with adequate controls, if a pill is superior to a placebo, then presumably it is for reasons unrelated to whether the patient expects the pill to be effective or is conditioned to respond to pills in general (e.g., see Hentschel, Brandstätter, Dragosics, Hirschl, Nemec, et al., 1993). The development of the randomized placebo control group will be reviewed and the logic of the design discussed in the following section.

The second means to establish specificity is to establish that the medical treatment operates through its intended mechanism. Administration of antibiotics leads to a decrease in *H. Pylori*, which subsequently leads to healing of the ulcer, lending support for the explanation and the mechanism of change and thus lending support for specificity—the antibiotic works through the intended mechanism (see Hentschel et al., 1993). Indeed, much of Pasteur's research was focused on explanation, mechanism, and specificity. Studies of the mechanisms of disease and the effects of treatment on the intervening biological systems often precede the clinical trials that are used to establish efficacy. There are, however, salient instances in which a drug is known to be effective but for unknown reasons. *Acetylsalicylic acid* (commonly known as aspirin) was used as an analgesic, anti-inflammatory, and antipyretic (fever reducer) before its biological mechanisms were understood.

Adaptation of the Medical Model to psychotherapy is a controversial project, which in many ways is the subject of this volume. As we will see, the development of psychotherapy as a treatment for mental disorders is entwined with the development of medicine. Medicine, of course, is the predominant force and psychotherapy is subordinate.

Evidence-Based Medicine

The development of the Medical Model and the genesis of "modern medicine" without much argument resulted in positive health outcomes, including cures of many diseases and prevention of others. To wit, small pox has been eradicated, poliomyelitis is prevented by vaccine, deaths due to post-surgical infection are rare, and antibiotics are able to treat most bacterial infections. Nevertheless, materialism and specificity as the ontological bases of medicine and the progress made by discrediting charlatans and creating a laboratory science of microbiology did not directly translate into implementation of treatments that resulted in optimal outcomes for patients. One hundred twenty-five years after Mesmer's treatments were subjected to examination and more than 50 years after Pasteur debunked spontaneous generation and established the germ theory of disease, medicine clung to many "primitive" practices. Prior to the First World War and the influenza epidemic of 1918, the typical medical school in the United States was unaffiliated with a college or university, was staffed by part-time faculty whose salaries were paid directly from student fees, was populated by students who had not taken any science courses, let alone attended college, and depended on a curriculum in which students never examined or treated patients and infrequently used laboratory equipment (Barry, 2004). In 1910, the Flexner report changed the nature of medical education in the United States and Canada, and in a relatively short period of time medical education became rigorous, competitive, and scientific. Nevertheless, little was known about the efficacy of many medications and procedures—indeed, it was not until the 1950s that the randomized placebo control group design was developed, and it was not until 1980 that the Food and Drug Administration (FDA) required such designs be used to approve drugs in the United States, as discussed in the next section.

Numerous examples can be found to document how medical practice has ignored accumulating evidence. For our purposes, the case of streptokinase, an enzyme that dissolves clots, as a treatment for acute myocardial infarction is illustrative (Hunt, 1997). Clinical trials of streptokinase began as early as 1959, but the results, due to small sample sizes, were inconclusive, as some found a significantly better outcome than the placebo control group while others did not. However, as early as 1969 there was sufficient evidence, had the trials been meta-analyzed, to conclude that this intervention was effective. Iain Chalmers, an early advocate of meta-analyses as a means to make conclusions that could be translated into medical practice, made the following observation:

> Streptokinase was the classic example. The meta-analyses showed clearly that the effect on mortality was statistically significant, but the experts in cardiology and the textbook authors whose opinions dominated the field weren't even beginning to recommend it until the late 1980s, and then only little by little.
>
> (quoted in Hunt, 1997, p. 87)

From the time the evidence was persuasive to the time streptokinase was accepted as standard practice following FDA approval in 1987, it is estimated that tens of thousands of patients died because they were not administered streptokinase.

The streptokinase example is one of many that led to the initiation of a movement to ensure that research evidence was translated into practice. This movement, called *evidence-based medicine,* initiated in the United Kingdom and Canada, emphasizes systematic and analytic reviews of evidence and the use of that evidence by clinicians. In 2001, the Institute of Medicine in the United States adopted the following definition, following closely from Sackett, Straus, Richardson, Rosenberg, and Haynes (2000): "Evidence-based practice is the integration of best research evidence with clinical expertise and patient values" (p. 147). This definition has been described as a "three legged stool," in that the use of evidence (first leg) is to be balanced with the expertise of the clinician (second leg) and characteristics and context of the patient (third leg). Nevertheless, an examination of the seminal book on evidence-based medicine, *Evidence-based Medicine: How to Practice and Teach EBM* (Sackett et al., 2000) reveals that the focus is on evidence related to the quality of diagnostic tests and effectiveness of treatments.

Intimately tied to the evolution of modern medicine is the development of methods that could establish specificity, most importantly the randomized double-blind placebo control group design. Consequently, our story now turns to the history of this design.

Randomized Designs as the "Gold Standard"

Randomized designs were needed by medicine to discriminate effects due to the purported active ingredients from those due to the "mind," such as hope, expectation, and relationship with the administrator of the substance or procedure. What is now known as the double-blind randomized placebo control group design, which is the "gold standard" for FDA approval of drugs, is a relatively recent invention. The history of the development of this design is critical to understanding the current status of psychotherapy as well as medicine and will reveal some important aspects of the therapeutic process that were omitted.

The Development of Randomization and Comparison Designs

Three strands, according to Danziger (1990), were intertwined to develop the notion of control group designs. The first strand emanated from Wilhelm Wundt, who established experimentation in psychology. In Wundt's laboratory, he and his students were *observers,* as they conceived of themselves as trained scientists who could report on and interpret aspects of the mind, much in the way that a physicist would interpret the photographic trace of a particle in a cloud chamber. Wundt and the students would design experimental protocols and manipulate various stimuli to record the effects, which were based on reports of internal perception (i.e., one type of introspection). The stimulus/response contiguity was the predominant model in experimental physiology at the time.

The responses reported by the Wundt's observers were typically "judgments of size, intensity, and duration of physical stimuli, supplemented at times by judgments of their simultaneity and succession" (Danziger, 1990, p. 35) and were used to derive general laws, mainly of sensation and perception.

At around the time of Wundt's laboratory experiments, the notion of "subjecting" lay individuals to various conditions can be traced to experimental studies of hypnosis in France and constitutes the second strand. These studies differed in an important way from Wundt's—the French scientists were the experimenters and the patients were *subjects*, a clear departure from the Wundtian tradition in which the scientists were subjected to experiments and also were observers (and authors of the research reports). That is, in the French context the role of the experimenter (the observer) and the role of the subject were separated. The change in role allowed the observation of classes of subjects who were not able to report internal states (e.g., children) and/or whose reports were suspect (e.g., people with mental illnesses). The paradigm, largely steeped in the French medical context, inevitably evolved into clinical research in that "healthy subjects" were compared to abnormal subjects with the goal of discovering essential differences between the two classes (Danziger, 1990). Nevertheless, in these experiments, the experimenter, a physician, had a professional relationship with the patients. It should be noted, for historical accuracy, sporadic examples of comparisons of various samples existed before the French physician studies (e.g., James Lind's experiments with scurvy in the eighteenth century), but the idea of "subjecting" participants to treatments appears to be derived from this French tradition.

The third strand involved "applicants," rather than observers or subjects, and the "applicants" were not abnormal, at least at the origin of this strand. The applicants were volunteers who paid to have their "mental faculties" tested by Francis Galton in England, many at the International Health Exhibition in London in 1884. During this period, phrenology was widely accepted as a means of assessing mental abilities and there was keen interest in knowing where one stood in *relation* to others. To accomplish such comparisons, Galton and other British social statisticians, such as Karl Pearson, needed to quantify mental ability and to locate that quantity in a distribution of scores—the important determination was how one's score *deviated* from the average (Danziger, 1990; Desrosières, 1998). In this approach, the relationship between investigator and subject was minimal: "For the Galtonian investigator the individual subject was ultimately 'a statistic'" (Danziger, 1990, p. 58). The British statistical approach contributed the critical concepts of measurement of unobservable characteristics (in this case, mental abilities) and statistical distributions of such characteristics, critical components of analysis of the observation in randomized control group designs. These contributions were made in the context that led to what was considered normal or above average mental abilities and thus logically to a class of people who were mentally defective (i.e., those who were not normal or above average). Unfortunately, this led as well to calibration of "genetic worth," which using the principles of Charles Darwin's (Galton's cousin) theory of evolution, spawned the field of eugenics (see Desrosières, 1998).

Wundt introduced laboratory methods in psychology and attempted to extract general rules. The French researchers devised designs in which the experimenter subjected research participants to various conditions and compared abnormal to normal persons. The British social statisticians provided the statistical theory related to deviations from the mean. These were all critical components of clinical trials in medicine and psychotherapy, but the missing component to this mix was randomization. The impetus for that critical component came, in part, from the desire to provide pragmatic knowledge to various consumer groups. Academic psychologists deemed education an apt context to demonstrate the utility of their nascent discipline. In the early 1920s, the treatment group methodology was "being sold to American school superintendents as the 'control experiment' and touted as a key element in comparing the 'efficiency' of various administrative measures" (Danziger, 1990, p. 114). Shortly thereafter, McCall (1923) published *How to Experiment in Education*, which introduced control group experimentation in education and discussed the notion of randomization. At about the same time, Sir Ronald Fisher took a position at an agricultural station where he developed the analysis of variance and various other procedures for comparing crop yields (Gehan & Lemak, 1994). Fisher's work in randomized experimental designs and the analysis of data derived from such designs was absolutely stunning—arguably the design and analysis of every clinical trial in medicine, psychology, and education is based on methods developed by Fisher (Danziger, 1990; Shapiro & Shapiro, 1997b) or derived from his work. Fisher's publications, most prominently *The Design of Experiments*, which appeared in 1935, became particularly useful to medical researchers eager to show the efficacy of various medications, although one additional component, the placebo control, was needed (Gehan & Lemak, 1994).

Introduction of Placebo Controls to Rule Out Nuisance Variables

The goal of modern medicine was to establish that the benefits of any medical treatment were due to the physiochemical properties of the medication and not to the patient's expectations, hopes, or other psychological processes, thereby establishing the specificity of the purported active ingredients of the medication. To rule out threats due to these psychological factors, researchers in the late 1930s began to use double-blind placebo studies in the United States and the United Kingdom, but the method did not take root, apparently because placebo carried a negative connotation (Gehan & Lemak, 1994; Shapiro & Shapiro, 1997a, b). Gradually however, the acceptance of the randomized double-blind placebo design spread. Harry Gold, a pharmacologist and one of those given credit for the development of the placebo control group design in the United States, participated in several conferences at Cornell University on the subject in the late 1940s and early 1950s; he became the first professor of *clinical pharmacology*, a new discipline. As noted by Shapiro and Shapiro (1997b):

> Gold advocated a comparison between "an allegedly potent agent and a blank of such physical properties as to render a distinction between the two impossible except through some pharmacologic potency which may exist. . . . [the recommended] double-blind procedure which calls for an investigation in which neither the patient nor the doctor is aware of the identify of the two agents until the results are in and analyzed. This is imperative to avoid the influence of subconscious bias . . ." (Gold, 1954, p. 724). The statement by Gold culminated twenty years of pioneering study of methods with which to reliably and validly evaluate the effectiveness of new drugs.
>
> (p. 148)

By 1980, the FDA required that evidence for the effectiveness of a drug be obtained from randomized double-blind placebo trials—historically speaking, a relatively recent development (see Figure 1.1).

The importance of the randomized double-blind placebo control group design methodologically and conceptually should not be underestimated. It took more than 300 years from Descartes' dualism of mind and body and nearly 200 years from the time that Mesmer was discredited on specificity claims to the institutionalization of a design that could rule out psychological threats to the establishment of the specific effects of substances on the body (see Figure 1.1).

Before leaving the short history of experimental designs, it is worth reiterating that there are two critical features of the randomized double-blind placebo control group design. The first is that the placebo administered as a control for psychological factors should be indistinguishable from the treatment in all respects. For trials of medications, the pharmaceutical industry manufactures placebos that are identical to the purportedly active medications in taste, shape, color, and form. One of the problems, as will be discussed in later chapters, is that subjects will try to guess which condition they are in and will use any cues available (e.g., the presence or absence of side effects).

The second critical feature of the randomized double-blind placebo control group is related to blinding. In actuality, the "double-blind" moniker refers to a triple-blind: the administrator of the intervention, the patient, and the evaluator, throughout the study, are ignorant of which treatment (medication or placebo) the patient is receiving. Any deviation from the blind could result in bias, either directly (e.g., by an evaluator who might unconsciously score a protocol to favor the medication) or through cues provided to the patient (e.g., greater enthusiasm when delivering the medication than when delivering the placebo). Issues in blinding will be discussed in subsequent chapters.[1]

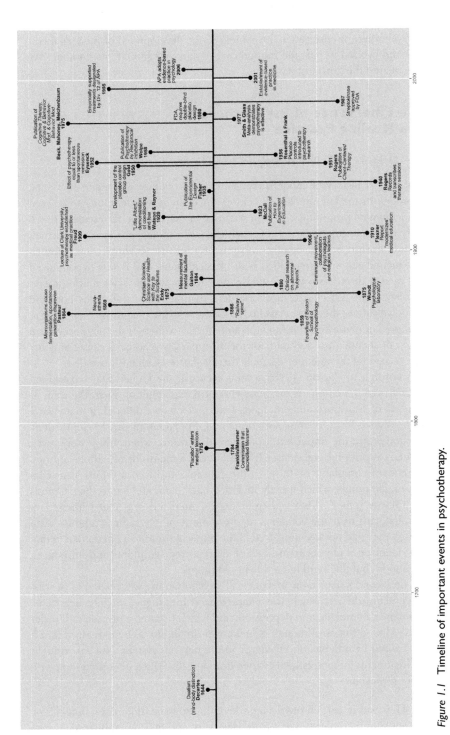

Figure 1.1 Timeline of important events in psychotherapy.

Psychotherapy emerged in the context of the development of modern medicine and utilized in part the randomized design to legitimate its standing. We now turn to the third history.

The Emergence of Psychotherapy as a Healing Practice

The Origins of Talk Therapy in the United States

In the short history of modern medicine, little mention was made of mental disorders. In the late nineteenth century, medicine was attempting to be seen as a legitimate profession based on scientific principles, and as discussed previously, medicine emphasized physiochemical (i.e., somatic) processes. Medicine's attitude toward mental health problems was one of psychophysical parallelism: mental states corresponded with physical states and it was hypothesized that mental disorders were caused by some (unknown) physiochemical process (Caplan, 1998). Of course, most disorders, mental or physical, at the time had unknown causes; they were classified as *functional* (cause unknown) as opposed to *structural* (i.e., cause known). Attempts were made to discover the physiochemical causes of mental disorders and, for the most part, psychosocial causes and any type of mental therapeutics (e.g., talk therapy) were assiduously avoided.

According to Caplan (1998), several events in the United States conspired to challenge the emphasis on physiochemical explanations. First, the train as a means of transportation emerged. Trains, of course, differed in many ways from previous forms of transportation, but for purposes of the development of psychotherapy, the important aspect was that trains, when things went awry, created catastrophic collisions, which produced a multitude of various injuries. A frequent complaint of those in the collisions involved a diffuse constellation of symptoms, which usually included back pain, and led to the diagnosis of "railway spine." What was troubling for medicine was that witnesses on the platforms near the collisions reported many of the same symptoms even though they had not been involved in the physical trauma, a phenomenon that cast doubt on a physiochemical cause of reported symptoms and introduced the notion that the mind has a role in symptoms.

The second perspicuous precursor of psychotherapy was related to the disorder neurasthenia, which was characterized by fatigue, anxiety, headache, impotence, neuralgia, and depression, and which became a prevalent disorder in the United States. Although of unknown origin, it was hypothesized that it was caused by a depletion of energy in the nervous system. Not surprisingly, the treatments for neurasthenia varied dramatically, which interested some prescient physicians:

> How was it, certain physicians asked, that so many different modalities of somatic therapies ranging from electricity and hydrotherapy to diet, rest,

nutrition, and medication could achieve identical results? Might they not share a common ground? Deducing from the variegated experiences of a wide array of somatic treatments, the Boston neurologist Morton Prince declared, "I think if these treatments are carefully analyzed it will be found that there is one factor common in them all, namely, the *psychical* element."

(emphasis added, Caplan, 1998, p. 45)

Needless to say, the introduction of the psyche in medical circles was not well received.

The third precursor to psychotherapy was development in various contexts of "mind cures." In the mid- to end of the nineteenth century, as medicine concentrated on the physiochemical, an increasing number of Americans turned toward practices that healed through the mind, most popular of which were Christian Science and the New Thought movement. Although these movements may seem to be relics of the past or marginalized religious practices, they were immensely popular (Caplan, 1998; Taylor, 1999). Christian Science, with only about 9,000 members in 1890, had more than 50,000 by 1906 (Caplan), which perhaps seems a modest number, but Christian Science was only one of many institutions that claimed to physically heal through mind, faith, or spirituality. Cushman (1992) attributes the popularity of these movements to the lack of a spiritual core in America and the desire to break free of the rigidity of a Victorian society (see also Taylor, 1999).

At first, medicine deliberately dismissed these movements, for the most part, as unscientific attempts to cure illnesses, whether physical or mental. Legitimacy lagged popularity, but gradually the involvement of American psychologists lent credibility to the idea of talk therapy as distinct from the religious movements. The Boston School of Psychopathology, initiated in 1859, which was an informal group of investigators, including the psychologists William James and G. Stanley Hall as well as neurologists and psychiatrists, was to become the epicenter of the new talk therapy. In 1906, the Emmanuel Movement was initiated as a collaboration between physicians who recognized the importance of the psyche and Christian ministers who recognized the moral aspect to behavior; lectures and services were followed by the administration of "therapy" to patients (Caplan, 1998; Taylor, 1999). The particularly threatening aspect of the Emmanuel Movement for medicine was that *patients* were being *treated* by psychical methods and often by non-physicians.

The manifestation of physical symptoms in the absence of physical cause, the efficacy of various incompatible treatments for a prevalent disorder, and the increasing popularity and legitimacy of talk therapies for physical and mental disorders were problematic for the emerging modern medical profession. And thus a dilemma for medicine: reject the emerging psychotherapeutics because it treated psychic disorders with non-medical means (viz., talk) or absorb the lucrative professional practice of mental therapeutics. Interestingly, talk therapies in America at this period had a connection with those interested in Mesmer's cures, which surely aroused the suspicions of physicians (Caplan, 1998; Cushman, 1992). Given the context, it is not surprising that medicine resisted acknowledging mental factors in the etiology, pathology, and treatment of mental disorders, and efforts were made to discredit mental therapeutics. On the other hand, some psychologists, although not all by any means, were interested in such treatments and their mechanisms: "As early as 1894, [William] James publicly assailed a proposal to proscribe the practice of mental healing, 'What the real interest of medicine requires,' James proclaimed, 'is that mental therapeutics should *not* be stamped out, but studied, and its laws ascertained'" (Caplan, 1998, p. 63).

In the end, medicine could not allow patients to be treated outside of the medical authority and it exerted its professional privilege to conduct psychotherapy. The sentiment was expressed by prominent physician John K. Mitchell, "Most earnestly should we insist that the *treatment* of a patient, whether it be surgical, medical, or psychic, should for the safety of the public, be in the hands of a doctor" (Caplan, 1998, p. 142). What was missing was a cogent theory of mental disorder and that would soon be provided.

Theoretical Orientations

Freud and the Origins of Psychodynamic Psychotherapy

When Sigmund Freud gave his lectures at Clark University in 1909, talk therapy was established as a legitimate medical practice in the United States, but he provided the missing theoretical coherence and all the better that it was provided by a physician and in the medical context. Within six years, psychoanalysis had become the predominant form of psychotherapy in the United States: "Psychoanalysis appeared to be more proper and civilized than mind cure, more scientific than Christian Science and positive thinking, and more medical than advertising" (Cushman, 1992, p. 38).

Sigmund Freud, in his practice as a physician, became involved with the treatment of hysterics. He proposed that a) hysteric symptoms were caused by the repression of some traumatic event (real or imagined) in the unconscious; b) the nature of the symptom was related to the event; and c) the symptom could be relieved by insight into the relationship between the event and the symptom. Moreover, from the beginning (as in his discussion of Anna O.), sexuality became central to the etiology of hysteria, with many symptoms associated with early sexual traumas. Freud experimented with various techniques to retrieve repressed memories, including hydrotherapy, hypnosis, and direct questioning, eventually promoting free association and dream analysis. From these early origins of psychoanalysis, the components of the Medical Model were apparent: a disorder (hysteria), a scientifically based explanation of the disorder (repressed traumatic events), a mechanism of change (insight into unconscious), and specific therapeutic actions (free association).

During his lifetime, Freud and his colleagues differed on various aspects related to theory and therapeutic action, creating irreconcilable rifts with such luminaries as Joseph Breuer, Alfred Adler, and Carl Jung, the latter two of whom were expelled from Freud's Vienna Psychoanalytic Society. The Medical Model is characterized by insistence on the correct explanation of a disorder and adoption of the concomitant therapeutic actions that are responsible for the patient benefits. Freud insisted that his theory was correct and that his treatments were specific and supported by scientific evidence. Although from a current vantage point, the empirical bases of Freudian psychoanalysis and competing systems (e.g., Adler's individual psychology or Jung's analytic psychology) seem to be tenuous, at best, there are claims that neuroscience has corroborated many psychodynamic constructs and theory (e.g., Westen, 1998). Regardless of the debates about the scientific merit of psychodynamic concepts, it should be realized that Freud's complex theories were introduced prior to Flexner's report and the reformation of medicine that resulted; that is, the substance and bases for Freud's claims were suitable for the period in which they occurred.

One critical point for our history of psychotherapy is related to the degree to which psychotherapy for the first half of the twentieth century was the province of medicine. As we have seen, psychotherapy was already incorporated into medicine at the turn of the century and Freud, a physician, provided an explanation acceptable to the medical profession. Moreover, admittance to psychoanalytic institutes and the practice of psychoanalysis was limited primarily to physicians, further defining psychotherapy as a medical practice. Interestingly, Freud himself trained lay (i.e., non-physician) analysts, the most notable of whom was Theodore Reik, who was charged with the crime of practicing medicine without a license. Although Reik was acquitted, upon Freud's death, access to the psychoanalytic institutes for non-physicians, including psychologists, was further restricted (VandenBos, Cummings, & DeLeon, 1992). As noted by Jerome Frank (1992), until mid-century, in the research context particularly, "The division of labor by discipline was unquestioned: Psychologists did intelligence testing and assessment of personality, usually the Rorschach test; social workers did the interviewing; and psychiatrists conducted therapy" (p. 392).

An Alternative to Psychodynamic Approaches: The Rise of Behaviorism

Behavioral psychology emerged as a parsimonious explanation of behavior based on objective observations. Ivan Petrovich Pavlov's work on classical conditioning detailed, without resorting to complicated mentalistic constructs, how animals acquired a conditioned response, how the conditioned response could be extinguished (i.e., extinction), and how experimental neurosis could be induced. John B. Watson and Rosalie Rayner's "Little Albert Study" established that a fear response could be conditioned by pairing a stimulus of fear (viz., loud noise) with a previously unconditioned stimulus (viz., a white rat that Albert had played with without fear) so that the unconditioned stimulus (i.e., the rat) elicited the fear response (i.e., became a conditioned stimulus; Watson & Rayner, 1920). Although Watson and Rayner did not attempt to alleviate Albert's fear, Mary Cover Jones (under the supervision of Watson) demonstrated that the classical conditioning paradigm could be used to desensitize a boy's fear of rabbits by gradually increasing the proximity of the stimulus (i.e., the rabbit) to the boy in a pleasant state, which was established with Albert's favorite food.

A major impetus to behavioral therapy was provided by Joseph Wolpe's development of systematic desensitization. Wolpe, who like Freud was a medical doctor, became disenchanted with psychoanalysis as a method to treat his patients. Based on the work of Pavlov, Watson, Rayner, and Jones, Wolpe studied how eating, an incompatible response to fear, could be used to reduce phobic reactions of cats, which he had previously conditioned. After studying the work on progressive relaxation by physiologist Edmund Jacobson, Wolpe recognized that the incompatibility of relaxation and anxiety could be used to treat anxious patients. His technique, which was called systematic desensitization, involves the creation of a hierarchy consisting of progressively anxiety-provoking stimuli, which are then imagined by patients, under a relaxed state, from least to most feared. His seminal book *Psychotherapy by Reciprocal Inhibition*, in which he explicated how classical conditioning could be used as a psychological treatment, was published in 1958—at about the same time the medical barrier was lowered and psychologists began to practice psychotherapy more prevalently.

Although the explanation of anxiety offered by the psychoanalytic and classical conditioning paradigms differ dramatically, systematic desensitization has many structural similarities to psychoanalysis. It is used to treat a disorder (phobic anxiety), is based on an explanation for the disorder (classical conditioning), imbeds the mechanism of change within the explanation (desensitization), and stipulates the therapeutic action necessary to effect the change (systematic desensitization). So, although the psychoanalytic paradigm is saturated with mentalistic constructs whereas the behavioral paradigm generally eschews intervening mentalistic explanations, they are both systems that explain maladaptive behavior and offer therapeutic protocols for reducing distress and promoting more adaptive functioning. Proponents of one of the two systems would claim that their explanations and protocols are superior to the other. Indeed, Watson and Rayner (1920) were openly disdainful of any Freudian explanation for Albert's fears:

> The Freudians twenty years from now, unless their hypotheses change, when they come to analyze Albert's fear of a seal skin coat—assuming that he comes to analysis at that age—will probably tease from him the

recital of a dream which upon their analysis will show that Albert at three years of age attempted to play with the pubic hair of the mother and was scolded violently for it.

(p. 14)

The behaviorists claimed that they rejected the Medical Model. However, it was the biological bases of mental illness that was antithetical to their theoretical position, as behaviorists at this period in time considered the child a *tabla rasa* onto which experience writes and, therefore, problems of adult living, including mental illness, are consequences of the learning history of the individual. Nevertheless, the idea of treating a particular problem, say a simple phobia, specifically with a particular treatment, say Wolpe's systematic desensitization, was critical to the behavioral paradigm.

As cognition gained a more prominent position in experimental psychology, several psychotherapy theoreticians and researchers, some of whom were trained as analysts or who were steeped in psychodynamic theory and practice and others of whom came from a behavior or social learning perspective, developed models of cognitive therapy. It is debatable whether the contributions of these luminaries, including Albert Ellis, Aaron Beck, Michael Mahoney, and Donald Meichenbaum, represented a subsystem of behavior therapy, which had become increasingly pragmatic and less tied to experimental paradigms (Fishman & Franks, 1992), or should be classified as a distinct paradigm (Arnkoff & Glass, 1992). As we shall see, the issue of treatment distinctiveness and evolution of treatment paradigms will reappear in several prominent instances in this volume. For the purposes of this book, the term cognitive-behavior therapy (CBT) will be used to refer to behavioral and cognitive therapies, although in some instances CBT will be used to refer to a very specific treatment modality. Indeed, as discussed in several places, the definition of CBT is ambiguous and there are disagreements about whether a particular treatment is or is not CBT.

Humanism as a Third Force

In the context of post–World War II modernism and attempts to make meaning of life given the ravages of war and the Holocaust, psychotherapy developed a third force (after psychoanalysis and behavioral therapy) derived from the humanistic philosophers (e.g., Kierkegaard, Husserl, and Heidegger). Humanistic approaches have in common a) a phenomenological perspective (i.e., therapy must involve understanding the client's world); b) an assumption that humans seek growth and actualization; c) a belief that humans are self-determining; and d) a respect for every individual, regardless of their role or actions (Rice & Greenberg, 1992). The best known of the original humanistic therapies are person-centered therapy (Carl Rogers, as discussed e.g., in *Client-Centered Therapy*, 1951a), Gestalt Therapy (Frederick "Fritz" Perls), and existential approaches (e.g., Rollo May and Victor Frankl). Humanistic approaches emanated from distinctly non-medical origins and non-experimental traditions, having roots more in philosophy than in science and medicine.

Status of Various Psychotherapies

Although dividing up the psychotherapy universe into three forces, psychodynamic, cognitive-behavioral, and humanistic, is arbitrary, it is revealing to ask, "What is the relative status of these forces?" Status, of course, is an ambiguous term, but three sources of information relative to the question are available: texts and other artifacts, psychotherapy practice, and research foci.

In a report on National Public Radio's *All Things Considered* (June 2, 2004) on the treatment of a woman suffering social phobia, Alix Spiegel began by stating, "Cognitive-behavioral therapy is the fastest growing and most rigorously studied form of psychotherapy. It is fast becoming what people in America mean when they say they are getting therapy." And it is not only the media that give primacy to some treatments over others. The *Oxford Textbook of Psychotherapy* (Gabbard, Beck, & Holmes, 2005), a comprehensive and voluminous treatment of the subject, indicated that the editors "tried to ensure that the diverse psychotherapeutic strategies were represented in a balanced way in each chapter," but the 534-page text discusses primarily cognitive-behavioral and psychodynamic approaches—humanistic approaches and their developers were mostly ignored (Wampold & Imel, 2006). As noted by Rice and Greenberg (1992), "During the last two decades . . . the humanistic psychotherapy approaches have become increasingly separated from mainstream theoretical psychology, especially in North America" (p. 214).

The types of treatments delivered by therapists constitute another indicator of the status of psychotherapies. Every 10 years, Norcross and colleagues survey psychologists with regard to a number of practices, including type of treatment provided (see Norcross & Karpiak, 2012; Norcross, Karpiak, & Santoro, 2005, for the most recent surveys of clinical psychologists). The results of the survey show a remarkable rise in the proportion of clinical psychologists who report that their orientation was *cognitive*: in the 1960s and 1970, virtually no clinical psychologist reported that they were cognitively oriented, whereas in the most recent survey (viz., 2010), about one-third do so. If one combines cognitive with *behavioral*, which has been steadily rising from 8 percent in 1960 to 15 percent in 2010, then 45 percent of clinical psychologists in the United States report that their primary orientation is either *cognitive* or *behavioral* (Norcross et al., 2012). On the other hand, the proportion that report a *dynamic* or *eclectic/intregrative* orientation has decreased from 35 percent and 36 percent, respectively, in 1960 to 18 percent and 22 percent in 2010, respectively. All other orientations, including Rogerian, humanistic, systems, and interpersonal, among others, were only endorsed by 14 percent of the clinical psychologists responding in the 2010 survey. Of course, psychotherapy is not solely practiced by clinical psychologists, but it appears, nevertheless, that not only have humanistic approaches been abandoned (or perhaps have abandoned) mainstream theoretical psychology, as Rice and Greenberg (1992) suggested, but psychotherapists (at least psychologists) have abandoned these approaches as well.

The third source of information, which is derived from research foci, is discussed in the next section, where a history of developments in psychotherapy research is presented. The conclusion here, however, is that cognitive behavioral treatments clearly enjoy an elite status; however, many practicing therapists indicate that they are delivering eclectic or integrative forms of psychotherapy.

Research Methods, Psychotherapy Efficacy, and the Ascendancy of Treatments for Disorders

The need to demonstrate the efficacy of psychotherapy in general and various treatments specifically shaped the development of psychotherapy. Research methods played an important role in this development, as more advanced methods were needed to demonstrate the effects of psychotherapy.

Research Methods Driven by a Need to Demonstrate Efficacy

Research methods in psychotherapy have paralleled those of medicine. A clear example is found with Freud, who considered himself a scientist but preferred clinical findings of his treatments to results of statistical analyses of data. This was not surprising given the state of such methods in the early twentieth century. In the case method used by Freud, only trained psychoanalysts could be "objective and impartial observers" to determine the outcomes of a specific treatment. The case methods used by Freud and colleagues documented that their treatments were remarkably successful but created much doubt by those outside of the psychoanalytic community (Strupp & Howard, 1992). Indeed, one of the continuing criticisms of psychoanalytic approaches has been the lack of objective verification of outcomes.

The first direct observation of psychotherapy emanated from the humanistic tradition, which is somewhat surprising given the phenomenological bent of this school. While advocates of other approaches, particularly the psychoanalysts, were loathe to invade the sanctity of the interview room, in the 1940s Carl Rogers and his group prepared transcripts of sessions from audio tapes, a technology that was evolving at the time (Rice & Greenberg, 1992). From this source material, Rogers and his research group generated hypotheses that were to be tested by the evolving research methods being developed in education and psychology (see, e.g., Rogers, 1951b). Rogers as well as researchers at the Menninger Foundation and the University of Pennsylvania examined whether psychotherapy resulted in changes in personality. Generally samples were small, treatments were not well defined, disorders were not assessed and codified, and outcomes were not well specified or operationalized (Goldfried & Wolfe, 1996; Strupp & Howard, 1992).

Not long after Rogers first began his program of research, Hans Eysenck published a series of articles and books (Eysenck, 1952, 1961, 1966) in which he claimed that the rate of recovery of patients receiving psychotherapy was equal to the rate of spontaneous remission, a damning indictment of the effects of psychotherapy. The issue of psychotherapy effectiveness will be presented in Chapter 4, including an elaboration of the history related to the issue. It should be noted here, however, that the term "psychotherapy" was used by Eysenck to refer to psychodynamic, humanistic, and eclectic treatments; behavior therapy in his view was distinct from these treatments as it was based on learning theory (i.e., scientific principles). In Eysenck's view, behavior therapy should be preferred to the alternatives treatments (see Wampold, 2013).

Eysenck's claims generated much debate (see Chapter 4) and also instigated increased rigor relative to the research designs employed to test the effects of various psychotherapies (Wampold, 2013). The randomized design, developed in the 1920s and 1930s, as well as the placebo control group design, developed in the 1950s, offered psychotherapy researchers designs that had the potential to answer the question of whether psychotherapy was effective. In 1956, Rosenthal and Frank recommended the use of placebo-type controls in psychotherapy research in order to establish the specificity as well as efficacy of psychotherapy:

> It may be possible to study the possible specific effects of any particular form of therapy by the use of a matched control group participating in an activity regarded therapeutically inert from the stand point of the theory of the therapy being studied. That is, it would not be expected to produce the effects predicted by the theory. The "placebo psychotherapy" in a sense would be analogous to placebos in that it would be administered under circumstances and by persons such that the patients would be expected to be helped by it.
>
> (pp. 299–300)

Although the use of placebo control groups in psychotherapy research is problematic (see Chapter 8), historically Rosenthal and Frank's recommendation was emblematic of psychotherapy's close connection with medicine. Psychotherapy was adopting models of research that were used by medicine to demonstrate the effects of medications, thereby conceptualizing psychotherapy as a medical treatment. This is a trend that has increased over the decades such that beginning in the 1980s psychotherapy began to label its outcome research as *clinical trials* as it sought to establish the viability of particular treatments for particular disorders. The use of placebo-type control groups in psychotherapy research was an attempt to show that psychotherapies, like drugs, were specific, which as we have seen, is a distinguishing feature of modern medicine.

Purportedly, the superiority of a particular psychotherapy to a placebo establishes the specificity of the treatment but also established the legitimacy of the psychotherapy enterprise.

The next important development in psychotherapy research turns the tables, as it originates in psychotherapy research (as well as in education) and was "exported" to medicine. As will be seen more fully in Chapter 4, one of the issues that emanated from Eysenck's claims was how the results of multiple studies should be aggregated, as the conclusions were closely tied to the method, particularly the manner in which studies were included and excluded and how the results of the included studies were synthesized. Mary Lee Smith and Gene Glass, in 1977, published a meta-analysis of all studies that compared a psychotherapeutic approach to some type of control group, thereby demonstrating the utility of the method of meta-analysis, which will be described more completely in Chapter 3. Subsequently, meta-analysis has become the standard method of aggregating research results in education, psychology, and medicine. Importantly for psychotherapy, Smith and Glass (1977; Smith, Glass, & Miller, 1980) found that psychotherapy was indeed efficacious, a conclusion that will be examined fully in Chapter 4.

An issue addressed by Smith and Glass, but one that was not resolved, was so indigenous to modern medicine that it does not get addressed explicitly. No one asks, "Does medicine work?" but rather, "Which treatment works best for this particular disorder?" Post Smith and Glass, psychotherapy turned, à la medicine, to identifying particular treatments that were effective for treating particular disorders (see Chapter 5). To address this issue, first treatments were to be standardized, accomplished with treatment manuals, after which the standardized treatments could be tested and compared.

Psychotherapy Treatment Manuals

A treatment manual contains "a definitive description of the principles and techniques of [the] psychotherapy . . . [and] a clear statement of the operations the therapist is supposed to perform (presenting each technique as concretely as possible, as well as providing examples of each)" (Kiesler, 1994, p. 145). The purpose of the treatment manual is to create standardization of treatments, thereby reducing variability in the independent variable in clinical trials, and to ensure that therapists deliver correctly the specific ingredients that are characteristic of the theoretical approach. With regard to the latter point, manuals enable "researchers to demonstrate the theoretically required procedural differences between alternative treatments in comparative outcome studies" (Wilson, 1996, p. 295). Credit for the first treatment manual usually is attributed to Beck, Rush, Shaw, and Emery (1979), who delineated cognitive-behavioral treatment for depression. The proliferation of treatment manuals since the Beck et al. manual in 1979 has been described as a "small revolution" (Luborsky & DeRubeis, 1984). Treatment manuals have become required for the funding and publication of outcomes research in psychotherapy: "The treatment manual requirement, imposed as a routine design demand, chiseled permanently into the edifice of psychotherapy efficacy research the basic canon of standardization" (Kiesler, 1994, p. 145).

The treatment manual, as a research operation, is imbedded in the Medical Model. The typical components of the manual, which include defining the target disorder, problem, or complaint; providing a theoretical basis for the disorder, problem, or complaint; as well as the change mechanism; specifying the therapeutic actions that are consistent with the theory; and the belief that the specific ingredients lead to efficacy, are identical to the components of the Medical Model.

Empirically Supported Treatments

The second development in psychotherapy research related to the issue of treatments and disorders was the idea of "empirically supported treatments" (ESTs). The emphasis in the 1990s on managed care in medicine and related health areas, including mental health, created the need to standardize treatments and provide evidence of efficacy. As diagnosis-related groups (DRGs), which allowed fixed payment per diagnosis, became accepted in the medical community, psychiatry responded with psychopharmacological treatments (i.e., drugs) for many mental disorders; the Medical Model in medicine was making significant inroads in the treatment of mental disorders. A task force of Division 12 (Clinical Psychology) of the American Psychological Association (APA) reacted in a predictable way: "If clinical psychology is to survive in this heyday of biological psychiatry, APA must act to emphasize the strength of what we have to offer—a variety of psychotherapies of proven efficacy" (Task Force on Promotion and Dissemination of Psychological Procedures, 1995, p. 3). Accordingly, to identify treatments that would meet the criteria of being empirically validated (the term originally used), the task force developed criteria, which if satisfied by a treatment, would result in the treatment being included on a list published by the task force. Although the criteria have evolved, they originated from the criteria used by the FDA to approve drugs. The criteria essentially stipulated that a treatment would be designated as empirically validated for a particular disorder provided that at least two studies showed superiority to groups that attempted to control for general effects and were administered to a well-defined population of clients (including importantly the clients' disorder, problem, or complaint) using a treatment manual.

The first attempt to identify treatments that satisfied the criteria netted 18 well-established treatments (Task Force on Promotion and Dissemination of Psychological Procedures, 1995). Revisions to the list were made subsequently (Chambless et al., 1996; 1998) and included such treatments as cognitive behavior therapy for panic disorder, exposure treatment for agoraphobia, behavior therapy for depression, cognitive therapy for depression, interpersonal therapy for depression, multicomponent cognitive-behavioral therapy for pain associated with rheumatic disease, and behavioral marital therapy for marital discord. A special issue of the *Journal of Consulting and Clinical Psychology* was devoted to a discussion of ESTs and the identification of empirically supported treatments for adult mental disorders, child and adolescent disorders, health related disorders (viz., smoking, chronic pain, cancer, and bulimia nervosa), and marital distress (Baucom, Shoham, Mueser, Daiuto, & Stickle, 1998; Beutler, 1998; Borkovec & Castonguay, 1998; Calhoun, Moras, Pilkonis, & Rehm, 1998; Chambless & Hollon, 1998; Compas, Haaga, Keefe, Leitenberg, & Williams, 1998; Davison, 1998; DeRubeis & Crits-Christoph, 1998; Garfield, 1998; Kazdin & Weisz, 1998; Kendall, 1998).

With ESTs, psychotherapy had taken another step toward adopting the Medical Model. First, the criteria clearly orient psychotherapy to disorder, problem, or complaint: "We do not ask whether a treatment is efficacious; rather, we ask whether it is efficacious for a specific problem" (Chambless & Hollon, 1998, p. 9). Although use of the *Diagnostic and Statistical Manual* (DSM) as the nosology for assigning disorders was not mandated, Chambless and Hollon indicated the DSM has "a number of benefits" for determining ESTs; indeed those who have reviewed research in order to identify ESTs typically use the DSM to organize the review (e.g., DeRubeis & Crits-Christoph, 1998).

The requirement that only treatments administered with a manual are certifiable as an EST further demonstrates a connection between ESTs and the Medical Model because, as discussed above, manuals are intimately tied to the Medical Model. The lists of empirically supported treatments were dominated by behavioral and cognitive-behavioral treatments, with a few exemplars of psychodynamic-derived treatments and no humanistic treatments, which may reflect the fact that behavioral and cognitive-behavioral treatments are easier to manualize than are humanistic or psychodynamic treatments and fit more neatly into the clinical trial paradigm.

A third perspicuous aspect of the EST movement is the criteria, which were patterned after the FDA drug-approval criteria that require that evidence is needed relative to specificity as well as efficacy. According to the EST criteria, specificity is established by demonstrating superiority to pill or psychological placebo or by showing equivalence to an already-established treatment. Clearly, specificity, a critical component in the Medical Model of psychotherapy, undergirds the EST movement.[2] Indeed, the motivation to adopt a Medical Model in order to bolster the status of psychotherapy was evident from the beginning:

> We [The Task Force] believe establishing efficacy in contrast to a waiting list control group is not sufficient. Relying on such evidence would leave psychologists at a serious disadvantage vis-a-vis psychiatrists who can point to numerous double-blind placebo trials to support the validity of their interventions.
>
> (Task Force on Promotion and Dissemination
> of Psychological Procedures, 1995, p. 5)

Essentially, the adoption of the EST scheme created a Medical Model of psychotherapy. In medicine, the Medical Model involves a) disease or illness, b) biological explanation, c) mechanism of change, d) therapeutic actions, and e) specificity. The only modification needed for the psychotherapy version is that the biological explanation is transformed to a psychological explanation. ESTs require a disorder and a treatment manual that outlines the psychological explanation of the disorder, the mechanism of change, and the therapeutic actions. Specificity, although not formally required in the EST criteria, is clearly claimed by advocates of particular treatments. Proponents of a particular treatment will argue that the specific actions specified in that treatment are remedial for the disorder through the pathways specified in the theoretical underpinning of the treatment. As will be discussed throughout this book, specificity in psychotherapy, for theoretical and methodological reasons, is a problematic concept.

An extension of the EST movement has been a recent trend in which ESTs have been compared to medications for particular disorders. In most instances, psychotherapy is as effective as medications approved by the FDA for several mental disorders, which not only adopts a Medical Model with regard to methodological rigor but establishes the effectiveness of the treatments by using medical standards. Barlow (2004) suggested that treatments for particular disorders that have been established as effective should be designated as *psychological treatments* to differentiate them from generic psychotherapy; the former being established treatments within health delivery systems (i.e., reimbursable by third-party payers) and the latter, which "is often used outside of the scope of health care systems" (p. 869).

Evidence-Based Practice in Psychology

In 2006, the APA defined evidence-based practice in psychology (EBPP) as "the integration of the best available research with clinical expertise in the context of patient characteristics, culture, and preferences" (APA Presidential Task Force on Evidence-Based Practice, 2006, p. 271; see also Wampold, Goodheart, & Levant, 2007), which was clearly modeled after the three-legged Institute of Medicine definition discussed earlier, although a careful reading will show that psychology emphasized clinical expertise and patient characteristics more fully than did medicine. According to the APA, the best research evidence refers to "scientific results related to intervention strategies, assessment, clinical problems, and patient populations in laboratory and field settings as well as to clinically relevant results of basic research in psychology and related fields" (p. 274). Often one reads about "evidence-based treatments," but no such term *officially* exists and intentionally the APA avoided the terminology. Rather the intent of the APA was to indicate that evidence about treatment efficacy and effectiveness is only one potential out of many sources of evidence that can be used to deliver effective mental health services. With regard to interventions, APA noted that the "validity of conclusions . . . is based on a general progression from clinical observation through systematic reviews of randomized clinical trials, while also recognizing gaps and limitations in the existing literature and its applicability to the specific case at hand" (p. 284). Moreover, "evidence-based practice requires that psychologists recognize the strengths and limitations of evidence obtained from different types of research" (p. 275). Clearly, if a treatment has been shown to be demonstrably superior to another treatment, then that is important evidence to be considered in an evidence-based practice. "It was not the charge to TF [Task Force] to designate certain treatments as being privileged by certain forms of evidence—EBPP is distinct from notions such as empirically supported treatments (ESTs) and practice guidelines (APA, 2002) and consequently terms such as 'evidence-based treatments' are not indigenous to EBPP as defined by the APA" (Wampold et al., 2007).

Clinical expertise, according to the APA "is used to integrate the best research evidence with clinical data (e.g., information about the patient obtained over the course of treatment) in the context of the patient's characteristics and preferences to deliver services that have a high probability of achieving the goals of treatment" (p. 284). Thus, a critical component of clinical expertise is the use of the best available research evidence in the design and delivery of services. But clinical expertise is much more than using evidence and includes according to the APA: a) assessment, diagnostic judgment, systematic case formulation, and treatment planning; b) clinical decision-making, treatment implementation, and monitoring of patient progress; c) interpersonal expertise; d) continual self-reflection and acquisition of skills; e) appropriate evaluation and use of research evidence in both basic and applied psychological science; f) understanding the influence of individual and cultural differences on treatment; g) seeking available resources (e.g., consultation, adjunctive or alternative services) as needed; and h) having a cogent rationale for clinical strategies. Clinical expertise is not incompatible with evidence but instead involves the careful use of research evidence to make decisions regarding treatment in all respects.

The third leg of the stool considers characteristics of the recipient of the mental health services and the social and cultural context in which they live. According to the APA, evidence-based practice recognizes that "services are most effective when responsive to the patient's specific problems, strengths, personality, sociocultural context, and preferences" (p. 284). Important variables to consider are functional status, readiness to change, social support, developmental history, sociocultural context, current environmental context, and the personal preferences and values of the patient.

Despite the efforts of APA in EBPP to avoid the focus on treatments, evidence-based practice in mental health is often interpreted to refer to *treatments* exclusively. It is not unusual to see variants of the term "evidence-based" treatments appear; for example, Weisz, Jensen-Doss, and Hawley (2006) referred to "evidence-based youth psychotherapies." Division 12 of the APA, the Society of Clinical Psychology, emphasizing that EBPP included research evidence, has chosen to emphasize "research evidence for psychological treatments" by compiling lists of "research-supported psychological treatments" (see http://www.psychologicaltreatments.org/). The criteria for "strong research" and "moderate research support" are identical to the original EST criteria and indeed, according to the website, the list of treatments "is an updated, online version of the original list of empirically-supported treatments," organized by disorders.

There is a countervailing initiative to the treatment for disorder scheme, which grew out of displeasure with the DSM classification scheme, the infeasibility of mastering a different treatment for each disorder, and the similarities among various related disorders. Barlow and colleagues have developed *transdiagnostic* treatment protocols:

> We have now developed a treatment protocol to target what we hypothesize to be the three main components of the major emotional disorders . . . namely, restructuring faulty cognitive appraisals, changing action tendencies associated with the disordered emotion, and preventing emotional avoidance and facilitating emotional exposure.
>
> (Moses & Barlow, 2006, p. 148)

Having discussed the development of psychotherapy theoretically, contextually (i.e., in relation to medicine), and empirically we now turn to an analysis of progress and omissions in this account.

Progress and Omissions

The triumphs of medicine have been many: the extension of life, the eradication of various diseases, vaccinations against many infectious diseases, and viable treatments for management of chronic diseases. The development of research methods, particularly randomized designs and the placebo control group, aided the material stance of medicine, are indispensable tools, particularly for determining specificity, which leads to the approval of drugs that are effective for particular disorders.

Psychotherapy, whose history is entwined with medicine, also has progressed. Originating in the United States in secular and spiritual spheres, psychotherapy was legitimized by an association with medicine. When criticized as ineffective, the randomized design and meta-analyses were sufficiently powerful to demonstrate the effectiveness of psychotherapy and retain its respectability. Arguably, psychotherapy avoided being relegated to the periphery of the health delivery systems, in the United States and many other countries, to a large extent because of the evidence collected that demonstrated that the treatments were effective for particular disorders. As an accepted treatment in many contexts, psychotherapy has benefited patients for more than 100 years and the contributions to the mental health of the citizens of the United States and many other countries should not be underestimated.

But progress comes with a cost. The omissions enumerated briefly in the remainder of the chapter become the focus of much of this volume.

Spiritual and Humanistic Aspects

In the United States, the origins of psychotherapy were in spiritual and religious realms. The association of psychotherapy with the medical profession at the beginning of the twentieth century diminished those influences. Before Freud's visit to Clark University, the physicians, clergy, and psychologists associated with the Emmanuel Movement addressed "physical, mental, and spiritual health" (Caplan, 1998, p. 123), but spiritual health was sloughed off as the emphasis shifted to treatments for particular disorders and a focus on symptoms (Taylor, 1999). The humanistic psychotherapies, which addressed many issues related to spirituality and being, enjoyed a brief period of popularity mid-century and vestiges remain in treatments such as Motivational Interviewing (Miller & Rollnick, 2012) and Emotionally Focused Therapy (Greenberg & Watson, 2005). However, they are now mostly out of the mainstream in terms of what is practiced and what is deemed respectable in research and other scholarly sources. While a majority of Americans consider themselves religious or spiritual, psychotherapy, for the most part, has become a secular and amoral healing practice.

Related to the spiritual aspects of psychotherapy was the dismissal of the experience of the person receiving the psychotherapy and a focus on the pathology of the patient instead. The development of the randomized design displays a transition from a close relationship between the experimenter and those experiencing a stimulus (viz., Wundt and his students) to the physician-patient relationship (viz., the French physicians and their "subjects") to the subject as a stranger (viz., British empirical investigations of mental faculties) to the double-blind design. The British social statisticians also introduced the notion of using a continuous distribution of a trait to designate abnormality, which forms the basis of most clinical trials in psychotherapy in which symptoms measured on a continuous scale constitute the outcome measure. This represents a change from examining concepts of self in relation to the ideal self and changes in personality, which were an integral part of the first empirical investigations in the humanistic tradition (see Rogers, 1951b). The notion of psychotherapy as an opportunity to grow or as an opportunity to make meaning is not considered in any substantial manner in the current empirical investigations of psychotherapy.

Culture and Context

At the beginning of the twentieth century, there were seven historically black medical colleges, but as a consequence of the recommendations of the Flexner report in 1910, most were forced to close (three survived, Howard University,

Meharry Medical College, and Morehouse College), as they had insufficient support to meet the standards that were required post-Flexner, and, as a consequence, opportunities to train African American physicians were restricted, which in turn restricted African Americans' access to medical services. The disappearance of these medical schools was emblematic of a profession that was essentially, in terms of practitioners, the province of European American males of substantial means. Culture and context were ignored for the most part, while emphasis was placed on treatment and scientific discovery of universal biological processes. That there are significant health disparities in the United States for various groups can be seen, in part, as a legacy of the focus on disease rather than the person in the context of society's issues with race, ethnicity, and social class.

Again, psychotherapy's close relationship created if not a mirror image, then at least a replica, of the general disregard of culture and context in medicine. In a review of 100 years of American psychotherapy, Mays and Albee (1992) began by noting, "Let us begin with a demographic fact: Members of ethnic minority groups are neither major users of traditional psychotherapy nor purveyors of psychotherapy in anything like their proportion in the population" (p. 552). The focus on the treatment/disorder matrix to the exclusion of other factors is nowhere more apparent than in a special issue of the *Journal of Consulting and Clinical Psychology* (Kendall, 1998) on ESTs—in methodological articles and reviews of ESTs in child, adolescent, adult, family and marital, and health, only two articles mentioned culture, ethnicity, or race as an important consideration (viz., Baucom et al., 1998; Kazdin & Weisz, 1998) and then not prominently.[3] In the past decade, there has been a renewed interest in multicultural counseling and the delivery of services to diverse populations. The APA, in its discussion of evidence-based practice in psychology, emphasized patient characteristics and context (APA Presidential Task Force on Evidence-Based Practice, 2006), but these are relatively recent developments. Even when culture is considered, the intervention remains paramount (see Lau, 2006; Huey, Tilley, Jones, & Smith, in press). In this volume, culture and context are inextricably blended with all aspects of the therapy enterprise.

The Common Factors and the Process of Psychotherapy

From the beginning of psychotherapy, there has been a focus on treatment differences. As noted somewhat glibly by Norcross and Newman (1992):

> Rivalry among theoretical orientations has a long and undistinguished history in psychotherapy, dating back to Freud. In the infancy of the field, therapy systems, like battling siblings, competed for attention and affection in a "dogma eat dogma" environment . . . Mutual antipathy and exchange of puerile insults between adherents of rival orientations were much the order of the day.
>
> (p. 3)

Freud insisted his treatments were proper; those of Adler, Jung, and his other one-time disciples were flawed. The behaviorists held the Freudians in low regard and considered them fabricators of unscientific mentalistic constructs. The humanists thought that Freudians and behaviorists took pessimistic or mechanistic views of human development and found hope in the self-actualizing nature of humans. The advent of clinical trials and the establishment of ESTs have only exacerbated the efforts to identify some treatments as privileged.

Early in the history of psychotherapy, there was a countervailing, although weak force, that claimed that the efforts to establish *the* best treatment (or for that matter, a class of better treatments) were misguided. In 1936, Saul Rosenzweig noticed that despite the differences among the various therapies of that time, the outcomes were generally similar:

> The proud proponent, having achieved success in the cases he mentions, implies, even when he does not say it, that his ideology is thus proved true, all others false. . . . [However] it is soon realized that besides the intentionally utilized methods and their consciously held theoretical foundations, there are inevitably certain *unrecognized* factors in any therapeutic situation–factors that may be even more important than those being purposefully employed.
>
> (p. 412)

Referring to a race in *Alice and Wonderland* in which contestants started when they wanted and ended when they wanted, Rosenzweig used the metaphor "At last the Dodo bird said, 'Everybody has won and all must have prizes'" to refer to the competition among the various psychotherapies. The general equivalence of the benefits of psychotherapy has been called the *Dodo bird effect*. Rosenzweig's unrecognized factors have become known as *common factors*, as they are aspects of therapy that are common to all, or at least most, psychotherapies, and include such aspects of therapy as hope, expectation, relationship with the therapist, belief, and corrective experience.

Over the years, there have been several theoretical presentations of the common factors. The various common factor models, which will be discussed in the next chapter, have nevertheless existed on the periphery, with their greatest acceptance coming during the period when humanistic treatments, with which they were most closely aligned, were also relatively popular. Attributing potency to common factors is analogous to saying that medications are potent because of the placebo effect, which of course would be most detrimental to the fundamental assumption of modern medicine. Advocates of particular treatments have assiduously resisted the common factor explanation. Indeed, acceptance of common factors as the cause of the benefits of psychotherapy would collapse the entire scaffolding of the theoretical bases of modern psychotherapy as conceptualized by the field and presented to the public. Consequently, the field of psychotherapy has attempted to establish the primacy of *treatment* and has attempted, through the use of placebo-type control groups and other designs, to rule out common factors as the critical component explaining the benefits of psychotherapy (see Chapter 8).

Closely aligned with the common factor models were attempts to describe and test hypotheses related to the process of psychotherapy—what happens in psychotherapy sessions and how do these events lead to patient change. The history of process research can be traced to Rogers' sound recordings and transcripts of client-centered therapy (see e.g., Rogers, 1951b) but has become quite diffuse. Some of the process aspects were bolstered by various theories, such as interpersonal theory (e.g., Benjamin, 1994; Kiesler, 1996, Leary, 1955), that were either focused on change in a particular type of therapy (e.g., Greenberg & Webster, 1982) or were pan-theoretical (e.g., Hill, 1986). Others were descriptive of the process of therapy or were focused on critical aspects, such as task analyses of change episodes (Greenberg, 2007), for example. Nevertheless, process research has decreased over the years, particularly in the age of ESTs (Goldfried & Wolfe, 1996).

The Therapist as an Agent of Change and Patients as Active Participants

The final omissions in psychotherapy revealed by this brief history are related to the therapists and the patients. Consider the role of the providers of service in the development of randomized control group design. Recall that the randomized design in education was a means to test the effectiveness of educational programs. The customers were educational administrators who possessed both money and power, whereas the providers of the programs were teachers, predominantly low-paid and low-status women (Danziger, 1990)—consequently, there was little interest in the effect that the teacher had on student achievement. R. A. Fisher, when he applied his statistical expertise to the field of agriculture, was focused on soil, fertilizers, and plant varieties. The farmers were presumably able to apply the agricultural practices uniformly, and thus optimal agriculture involved using optimal farming practices.

In medicine, the variability in outcomes attributable to the physician was considered unimportant as well—well, more accurately, such variability was an anathema. Recall that medicine was interested in the specific effects of drugs and procedures. Mesmer was discredited not because his treatments were ineffective but because the theoretically postulated animal magnetism explanation was flawed; indeed, the commission attributed in part the success of the treatment to Mesmer's charisma. In the placebo control group design, there is a blind to rule out effects due to the provider of the treatment. Clearly, variability attributable to physicians is uninteresting and, for medicine, problematic. Interestingly, in the test of Mesmer's treatment, Mesmer was opposed to having Charles Deslon, a former student and assistant, administer the animal magnetic treatments, as Mesmer felt that Deslon was not competent do so; the Royal Commission's and medicine's response was that the treatment per se should be sufficient to benefit the patient through the ingredients and any benefit due to the charisma, warmth, or skill of the physician was irrelevant.

The focus on treatments and the avoidance of provider effects in education, agriculture, and medicine was extended to psychotherapy, where therapists similarly were ignored as an important source of variation in outcomes (Wampold & Bhati, 2004). In Chapter 6, the implications of ignoring therapist effects in psychotherapy will be discussed more fully and, as well, the variability in outcomes due to the psychotherapist will be estimated.

A similar omission is related to the role of patients. In each of the venues where randomized designs were used, the units receiving the treatment were assumed to be passive subjects. In medicine, what is important is whether serum levels of the medication are sufficient to be remedial, and the patient's involvement in the treatment (e.g., the patient's beliefs) is for the most part irrelevant. Indeed, the randomization of patients in clinical trials is used to make various patient variables comparable across the groups, thereby ruling out patient confounds. Although psychotherapy has examined patient variables to a greater extent than medicine, the gradual increased attention to the outcomes of treatments in clinical trials of psychotherapy has led to a de-emphasis of patient variables, which has troubled those who argue that the patient is a critical component of the therapy (e.g. Bohart & Tallman, 1999; Duncan, Miller, & Sparks, 2004).

Summary

In this chapter we have reviewed the history of psychotherapy practice and the methods used to investigate psychotherapy. Clearly, the development of psychotherapy, as practiced and studied, is closely entwined with medicine. Psychotherapy has progressed and is now considered a legitimate practice in health systems throughout the world. As with any progression, important aspects get left out. The contention of this volume is that several important aspects of psychotherapy have been ignored, to the detriment of understanding how psychotherapy works, to policy, and to practice.

Notes

1. There is an interesting coincidental convergence of language worth noting, if only for its curiosity. "Gold," fittingly, figures prominently in three ways. First, *Harry Gold* was instrumental in developing the randomized double-blind placebo control group design, which has become the *"gold standard"* for establishing the effectiveness of psychotherapy as well as medicines. Where did the term "blinding" come from? Blinding is a term coined by Gold, based on television advertisements that used the "blindfold test" to demonstrate the superiority of one brand of cigarette over the competitor—the "subject" was blindfolded and, after smoking both cigarettes,

proclaimed his preference for *Old Golds*, a popular cigarette brand of the times (Shapiro & Shapiro, 1997b).

2. Interestingly, some of those involved with the empirically supported treatment movement have recommended dropping the specificity requirement: "Simply put, if a treatment works, for whatever reason . . . then the treatment is likely to be of value clinically, and a good case can be made for its use" (Chambless & Hollon, 1998, p. 8). Nevertheless, treatments that could demonstrate specificity as well as efficacy would be "highly prized," indicating the continued belief that specificity remains central, as will be discussed later in this chapter.

3. One has to be careful about the use of the term culture. Psychotherapy typically has not been examined as a healing practice imbedded in a particular culture nor was it of interest how it "works" with other cultures, even in those instances when it was applied to other groups. An assumption is that psychotherapy was developed in a European and European American context in the United States and Europe. A careful analysis yields further distinctions, as it has been claimed that psychotherapy derived from the Freudian tradition is influenced by Ashekenic Jewish traditions, particularly Jewish mysticism (Kabbalah). Gestalt and some humanistic therapies were similarly influenced by Jewish experience (e.g., the Holocaust) and traditions. On the other hand, behavioral treatments, less reflective and more instrumental, were more in line with "white" (i.e., Christian) European American culture (Langman, 1997).

Chapter 2

The Contextual Model

Psychotherapy as a Socially Situated Healing Practice

As mentioned in Chapter 1, Saul Rosenzweig, who was the progenitor of the term "common factors," proposed that they were what produced the benefits of psychotherapy (Duncan, Miller, Wampold, & Hubble, 2010). He described several factors that he suggested were responsible for the benefits of psychotherapy. Subsequently, many others have taken up the challenge to describe exactly what the common factors are and how they work. In this chapter, we review alternatives to understanding psychotherapy from a specific theoretical orientation but focus primarily on one such model, the Contextual Model. However, before turning to these alternatives to a Medical Model, there are some definitional and philosophical issues that are necessary to understanding and interpreting psychotherapy evidence.

Definitions and Terminology

Definition of Psychotherapy

The definition of psychotherapy used here is not controversial and is consistent with either the Medical Model or the Contextual Model that will be examined subsequently. The following definition is used in this book:

> Psychotherapy is a primarily interpersonal treatment that is a) based on psychological principles; b) involves a trained therapist and a client who is seeking help for a mental disorder, problem, or complaint; c) is intended by the therapist to be remedial for the client disorder, problem, or complaint; and d) is adapted or individualized for the particular client and his or her disorder, problem, or complaint.

Psychotherapy is defined as an interpersonal treatment to rule out psychological treatments that may not involve an interpersonal interaction between therapist and client, such as bibliotherapy, systematic desensitization based on tapes that the client uses in the absence of a therapist, or Internet-mediated therapy where the client does not interact with the therapist. The adjective *primarily* is used to indicate that therapies employing adjunctive activities not involving a therapist, such as bibliotherapy, listening to relaxation tapes, or performing various homework assignments, are not excluded from this definition.

Presumably psychotherapy is a professional activity that involves a minimum level of skill and consequently the definition requires that the therapist be professionally trained. Because the relationship between training and outcome in psychotherapy has not been established, the amount of training is not specified, but here it is assumed that the training be typical for therapists practicing a given form of therapy and that the client believes the therapist has sufficient training to assist the client.

Psychotherapy has traditionally been viewed as remedial, in that it is a treatment designed to remove or ameliorate some client distress, and, therefore, the definition requires that the client have a disorder, problem, or complaint. Thus, prevention programs or interventions are not considered psychotherapy. This definition of psychotherapy includes a client *seeking help*, which helps rule out various interventions that are delivered to people who are not seeking assistance, as would be the case when it is determined that someone is at risk of developing a disorder and an intervention is delivered whether or not the patient has developed distress or desires to participate in a psychosocial process (e.g., critical incident stress debriefing for those who have been traumatized).

Treatments that do not have a psychological basis are excluded. It may well be that non-psychological treatments are beneficial when both the client and the practitioner believe in their efficacy. Treatments based on the occult, indigenous peoples' cultural beliefs about mental health and behavior, new age ideas (e.g., herbal remedies), and religious practices (e.g., prayer or faith healing) may be efficacious through some of the mechanisms hypothesized in the Contextual Model, but they are not psychotherapy and will not be considered in this book. This is not to say that such activities are not of interest to social scientists in general and psychologists in particular; simply, psychotherapy, as considered here, is limited to therapies based on psychological principles. It may turn out that psychotherapy is efficacious because Western cultures value the activity rather than because the specific ingredients of psychotherapy are efficacious, but that does not alter how psychotherapy is defined here.

Importantly, it is required that the therapist intends the treatment to be effective. In the Contextual Model, therapist belief in treatment efficacy is necessary. In Chapter 5, evidence that belief in treatment is related to outcome will be discussed.

In the definition, the term *client* is used, although in some contexts the term *patient* is customary, so the terms are used interchangeably, despite the fact that the latter connotes a Medical Model conceptualization.

Terminology

The presentation that follows depends on a careful distinction between various components of psychotherapeutic treatments and their related concepts. Over the years, various systems for understanding these concepts have been proposed by Brody (1980), Critelli and Neumann (1984), Grünbaum (1981), Shapiro and Morris (1978), Shepherd (1993), and Wilkins (1984), among others. As well, the terms are often used in an imprecise fashion, which adds to confusion about the evidence, and consequently terms are defined in this volume as precisely as possible and are not allowed to "wiggle" around as the evidence is presented. Although technical, the logic and terminology presented by Grünbaum (1981) is adapted to present the competing models because of its consistency and rigor. Here, we explain the notation and terms as well as substituting more commonly used terminology.

Grünbaum's (1981) exposition is as follows:

> The therapeutic theory ψ that advocates the use of a particular treatment modality t to remedy [disorder] D demands the inclusion of certain *characteristic* constituents F in any treatment process that ψ authenticates as an application of t. Any such process, besides qualifying as an instance of t according to ψ, will typically have constituents C *other than* the characteristic ones F singled out by ψ. And when asserting that the factors F are remedial for D, ψ *may* also take cognizance of one or more of the non-characteristic constituents C, which I shall denominate as "incidental."
>
> (p. 159)

An example of a therapeutic theory ψ could be psychodynamic theory; the particular treatment modality t would then be some form of psychodynamic therapy based on ψ. The treatment t would be applied to remediate some disorder D, such as depression. This treatment would contain some constituents F that are characteristic of the t and that are consistent with the theory ψ. At this point, it is helpful to make this concrete by considering Waltz, Addis, Koerner, and Jacobson's (1993) classification of therapeutic actions into four classes: a) unique and essential, b) essential but not unique, c) acceptable but not necessary, and d) proscribed. Waltz et al. provide examples, which are presented in Table 2.1, of these four therapeutic actions for psychodynamic and behavioral therapies. Grünbaum's (1981) characteristic constituents are similar to Waltz et al.'s unique and essential therapeutic actions. Forming a contingency contract is a unique and essential action in behavioral therapy (see Table 2.1) and it is characteristic of the theory of operant conditioning. A term ubiquitously used to refer to theoretically derived actions is *specific ingredients*. Thus, characteristic constituents, unique and essential actions, and specific ingredients all refer to essentially the same concept. For the most part, the term specific ingredients will be used in this book.

Table 2.1 Examples of Four Types of Therapeutic Actions

Psychodynamic Therapy	Behavioral Therapy
Unique and Essential Ingredients	
Focus on unconscious determinants	Assigning homework
Focus on internalized object relations as historical causes of current problems	Practicing assertion in the session
Focus on defensive mechanisms used to ward off pain of early trauma	Forming a contingency contract
Interpretation of resistance	
Essential But Not Unique	
Establish a therapeutic alliance	Establish a therapeutic alliance
Setting treatment goals	Setting treatment goals
Empathic listening	Empathic listening
Planning for termination	Planning for termination
Exploration of childhood	Exploration of childhood
Acceptable but Not Necessary	
Paraphrasing	Paraphrasing
Self-disclosure	Self-disclosure
Interpreting dreams	Exploration of childhood
Providing treatment rationale	
Proscribed	
Prescribing psychotropic medication	Prescribing psychotropic medication
Assigning homework	Focus on unconscious determinants of behavior
Practicing assertion in the session	Focus on internalized object relations as historical causes of current problems
Forming contingency contracts	Focus on defense mechanisms used to ward off pain of early trauma
Prescribing the symptom	Interpretation of resistance

Note. Adapted from "Testing the integrity of a psychotherapy protocol: Assessment of adherence and competence," by J. Waltz, M. E. Addis, K. Koerner, and N. S. Jacobson, 1993, *Journal of Consulting and Clinical Psychology, 61,* p. 625. Copyright 1993 by the American Psychological Association. Adapted with permission.

Grünbaum (1981) also referred to incidental aspects of each treatment that are not theoretically central. The common factor approach, which will be discussed later in this chapter, has identified those elements of therapy, such as the therapeutic relationship, which seem to be common to all (or most) treatments, and, therefore, these factors often are referred to as *common factors.* Common factors typically are incidental. However, there may be instances where a common factor, such as empathy, which may be incidental in exposure and response prevention for obsessive-compulsive disorder, is characteristic in other treatments, as is the case for Motivational Interviewing (MI) (see Miller & Rose, 2009). There also may be aspects of a treatment that are incidental (i.e., not characteristic of the theory) but not common to all (or most) therapies, although it is difficult to find examples of such aspects in the literature. Consequently, the term *common factors* will be used interchangeably with *incidental aspects*. In Waltz et al.'s (1993) classification, the "essential but not unique" and some of the "acceptable but not necessary" therapeutic actions (see Table 2.1) appear to be both incidental theoretically as well as common. For example, behavioral therapy and psychodynamic therapy, as well as most other therapies, include establishing a therapeutic alliance, setting treatment goals, a therapist who empathically listens, and planning for termination. Thus, incidental aspects and common factors are actions that are essential but not unique or are acceptable but not necessary. Because *common factors* is the term typically used in the literature, it will enjoy prominence in this book, although *incidental aspects*, which connotes that these ingredients are not theoretically central, will be used as well. The term common factors is misunderstood and even used in a pejorative manner, as we shall see.

There is one aspect of the terminology that, unless clarified, will cause continued confusion. If treatment t is *remedial for disorder D* (in Grünbaum's terms) then, simply said, the treatment is beneficial. However, there is no implication that it is the characteristic constituents (i.e., specific ingredients) that are causal to the observed benefits. Thus, the language of psychotherapy must distinguish cause and effect constructs (see Cook & Campbell, 1979). Specific ingredients and incidental aspects of psychotherapy are elements of a treatment that may or may not cause beneficial outcomes and thus are *putative* causal constructs. A psychotherapy treatment contains both specific ingredients and incidental aspects, both, one, or none of which might be remedial. The term *specific effects* will be used to refer to the benefits produced by the specific ingredients; *general effects* will be used to refer to the benefits produced by the incidental aspects (i.e., the common factors). If both the specific ingredients and the incidental aspects are remedial, then there exist specific effects (i.e., the ones caused by the specific ingredients) and general effects (i.e., the ones caused by incidental aspects). If the treatment is not effective, then neither specific nor general effects exist although specific ingredients and incidental aspects of psychotherapy are present. As an aid, the following is offered, where the arrows indicate causality:

specific therapeutic ingredients → specific effects
common factors (incidental aspects) → general effects

We choose to use the term *therapeutic elements* to denote those constituents that create the benefits of psychotherapy regardless of their status as specific ingredients or common factors.

The effects—specific effects and general effects—are not distinguishable. It is not simply a matter of imprecise observation—they are epistemologically identical. It is only the causes that differ. Of course, it might be that specific ingredients cause different effects (e.g., a decrease in symptoms) than do common factors (e.g., an increase in well-being), but that is a different, but very interesting, matter, and one that needs to be clarified. However, as noted above, some therapeutic elements that would typically be labeled common will be labeled specific in some treatments (e.g., empathy in MI) and thus their effects can be labeled specific or common. However, the general distinction is illustrative. Essentially, the goal of this book is to identify the therapeutic elements of psychotherapy by examining the research evidence—in simple terms, what makes psychotherapy work?

Having adopted certain terminology, it should be noted that the following terms used to describe specific ingredients and incidental factors as well as their effects are eschewed: active ingredients, essential ingredients, nonspecific ingredients, nonspecific effects, and placebo effects (except in the case of the effects of placebo medications—see Chapter 7). Active ingredients and essential ingredients, terms often used to refer to specific ingredients, inappropriately imply that the specific ingredients are remedial (i.e., there exists specific effects); whether specific ingredients produce effects or not is an empirical question. Nonspecific ingredients and nonspecific effects are avoided because they imply that the incidental factors or common factors are inferior to specific ingredients. Placebo effects, which are discussed in Chapter 7, often are denigrated as effects produced by pathways that are irrelevant to the core elements of a treatment. For example, the therapeutic alliance, a common factor that has been shown to have potent beneficial effects (see Chapter 7), is sometimes denigrated by referring to the effects it produces as nonspecific effects or placebo effects. The term "general effects" is used here because it is comparable linguistically and logically to its counterpart "specific effects."

We now turn to placing the two models that will be investigated in this book (viz., the Medical Model and the Contextual Model) at their proper level of abstraction.

Levels of Abstraction

As psychotherapy is an exceedingly complex phenomenon, levels of abstraction will be indeterminable, to some extent. Nevertheless, a short discussion of various levels is needed to understand the central thesis of this book. Four levels of abstraction will be presented here: therapeutic techniques, therapeutic strategies, theoretical approaches, and meta-theoretical models. These four levels are not distinct (i.e., the boundaries between them are ill-defined) and it would be impossible to classify each and every research question and theoretical explication into one and only one of the levels. Some studies have examined questions that do not fit neatly into one of the levels and some studies have examined questions that seem to span two or more levels. Nevertheless, it is necessary to understand how the thesis of this book, which contrasts the Medical Model with the Contextual Model, exists at a meta-theoretical level. At this level of abstraction, the vast array of research results produced by psychotherapy research create a convergent and coherent conclusion. The three levels of abstraction presented by Goldfried (1980), as well as a fourth, higher level are summarized in Table 2.2.

The highest level of abstraction discussed by Goldfried (1980) is the theoretical framework and the concomitant individual approaches to psychotherapy and their underlying, although sometimes implicit, philosophical view of human nature. In Grünbaum's (1981) terms, this is the level of the therapeutic

Table 2.2 Levels of Abstraction of Psychotherapy and Related Research Questions

Level of Abstraction	Examples of Units of Investigation	Research Questions	Research Designs
Techniques (i.e., specific ingredients)	Interpretations Disputing Maladaptive Thoughts In Vivo Exposure	Is a given technique or set of techniques necessary for therapeutic efficacy? What are the characteristics of a skillfully administered technique?	Component designs (dismantling and additive designs) Parametric designs Clinical trials with placebo controls Passive designs that examine the relationship between technique and outcome (within the corresponding treatment)
Strategies	Corrective experiences Activation for depressed patients	Are strategies common to all psychotherapies? Are the strategies necessary and sufficient for change?	Passive designs that examine the relationship between technique and outcome (across various treatments)
Theoretical Approach	Cognitive-behavioral Interpersonal approaches Psychodynamic	Is a particular treatment effective? Is a particular treatment more effective than another treatment?	Clinical Trials with no treatment controls Comparative Clinical Trials (Tx A vs. Tx. B)
Meta-Theory	Medical Model Contextual Model	Which Meta-theory best accounts for the corpus of research results?	Research synthesis

Note. Adapted from "Toward the delineation of therapeutic change principles," by M. R. Goldfried, 1980, American Psychologist, 35, pp. 991–999. Copyright 2001 by the American Psychological Association. Adapted with permission.

theory and the particular treatment modality t. Although Table 2.2 gives three examples of theoretical approaches to psychotherapy (viz., cognitive-behavioral, interpersonal, psychodynamic), by one estimate there are more than 500 approaches to psychotherapy if one considers the many variations proposed and advocated in the literature (Kazdin, 2000; see also Goldfried & Wolfe, 1996). At this level of abstraction, there is little agreement among researchers or practitioners. Advocates of a particular approach defend their theoretical positions and, to varying degrees, can cite research to support the efficacy of their endeavors. For example, recent reviews of research have found evidence to support behavioral treatments (Emmelkamp, 2013), cognitive and cognitive-behavioral treatments (Hollon & Beck, 2013; Tolin, 2010), psychodynamic approaches (Barber, Muran, McCarthy, & Keefe, 2013; Shedler 2010), and experiential treatments (Elliott, Greenberg, Watson, Timulak, & Freire, 2013). The plethora of research results emanating from clinical trials in which the efficacy of a particular treatment is established by comparisons to a no-treatment control or to another treatment is testimony to the importance of this level of abstraction (see Chapter 4 & 5). Unfortunately, the use of a particular approach seems to be divorced from this research, as noted decades ago, and which is probably as poignant now as it was then:

> The popularity of a therapy school is often a function of variables having nothing to do with the efficacy of its associated procedures. Among other things, it depends on the charisma, energy level, and longevity of the leader; the number of students trained and where they have been placed; and the spirit of the times.
>
> (Goldfried, 1980, p. 996)

The lowest level of abstraction involves the techniques and actions employed by the therapist in the process of administering a treatment. Well-articulated treatments prescribe the specific ingredients that should be used; consequently, techniques and approaches coincide, and, therefore, discussions of the efficacy of a particular treatment are related to the corresponding techniques. Psychodynamic psychotherapists make interpretations of the transference whereas cognitive-behavioral therapists dispute maladaptive thoughts. Advocacy for the theoretical bases of cognitive-behavioral treatments is also advocacy for the actions prescribed by the treatment. As presented in Table 2.2, various research designs have been used to test whether or not techniques, described at this level of abstraction, are indeed responsible for positive therapeutic outcomes.

According to Goldfried (1980), a level of abstraction exists between individual approaches and techniques, which he labels clinical strategies. Clinical strategies "function as clinical heuristics that implicitly guide [therapist] efforts during the course of therapy" (Goldfried, 1980, p. 994). Goldfried's purpose of identifying this intermediate level of abstraction was to show that therapeutic phenomena at this level would exhibit commonalities across approaches and possibly provide a consensus among the advocates of the various theoretical approaches. The two clinical strategies identified by Goldfried as generally common to all psychotherapeutic approaches are providing corrective experiences and offering direct feedback. A recent development at this level of abstraction is the identification of factors that are common for treatments shown to be effective for particular disorders (Beutler & Castonguay, 2006); these factors might include what generally would be specific ingredients (e.g., exposure for patients with avoidant anxiety disorders) or common factors (e.g., goal setting or the alliance). The research questions at this level of abstraction are concerned with identifying the common strategies and identifying whether they are necessary and sufficient for therapeutic change. Although innovative and potentially explanatory, the strategy level of abstraction has not produced much research, particularly in comparison with research devoted to establishing the efficacy of particular approaches.

The thesis of this book is situated at a level of abstraction beyond the theoretical perspectives that undergird the major approaches to psychotherapy. It is generally accepted that psychotherapy works (but just in case there is any doubt, this evidence will be reviewed in Chapter 4). But understanding the factors that are responsible for the benefits of psychotherapy has proved to be exceedingly difficult (Kazdin, 2009). In more mundane terms: What is it about psychotherapy that makes it so helpful? Explanations exist at each of the three lower levels of abstraction. During the course of presenting the research evidence, it will become clear that a) logical impediments to understanding causal mechanisms exist at each of these levels of abstraction, and moreover b) when viewed at these levels, the research evidence does not converge to an answer to the causality question. Consequently, a fourth level of abstraction is needed— theories about psychotherapeutic theories. In this book, two meta-theories are contrasted: the Medical Model and the Contextual Model.

In the previous chapter we discussed the Medical Model, in medicine and adapted for psychotherapy. In the remainder of this chapter we will present one particular alternative meta-theory to the Medical Model, although first we present several possible alternatives.

Alternatives to Specific Theories of Psychotherapy

According to Arkowitz (1992), dissatisfaction with individual theoretical approaches spawned three movements: a) theoretical integration, b) technical eclecticism, and c) common factors. Although the Contextual Model is a derivative of the common factors view, it is useful to be acquainted with the other alternatives.

Theoretical Integration

Theoretical integration is the fusion of two or more theories into a single conceptualization or the assimilation of various approaches into an existing approach
(Norcross & Goldfried, 1992, 2005). The origins of theoretical integration are
often credited to Thomas French, who gave an address to the American Psychiatric Association in which he drew parallels between psychoanalysis and
Pavlovian conditioning; his address did not receive an altogether welcoming
reception (French, 1933; see Norcross & Goldfried, 2005). Dollard and Miller's
(1950) seminal book *Personality and Psychotherapy: An analysis in Terms of Learning,
Thinking, and Culture* was perhaps the first true integration of two theories that
provided an explanation of behavior (in this case neuroses) (Arkowitz, 1992).
Because behavior therapy was not well developed at this time, Dollard and
Miller's work was considered theoretical and provided little direction for an
integrated treatment. Following the introduction of behavioral techniques (e.g.,
systematic desensitization), behavior therapists generally were more interested
in remarking on the differences rather than the similarities of the two theories.
Nevertheless, during the 1960s and 1970s, psychodynamic therapists shed the
orthodoxy of psychoanalysis and became more structured, more attentive to
coping strategies in the here-and-now, and more inclined to assign responsibility to the client (Arkowitz, 1992). At the same time, behavior therapists were
allowing mediating constructs, such as cognitions, into their models and began
to recognize the importance of factors incidental to behavioral theories, such
as the therapeutic relationship (for an integrative behavioral treatment in which
the therapeutic relationship is a specific therapeutic element see Functional
Analytic Psychotherapy; Kohlenberg & Tsai, 2007).

The softening of the orthodoxy of both psychodynamic and behavioral
approaches set the stage for Wachtel's (1977) integration of psychoanalysis and
behavior therapy, *Psychoanalysis and Behavior Therapy: Toward an Integration.* Wachtel, in this and other writings, demonstrated how psychodynamic and behavior
explanations could stand together to explain behavior and psychological disorders and how interventions from the two theories could facilitate therapeutic
change, both behavioral and intrapsychic. The essence of the integration was
nicely summarized by Arkowitz (1992):

> From the psychodynamic perspective, he [Wachtel] emphasized uncon-
> scious processes and conflict and the importance of meanings and fanta-
> sies that influenced our interactions with the world. From the behavioral
> side, the elements included the use of active-intervention techniques,
> a concern with the environmental context of behavior, a focus on the
> patient's goals in therapy, and a respect for empirical evidence. . . . Active
> behavioral interventions may also serve as a source of new insights
> (Wachtel, 1975), and insights can promote changes in behavior (Wachtel,
> 1982, pp. 268–269).

Since Wachtel's seminal work, psychotherapy integration has grown in popularity, with new integrations and refinements of others becoming accepted treatment modalities (Norcross & Goldfried, 2005). The central issue for psychotherapy integration is to avoid having the integrated theory become a unitary theory of its own and to generate hypotheses that are distinct from the theories on which the integration is based (Arkowitz, 1992). One could make a case that all psychotherapies, with some exceptions (e.g., pure exposure treatments for simple phobias, perhaps, although see Powers, Smits, Whitley, Bystritsky, & Telch, 2008), contain elements from a variety of perspectives and are thus integrative. In this way, integrated approaches can be added to the list of psychotherapies and generate conjectures not very different from "pure" treatments. Consequently, an integrated theory does not constitute a viable alternative to established treatments when it comes to understanding how psychotherapy works.

Technical Eclecticism

The guiding light of technical eclecticism is Paul's question: "What treatment, by whom, is most effective for this individual with that specific problem, under which set of circumstances, and how does it come about?" (Paul, 1969). Technical eclecticism is dedicated to finding the answer to Paul's questions for as many cells as possible in the matrix created by crossing client, therapist, and problem dimensions. The search is empirically driven and theory becomes relatively unimportant. The two most conspicuous systems for technical eclecticism are Arnold Lazarus' *Multimodal Therapy* (see e.g., Lazarus, 1981) and Larry Beutler's *Systematic Eclectic Psychotherapy* (Beutler & Clarkin, 1990; Beutler & Harwood, 2000; Beutler, Harwood, Kimpara, Verdirame, & Blau, 2011; Beutler, Harwood, Michelson, Song, & Holman, 2011). Essentially, technical eclecticism is focused on the lowest level of abstraction— techniques (see Table 2.2). As such, it involves one aspect of the Medical Model, specific treatments for specific disorders, but shies away from the explanatory aspects of the Medical Model. Consequently, it would be impossible to derive hypotheses that would differentiate technical eclecticism from a Medical Model bases for the efficacy of psychotherapy. Nevertheless, some of the empirical evidence generated by technical eclecticism has been applied at the strategy level of abstraction (Beutler & Baker, 1998; Beutler, Harwood, Kimpara, et al., 2011; Beutler, Harwood, Michelson, et al., 2011), which is discussed in Chapter 8.

Attention is now turned to the common factor approach, which forms the basis of the Contextual Model.

Common Factors

Since Rosenzweig proposed that common elements of therapy were responsible for the benefits of psychotherapy, attempts have been made to identify and codify the aspects of therapy common to all psychotherapies. The most comprehensive model of the common factors was first developed in the 1960s by Jerome Frank and presented in various editions of his book *Persuasion and Healing* (Frank, 1961, 1973; Frank & Frank, 1991). To a large extent, the Contextual Model is derived from Frank's model, with refinements to reflect psychological, evolutionary, clinical, and anthropological theory and research that has emerged in the last two decades.

Frank's Model

According to Frank and Frank, "The aim of psychotherapy is to help people feel and function better by encouraging appropriate modifications in their assumptive worlds, thereby transforming the meanings of experiences to more favorable ones" (1991, p. 30). Persons who present for psychotherapy are demoralized and have a variety of problems, typically depression and anxiety. That is, people seek psychotherapy for the demoralization that results from their symptoms rather than for symptom relief. Frank proposed that "psychotherapy achieves its effects largely by directly treating demoralization and only indirectly treating overt symptoms of covert psychopathology" (Parloff, 1986, p. 522).

Frank and Frank (1991) described the components shared by all approaches to psychotherapy. The first component is that psychotherapy involves an *emotionally charged, confiding relationship with a helping person* (i.e., the therapist). The second component is that the context of the relationship is a *healing setting*, in which the client presents to a professional, who the client believes can provide help and who is entrusted to work in his or her behalf. The third component is that there exists a *rationale, conceptual scheme, or myth* that provides a plausible explanation for the patient's symptoms. According to Frank and Frank, the particular rationale needs to be accepted by the client and by the therapist but need not be "true." The rationale can be a myth in the sense that the basis of the therapy need not be "scientifically" proven. However, it is critical that the rationale for the treatment be consistent with the world view, assumptive base, and/or attitudes and values of the client or, alternatively, that the therapist assists the client so that he or she is in accord with the rationale. Simply stated, the client must believe in the treatment or be lead to believe in it. The final component is a *ritual or procedure* that requires the active participation of both client and therapist and that it is consistent with the rationale that was previously accepted by the client (i.e., the ritual or procedure is believed to be a viable means of helping the client).

Frank and Frank (1991) discussed six elements that are common to the rituals and procedures used by all psychotherapists. First, the therapist combats the client's sense of alienation by developing a relationship that is maintained after the client divulges feelings of demoralization. Second, the therapist maintains the patient's expectation of being helped by linking hope for improvement to the process of therapy. Third, the therapist provides new learning experiences. Fourth, the clients' emotions are aroused as a result of the therapy. Fifth, the therapist enhances the client's sense of mastery or self-efficacy. Sixth, the therapist provides opportunities for practice.

Other Common Factor Models

There have been several other common factor models that have been developed to explain the benefits of psychotherapy, and a few prominent ones will be briefly described here. Goldfried (1980), as mentioned previously, sought to find a level of abstraction more general than techniques and suggested two possible principles that are common to all therapies: providing the client new and corrective experiences and offering the client direct feedback. The idea of common strategies was pursued by a joint task force of the Society of Clinical Psychology (Division 12 of the APA) and the North American Society of Psychotherapy Research that reviewed and extracted factors that were common to effective treatments for particular classes of disorders (viz., dysphoric disorders, anxiety disorders, personality disorders, and substance use disorders; Castonguay & Beutler, 2006). In 1986, Orlinsky and Howard developed a *generic model* of psychotherapy that included the following components: the therapeutic contract, therapeutic interventions, the therapeutic bond, the patient's self-relatedness, therapeutic realizations, and therapeutic outcomes. These components were hypothesized to be reciprocally related to each other within a social and treatment setting context (see Figure 8.1; Orlinsky & Howard). Castonguay (1993) was concerned that focusing on therapist actions ignored other common aspects of psychotherapy and generated three classes of common factors in psychotherapy. The first, which is similar to Goldfried's strategy level of abstraction, refers to global aspects of therapy that are not specific to any one approach (i.e., are common across approaches), such as insight, corrective experiences, opportunity to express emotions, and acquisition of a sense of mastery. The second class refers to aspects separate from treatment, including interpersonal and social factors, which then encompasses the therapeutic context and the therapeutic relationship (e.g., the working alliance). The third class involves other aspects of psychotherapy that influence outcomes, including client expectancies and involvement in the therapeutic process. In another common factor model, Sol Garfield, in *Psychotherapy: An Eclectic-Integrative Approach* (1995), attempted to base a common factor model on the research evidence.

Recognizing that lists of common factors could be generated with relative ease and frequency, researchers have attempted to bring a conceptual scheme to the common factors. Grencavage and Norcross (1990) reviewed publications that discussed commonalities among therapies and segregated commonalities into five areas: client characteristics, therapist qualities, change processes, treatment structures, and relationship elements. Lambert (1992) parsed the various factors that led to psychotherapy success into four categories, in order of their importance for producing therapeutic benefits: a) client/extracurricular factors; b) relationship factors; c) placebo, hope, and expectancy factors; and d) model technique factors. According to Lambert, the most important factor, client/extracurricular factors, involved characteristics of the client and events that occur outside of therapy. Quite clearly, much of what happens in therapy is due to the client's motivation, resources (e.g., social support), and personality structure as well as to events that transpire indirectly as a result of therapy (e.g., a depressed husband talks to his wife about his distress) or serendipitously (e.g., client's parent dies unexpectedly). The second most important aspect according to Lambert involves relationship factors, which include all of the aspects of being in a relationship with a genuine, empathic, and caring therapist who facilitates work toward solving problematic issues. The third factor, placebo, hope, and expectancy, is created as a function of seeking help from a professional in the healing context—the client believes that the therapy will helpful. Finally, according to Lambert, model/technique factors account for part of the success of psychotherapy. That is to say, the ingredients of the specific treatment are responsible for the some of the benefits of psychotherapy. A popular book entitled *Heart and Soul of Change* (Hubble, Duncan, & Miller, 1999) was organized around Lambert's scheme and promoted the power of the common factors.

The Contextual Model

The current version of the Contextual Model explicates three pathways that purportedly explain the benefits of psychotherapy. The model is grounded in what is known about humans and human healing—that is, the model is grounded in the social sciences, broadly speaking. The basic premise of the model is that the benefits of psychotherapy accrue through social processes and that the relationship, broadly defined, is the bedrock of psychotherapy effectiveness.

Humans are one of the few ultra-social species, labeled as *eusocial* species by E. O. Wilson, which include several insect species (e.g., ants and termites; Wilson, 2012). Eusocial species have an advantage over animals that "go it alone," as Wilson argues with respect to humans:

> A group with members who could read intentions and cooperate among themselves while predicting the actions of competing groups, would have an enormous advantage over others less gifted. There was undoubtedly competition among group members, leading to natural selection of traits that gave advantage to one individual over another. But more important for a species entering new environments and competing with powerful rivals were unity and cooperation within the group. . . . The primary and crucial difference between human cognition and that of other animal species, including our closest genetic relatives, the chimpanzees, is the ability to collaborate for the purpose of achieving shared goals and intentions. The human specialty is intentionality, fashioned from an extremely large

working memory. We have become the experts at mind reading, and the world champions at inventing culture.

(p. 224, 226)

In eusocial species, there are evolutionary forces acting at the group level as well as at the individual level (often referred to as multilevel selection; see Wilson, 2012, e.g.), which is to say that fitness is important for the group as well as for individuals. As an example, consider how the fishermen of Luarca Spain decided to take their small boats from their well-protected port on the Costa Verde to fish on foul-weather days. At an individual level, the fisherman would weigh the peril of being lost at sea in what is a notoriously dangerous coast versus gaining an economic advantage over the other fishermen by fishing on a day when others would not dare to venture out. The most skilled fisherman (i.e., the fittest, from an evolutionary perspective) would venture out more often than the others and thereby have an economic advantage over others. However, such behavior would build pressure for other fisherman to venture out as well, in order to compete; the escalating risk-taking puts the welfare of the fishing community at risk. Taking into account concern for the fishing community (and for the entire village, as fishing was the primary industry), the fisherman devised the following strategy, as illustrated in in Figure 2.1. On the

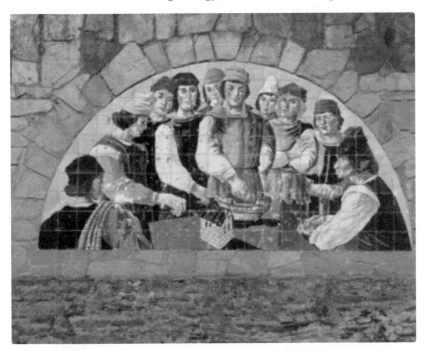

Figure 2.1 Fisherman of Luarca Spain making a group decision whether to fish on foul-weather days.

morning of stormy days, the fishermen gathered around a table on which a model house and a model boat were placed; each fisherman had a token, which they placed at either the house or the boat. If the majority of tokens were placed at the boat, then the fishermen were allowed to go fishing, although they could choose not to if they wanted to stay home. However, if the majority of tokens were placed at the house, it was agreed that there would be no fishing on that day. This strategy emphasized the value of the community that would provide an advantage to this fishing community vis-à-vis others that did not use a comparable cooperative strategy.

Although there is controversy about whether traits that lead to group cooperation (e.g., altruism) result from an evolutionary process at the group level, there is no doubt that eusocial species utilize cooperation to further the good of the group. Furthermore, there is little doubt about the prominence of sociality as a critical human characteristic. Lieberman and colleagues have investigated the neurological basis of sociality and concluded that "there is increasing evidence that our [i.e., human] dominance as a species may be attributable to our ability to think socially" (Lieberman, 2013, p. 7).

With regard to healing, cooperation in eusocial species is realized in what has been called "social immunity" (Cremer & Sixt, 2009). Of course, individuals have biological and behavioral strategies for avoiding pathogens and mitigating the effects of illness. However, eusocial species also have analogous disease defenses at the societal level that involve cooperation among individuals. For example, bees will quarantine a pathogen by surrounding it with workers ("social encapsulation," analogous to how immune cells work at the individual level) or, if bees are infected, workers will fan their wings to raise the temperature of the hive to help the infected bees fight the infection (Cremer & Sixt, 2009). Ants will actively seek out infected colony mates to rub up against so that a small dose of the pathogen is transferred to the uninfected ants, thereby immunizing the colony to the pathogen, in what has been termed "social immunization" (Konrad et al., 2012).

Humans have similarly evolved to heal through social means. All human civilizations, from the earliest records, have practiced some form of healing, with designated healers, elaborate explanations for illness, and healing rituals (Wilson, 1978; Shapiro & Shapiro, 1997b), as discussed in Chapter 1. There is compelling evidence that the facial expression of pain evolved to elicit the help of others (Williams, 2002). Physical as well as mental disease and well-being propagate through social networks—cardiac health, obesity, depression, loneliness, and happiness are socially contagious in the same way that influenza is physically contagious (Cacioppo, Fowler, & Christakis, 2009; Christakis & Fowler, 2007; Fowler & Christakis, 2009, 2010; Rosenquist, Fowler, & Christakis, 2011). Health and well-being are not simply conditions of an individual.

The point here is that a claim could be made that psychotherapy is a social healing practice. Or perhaps better said, psychotherapy utilizes evolved human propensities to help clients change (Wampold & Budge, 2012). Lieberman, in his review of the "hard wiring" of the social nature of humans, notes, "Antagonism between social and nonsocial thinking is really important because the more someone is focused on a problem, the more that person might be likely to alienate others around him or her who could help solve the problem. . . . *Our brains are designed to be influenced by others*" (emphasis added, 2013, p. 8). However simple as this point may seem, it is often ignored when explanations for the benefits of psychotherapy are discussed. The Contextual Model takes into account the social healing aspects of psychotherapy, with the relationship between the therapist and the client being paramount. However, exactly how psychotherapy works through social means is not a simple matter—there is much more than the logic that humans are social and, therefore, heal through social means. The Contextual Model posits three pathways through which psychotherapy exerts its influence on healing, as briefly described below (see Wampold, 2007; Wampold & Budge, 2012; Wampold, Imel, Bhati, & Johnson Jennings, 2006 for a more complete discussion of the Contextual Model).

A Relationship-Based Model of Psychotherapy—The Contextual Model

We present the basics of a tripartite model for how psychotherapy produces benefit in Figure 2.2. This model is designed to account for the benefit of all "bona fide" psychotherapies that meet the criteria discussed later in this chapter. Others may argue that there are additional benefits to specific therapies, an argument we examine in detail in Chapter 8.

Before the three pathways can be employed, the therapist and the client must form an initial bond. After the bond is formed, the therapist and patient create a "real" relationship, the first pathway to client change. Through explanation and treatment actions, expectations about therapy are created, which in and of themselves create a second process of change. The third pathway involves change that is a result of carrying out treatment actions. Each of these components is described below (see also Wampold & Budge, 2012).

The Initial Therapeutic Bond

Before the work of therapy can begin, an initial bond between the therapist and client needs to be created. Ed Bordin (1979), who was the intellectual force behind understanding the alliance construct, suggested that this initial bond is needed before the work of psychotherapy can be undertaken: "Some basic level of trust surely marks all varieties of therapeutic relationships, but when attention is directed toward the more protected recesses of inner experience, deeper bonds of trust and attachment are required and developed" (p. 254).

The formation of the initial bond is a combination of bottom-up and top-down processing. The bottom-up processing is essentially driven by the meeting of two strangers. Humans make very rapid determination (within 100

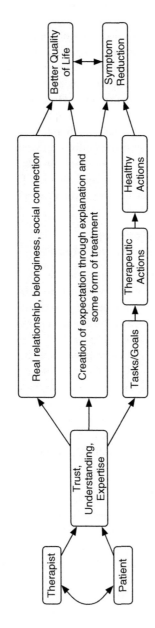

Figure 2.2 Contextual Model.

ms), based on viewing the face of another human, whether the other person is trustworthy or not (Willis & Todorov, 2006; see also Ambady, LaPlante, Nguen, Rosenthal, & Levenson, 2002; Ambady & Rosenthal, 1993; Albright, Kenny, & Malloy, 1988), suggesting that clients make very rapid judgments about whether they can trust their therapist or not. More than likely, clients make rapid judgments about the dress of the therapist, the arrangement and decorations of the room (e.g., diplomas on the wall), and other features of the therapeutic arrangement (Heppner & Claiborn, 1989).

Clients do not come to the therapy session *tabula rasa*, however, as they have expectations about the therapist and about therapy based on their attitudes and experiences with psychotherapy, what they might have been told about therapy from significant others, their motivation to change, their knowledge of the particular therapist, and so forth. However, as discussed earlier, generally speaking humans are predisposed to have a positive orientation toward healing, but only if the healing practice is consistent with their cultural traditions and accepted with a positive orientation. For the most part, Europeans or European Americans presenting to a physician practicing Western medicine will have a positive orientation toward the physician and the treatments employed; for many the same is true of psychotherapy, although likely not to the same degree. Recall, however, that the definition of psychotherapy used in this book assumes that the client presents voluntarily to psychotherapy to reduce distress, so in that sense only clients who have a modicum of belief in psychotherapy are considered here.

It seems safe to say that the initial interaction of client and therapist must establish sufficient engagement and a level of trust that the therapist will be able to help the client for therapy to begin. More clients drop out of therapy after the first session than at any other time and with each successive session fewer clients drop out (Connell, Grant, & Mullin, 2006; Simon & Ludman, 2010).

Pathway I: The Real Relationship

The real relationship between the therapist and the client refers to the fact that in the therapy room, two humans are having an intimate emotional relationship. The real relationship, with psychodynamic theoretical roots, is defined by Gelso (2014; see also Gelso, 2009) as "the personal relationship between therapist and patient marked by the extent to which each is genuine with the other and perceives/experiences the other in ways that befit the other" (p. 119). The real relationship is a based on genuineness, which is "the ability and willingness to be what one truly is in the relationship—to be authentic, open and honest" (Gelso & Carter, 1994, p. 297), and realistic perceptions, which are "those perceptions that are uncontained by transference distortions and other defenses" (p. 297). Moreover, there is evidence that basic psychological processes that are present in general social interactions such as synchrony in vocal tone (Imel et al., 2014) and nonverbal movement (Ramseyer & Tschacher, 2011) operate in psychotherapy and are related to treatment process and outcome.

Although the psychotherapeutic relationship is influenced by general social processes, it is an unusual social relationship. In psychotherapy, there is a contract that therapy will continue until treatment is completed, although the duration of therapy often is limited by third-party payers. Moreover, the interaction is confidential, with some statutory limits (e.g., child abuse reporting). Most importantly, psychotherapy is fundamentally different from naturally occurring relationships in which disclosure of difficult material not infrequently ruptures the social bond (e.g., disclosure of infidelity to a spouse). Indeed, in psychotherapy the client is able to talk about difficult material without the threat that the therapist will terminate the relationship.

Is this real relationship therapeutic? Or, is it simply an aspect of therapy that is superfluous—necessarily present but not therapeutic? The Contextual Model posits that the real relationship will be therapeutic in and of itself, to some extent. Research from a number of areas strongly suggests that human connection, whether it is called attachment (e.g., Bowlby, 1969, 1973, 1980), belongingness (e.g., Baumeister, 2005), social support (e.g., Cohen & Syme, 1985), or the lack of loneliness (e.g., Cacioppo & Cacioppo, 2012; Lieberman, 2013), is necessary for healthy functioning. Lieberman (2013) argues that social connection is as basic a need to humans as food or shelter. In fact, perceived loneliness is a significant risk factor for mortality, equal to or exceeding the risk factors for smoking, obesity, not exercising (for those with chronic cardiac disease or for healthy individuals), environmental pollution, or excessive drinking (e.g., see also Luo, Hawkley, Waite, & Cacioppo, 2012). Psychotherapy provides the client a human connection with an empathic and caring individual, which should be health promoting, especially for clients who have impoverished or chaotic social relations.

The critical processes in the real relationship depend on empathy. Empathy, a complex process by which an individual can be affected by and share the emotional state of another, assess the reasons for another's state, and identify with the other by adopting his or her perspective, is thought to be necessary for the cooperation, goal sharing, and the regulation of social interaction (de Waal, 2008; Niedenthal & Brauer, 2012; Preston & de Waal, 2002). Such capacities are critical to infant and child rearing, as children, who are unable to care for themselves, signal to the caregiver that care is needed, a process that is then put to use to manage social relations among communities of adult individuals (de Waal, 2008; Lieberman, 2013):

> At the core of the empathetic capacity lies a mechanism that provides the observer [the subject] with access to the subjective state of another [the object] through the subjects own neural and bodily representations. When the subject attends to the object's state, the subject's neural representations of similar states are automatically and unconsciously activated. The more similar and socially close two individuals are, the easier the subject's identification with the object, which enhances the subject's matching motor and autonomic responses. This lets the subject get "under the skin" of the

object, bodily sharing its emotions and needs, which in turn may foster sympathy and helping.

(de Waal, 2008, p. 286)

Ratings of therapist empathy are among the most consistent predictors of psychotherapy outcome available (Elliott, Bohart, Watson, & Greenberg, 2011; see also Moyers & Miller, 2013, and Chapter 7).

Despite concerns about the idea of a "real" relationship (Gelso, 2014), humanistic and some dynamic therapies, say of the relational perspective, emphasize the real relationship, whereas others, particularly the behavioral or cognitive behavioral therapies, do not. Indeed, the real relationship was the core of Rogerian therapy (Rogers, 1951a). Nevertheless, according to the Contextual Model, the real relationship should be related to outcome—the stronger the real relationship, the better the outcome of therapy—regardless of theoretical orientation. It would be expected that real relationship would have its effect on general well-being rather than symptom reduction.

Pathway 2: Expectations

What one expects in a certain situation has a strong influence on what the person experiences. Anticipating a great meal at a popular restaurant full of satiated patrons will bring a greater satisfaction that the same meal in a less appealing setting (for example related to wine pricing, see Plassmann, O'Doherty, Shiv, & Rangel, 2008). Many experiments have experimentally detected the effect of expectations. For instance, subjects who are led to believe that a highly bitter taste would not be as aversive as it actually was reported that the taste was not as bad as when they had accurate information about the taste. Moreover, the activation of the taste cortex mirrored the subjective reports indicating that the expectation of taste had objective as well as subjective effects, even though it has been thought that the taste cortex responds only to sensory input (Nitschke et al., 2006).

The effect of expectations has been studied in the context of the placebo, the literature about which is reviewed in Chapter 7. At this point, suffice it to say that the effect of placebos in experimental and medical contexts is quite robust (Benedetti, 2009, 2011; Price, Finniss, & Benedetti, 2008; Wampold, Minami, Tierney, Baskin, & Bhati, 2005), notwithstanding some claims otherwise (Hróbjartsson & Gøtzsche, 2001). Much of the effect of many medical procedures is to a large extent due to the placebo effect (Wampold et al., 2005), particularly psychotropic medications and most prominently antidepressants (Kirsch, 2002, 2009; Kirsch et al., 2008; Kirsch, Moore, Scoboria, & Nicholls, 2002). Although there are several explanations for the placebo effect, expectations appear to be prominently involved (Benedetti, 2009; Price et al., 2008).

Expectations in psychotherapy work in several possible ways. Frank (Frank, 1973; Frank & Frank, 1991) indicated that clients present to psychotherapy demoralized not only because of their distress but because they have attempted many times and in many ways to overcome their problems, all unsuccessfully—nothing seems to work. Taking action by seeking help of a psychotherapist is another form of seeking a solution, one that a client will often believe will be beneficial. The very act of arranging psychotherapy seems to be ameliorative, as much benefit is realized between the time the appointment is made and the first session (Frank & Frank, 1991; see also Baldwin, Berkeljon, & Atkins, 2009; Simon, Imel, & Steinfield, 2012). Greenberg, Constantino, and Bruce (2006) emphasize the importance of instilling hope in the initial sessions. The positive effect of believing that engaging in psychotherapy will provide hope that life will be better has been labeled as "remoralization" by Frank, and it is often mentioned as one of the prominent common factors.

However, expectations in therapy are also more specific than the general hopefulness created by engaging in psychotherapy. According to the Contextual Model, patients come to therapy with an explanation for their distress, formed from their own psychological beliefs, which is sometimes called "folk psychology" and is related to the concept of "theory of the mind" (Boyer & Barrett, 2005; Molden & Dweck, 2006; Thomas, 2001). These beliefs, which are influenced by cultural conceptualizations of mental disorder (Lillard, 1998) but also are idiosyncratic, are typically not adaptive in the sense that they do not allow for solutions. For instance, a person with social phobia may believe that his or her difficulties in social relations are due to their personal unattractiveness or their inability to mask their anxiety. In the former case, the client is not able to change their appearance and in the latter case their solution—to hide their anxiety—likely leads to increased anxiety and greater avoidance. Psychotherapy provides an explanation for the client's difficulties that is adaptive in the sense that it provides a means to overcome or cope with the difficulties (Wampold, 2007; Wampold & Budge, 2012; Wampold et al., 2006). The client comes to believe that participating in and successfully completing the tasks of therapy, whatever they may be, will be helpful in coping with his or her problems, which then furthers for the client the expectation that he or she has the ability to enact what is needed. The belief that one can do what is necessary to solve his or her problem has been discussed in various ways, including discussions of mastery (Frank & Frank, 1991; Liberman, 1978), self-efficacy (Bandura, 1999), or response expectancies (Kirsch, 1999).

Of course, every approach to psychotherapy has a different explanatory system for disorders, as Laska, Gurman, and Wampold (in press) describe in reference to post-traumatic stress disorder:

> Each [treatment] posits a specific mechanism of change based on a given scientific theory. For example, prolonged exposure (PE) for PTSD (Foa, Hembree, & Rothbaum, 2007) is conceptually derived from emotional processing theory (Foa & Kozak, 1986), and the specific ingredients of PE (viz., imaginal and in vivo exposure) (a) activate the "fear network,"

(b) whereby clients habituate to their fears, and thus, (c) extinguish the fear response. On the other hand, interpersonal therapy (IPT) for PTSD (Markowitz, Milrod, Bleiberg, & Marshall, 2009) is derived from interpersonal and attachment theory (Bowlby, 1973; Sullivan, 1953) and "focuses on current social and interpersonal functioning rather than exposure" (Bleiberg & Markowitz, 2005, p. 181).

What is important for creating expectations is not the scientific validity of the theory but the acceptance of the explanation for the disorder, as well as therapeutic actions that are consistent with the explanation (Wampold, 2007; Wampold & Budge, 2012; Wampold et al., 2006). The causes of mental disorders are notoriously difficult to determine (e.g., Roth, Wilhelm, & Petit, 2005) and for the sake of creating expectation are irrelevant. If the client believes the explanation and that engaging in therapeutic actions will improve the quality of their life or help them overcome or cope with their problems, expectations will be created and will produce benefits. As will be discussed in much detail in Chapter 7, the therapeutic alliance, which includes agreement about the goals and tasks of therapy, is predictive of outcome across treatment (Horvath, Del Re, Flückiger, & Symonds, 2011), suggesting that acceptance of the model presented to the client is indeed critical to the outcome of all therapies. At the origins of the concept of the alliance, Bordin (1979) hypothesized that the alliance was necessary to induce expectations, which then would be important for the benefits of psychotherapy.

There is a critical issue about treatment that needs to be clarified at this juncture. The pathway that involves expectations, as well as the third pathway discussed in the next section, involves a cogent explanation for the disorder and concomitant therapeutic actions (Laska et al., 2014; Wampold & Budge, 2012). Absent a treatment, there can be no agreement about the goals and tasks of therapy and a crucial component required for creating expectations is missing. It is not uncommon to read that common factors can be activated simply by discussing one's problems with an empathic listener; although such a "treatment" (sometimes called a "common factor" treatment) may be beneficial through the real relationship pathway, it is insufficient to fully activate the potential benefits of psychotherapy. Frank, as early as 1961, noted that all effective healing practices contain a "myth" and a "ritual." Said another way, one of the common factors is the systematic use of some set of specific ingredients, delivered in a cogent and convincing manner to the client and accepted by the client.

Pathway 3: Specific Ingredients

After there is agreement on the goals and tasks of therapy, the client engages in the therapeutic actions of the treatment; that is, the client "takes" the specific ingredients of the treatment. To many this is the potent part of psychotherapy. Indeed, there has been a distinction made between *psychological treatments*, that contain purported scientific specific ingredients, and generic psychotherapy that does not. Barlow (2004) noted that psychological treatments contain components common to all psychotherapies, such as "the therapeutic alliance, the induction of positive expectancy of change, and remoralization," but contain important "specific psychological procedures targeted at the psychopathology at hand" (p. 873). That is to say, the specific ingredient is what corrects the client's deficit in a way that makes treatment effective.

The Contextual Model indeed recognizes the importance of engaging in the therapeutic ingredients but for a different reason than that proposed by a Medical Model. Instead of positing a deficit that is remediated by a specific ingredient, the Contextual Model posits that the specific ingredients in all therapies induce the client to do something that is salubrious. That is, the client engages in some action that is health promoting in that the activity results in an increase in something healthy or a decrease in something unhealthy. For the most part, the effects of lifestyle variables, whether some form of exercise, increased social interaction, stress reduction, or religious and spiritual involvement, on mental health have been underestimated and often ignored (Walsh, 2011).

When considering how different types of therapies promote psychological health, it is useful to classify patient problems into broad classes of problems. Across disorders, many patients think about the world in dysfunctional ways. Cognitive therapies are focused on changing dysfunctional thoughts and core dysfunctional cognitive schemas, and certainly having more adaptive cognitions is "healthy." However, other therapies often address such issues, but use different terms (e.g., attachment styles developed early in life are similar schemas, in a broad sense) and dynamic therapists use very different procedures than cognitive-behavioral therapists, but likely the interventions of the latter also change cognitions. As discussed in Chapter 8, patients in many different therapies will have changes in dysfunctional thoughts as a result of the interventions. Many patients avoid objects (some phobias) or situations (e.g., social phobia) and many therapies address these issues by reducing the avoidance, often by exposure, which of course is beneficial to patient. As will be discussed in Chapter 8, it is difficult to design a treatment for avoidant patients that does not have some type of exposure, and the idea of "getting back on the horse" is one that is almost universally accepted in our culture (Anderson, Lunnen, & Ogles, 2010). As we have discussed previously (Wampold et al., 2010), even therapies that explicitly avoid discussion of traumatic events may have some elements of exposure. More broadly, many patients avoid difficult psychology material or are fearful of certain emotions; some treatments deal with these issues directly (e.g., Emotionally Focused Therapy, Greenberg, 2010, and Affect Phobia Therapy, McCullough & Magill, 2009). Across disorders, patients often have difficulty with interpersonal relationships and most treatments will address those issues, although not to the extent that treatments focused on this issue do (e.g., Interpersonal Psychotherapy, Klerman, Weissman, Rounsaville, & Chevron, 1984). Some therapies promote well-being by developing a stronger sense of self (e.g., Compassion Focused Therapy, Gilbert, 2010). Some patients come with a desire to reduce some type of behavior, such as alcohol or drug use, compulsive behaviors, or unnecessary worry. Patients typically have a constellation of these features and different therapies by their nature will focus on different ways to intervene, regardless of the primary diagnosis. Each therapy promotes psychological well-being and symptom reduction in some cogent manner. The difficulty for psychotherapy research (but fortunate for patients) is that aiding patients in one domain will generalize to other domains (see Chapter 8). It is difficult not to get better in any type of therapy without also thinking about the world in less dysfunctional ways; it is difficult not to get better in some sort of behavior therapy without feeling more positive about the self; it is difficult to reduce alcohol use and drug use without finding that interpersonal relationships have improved; and so forth. The broad argument of this volume is that while any number of therapies meet the topographical requirements of a psychotherapy outlined in the Contextual Model (see figure 2.2), the particular flavor of psychological activity is not necessarily a guide to how the treatment works mechanistically.

Summary

In this chapter, we defined terms so that key concepts were clear, as confusion often results in psychotherapy research because the terms are ambiguous. In this volume, we use the terms "specific effects" to denote the benefits of psychotherapy that are due to specific ingredients and "general effects" to denote the benefits due to common factors. We presented various alternatives to the Medical Model, with emphasis on the Contextual Model. The Contextual Model proposes that there are three pathways that create change in psychotherapy: the real relationship, expectations, and specific ingredients.

Chapter 3

Contextual Model Versus Medical Model
Choosing a Progressive Research Programme

According to Baker, McFall, and Shoham (2008), "The principal goals of clinical psychology are to generate knowledge based on scientifically valid evidence and to apply this knowledge to the optimal improvement of mental and behavioral health" (p. 68), a proclamation that, on the one hand, is so uncontroversially apparent that it should elicit universal agreement. On the other hand, this statement raises fundamental issues regarding the science of mental health services and the nature of evidence. No rational person argues against evidence as central to science. Isaac Asimov, when challenged to say what he believed in, replied:

> I believe in evidence. I believe in observation, measurement, and reasoning, confirmed by independent observers. I'll believe anything, no matter how wild and ridiculous, if there is evidence for it. The wilder and more ridiculous something is, however, the firmer and more solid the evidence will have to be.

Carl Sagan, in discussing science and pseudoscience, remarked, "I maintain there is much more wonder in science than in pseudoscience. And in addition, to whatever measure this term has any meaning, science has the additional virtue, and it is not an inconsiderable one, of being true."

Simply said, science utilizes evidence to discover truth. Unfortunately, the concepts of evidence and truth are vague. What constitutes evidence? Can truth be established? In the second half of the twentieth century, philosophers of science, including notably Karl Popper, Thomas Kuhn, Imre Lakatos, and Paul Feyerabend, were absorbed with these questions. Central to the discussion was the issue of demarcation of science and pseudoscience, with a desire to show that Freudian psychoanalysis and Marxist economics were pseudoscience, as well as to clarify what constitutes progress in science. These issues are still central to understanding the nature of psychotherapy, as Paul Meehl (1967, 1978) noted some three decades ago:

> Theories in "soft" areas of psychology lack the cumulative character of scientific knowledge. They tend neither to be refuted nor corroborated, but instead merely fade away as people lose interest.
>
> (Meehl, 1978, p. 806)

To understand the nature of science, philosophers of science developed various schemes that could "reconstruct" or explain how science has progressed. Despite the philosophical difficulties involved in the notions of evidence, truth, science versus pseudoscience, and so forth, some model of how science works must be adopted to interpret the evidence that is based on cumulative scientific knowledge rather than by popularity or politics. For the purpose of this volume, we use the reconstruction of Lakatos (Lakatos, 1970, 1976; Larvor, 1998; Serlin & Lapsley, 1985, 1993), whose work falls somewhere between conjectures and refutation proposed by Popper (also called critical rationalism; see Miller, 1994; Popper, 1963) and scientific revolutions described by Kuhn (Kuhn, 1962, 1970). Adoption of this particular reconstruction does not change the conclusion of this volume, as one could utilize any scheme, with the exception of radical constructivism, and the same conclusions would result. Simply put, Lakatos presents a reconstruction, which is eminently useful in making sense of psychotherapy evidence.

Philosophy of Science: Lakatos and Research Programmes[1]

Rarely, if ever, does a single experiment either confirm or refute a theoretical conjecture, despite the commonly held notion that theories cannot be proved but can be refuted by crucial experiments. According to the critical rational idea of refutation, a theory T must stipulate a priori what evidence, collected under what conditions, would demonstrate that T is false (Lakatos, 1970; Miller, 1994; Popper, 1963). The critical rational reconstruction rests on the *modus tollens*: If A, then B; if not B, then not A. In psychology, the evidence to falsify a hypothesis typically is given as a statement about population parameters of a distribution. Serlin and Lapsley (1985) laid out the strategy:

> On the basis of some theory T we derive the conclusion that a parameter . . . will differ for two populations [and let δ be the difference between the two parameters]. In order to examine this conclusion, we can set up a point-null hypothesis, H_0 $\delta = 0$, and test this hypothesis against the predicted outcome, $H_1 : \delta \neq 0$.
>
> (p. 74)

As much as we like to believe that as scientists we put theories to the test through refutation based on the *modus tollens*, such a notion misrepresents actual practice. Meehl, never one for restraint, severely criticized this idea: "The almost universal reliance on merely refuting the null hypothesis is a terrible mistake, is basically unsound, poor scientific strategy, and one of the worst things that ever happened in the history of psychology" (1978, p. 817).

A few examples taken from psychotherapy research will show the difficulties in making conclusions from single studies. Consider a study investigating a theoretical proposition related to cognitive-behavioral therapy for depression, the most widely disseminated and tested psychotherapy in existence. The purpose of the study was to "provide an experimental test of the theory of change put forth by A. T. Beck, A. J. Rush, B. F. Shaw, and G. Emery (1979) to explain the efficacy of cognitive-behavioral therapy (CT) for depression" (Jacobson et al., 1996, p. 295). To accomplish this goal, patients with major depression were randomly assigned to one of three treatment conditions: a) CT in its entirety, including behavioral activation (BA), automatic thought modification (AT), and modification of core schemas; b) BA and AT; and c) only BA. The authors made a specific prediction: "According to the cognitive theory of depression, CT should work significantly better than AT, which in turn, should work significantly better than BA" (p. 296). Contrary to expectations, the outcomes of the BA condition were comparable to CT at termination and follow-up:

> These findings run contrary to hypotheses generated by the cognitive model of depression put forth by Beck and his associates (1979), who proposed that direct efforts aimed at modifying negative schema are necessary to maximize treatment outcome and prevent relapse. These results are all the more surprising, given that they run counter to the allegiance effect (Robinson, Berman, & Neimeyer, 1990), which is quite commonly related to outcome in psychotherapy research.
>
> (Jacobson et al., 1996, p. 302)

The unexpected result led the authors to reconsider the mechanisms of change in CT but also to reconsider what was a legitimate treatment for depression: "If BA and AT treatments are as effective as CT and also are as likely to modify the factors that are thought to be necessary for change to occur, then not only the theory but also the therapy may be in need of revision" (p. 303). But neither the theory nor the therapy have been rejected or revised in any fundamental way. Is this an example of the flaws of "soft" psychology, as opposed to say astrophysics, where theories can be refuted by critical experiments? As many philosophers of science note, the romantic notion of a critical experiment changing the course of scientific thinking is a myth. A salient example is the attribution that the "famous" Michelson-Morely experiment definitively refuted the aether theory that attempted to explain propagation of forces at a distance, when in fact the existence of ether did not disappear from science for some years after the Michelson and Morely experiment, allowing time for the presentation of additional evidence and a reinterpretation of the data produced by the original experiment (Lakatos, 1970). Giving prominence to a single study as evidence for a theoretical proposition will surely be ambiguous if not misleading.

Another problem, noted prominently by Meehl (1978), is that testing a point-null hypothesis (e.g., H_0: $\delta = 0$) has a high likelihood of resulting in rejection if there is sufficient statistical power and the population parameter is not exactly zero, which is unlikely. Thus studies with large sample sizes will almost surely result in rejection of the null, a problem exacerbated in psychotherapy trials by multiple outcome measures or process studies with multiple variables. For example, Leichsenring et al. (2013) compared cognitive-behavioral treatment to psychodynamic treatment for social anxiety and found quite small differences between the two treatments. Some of the differences, despite being quite small, were statistically significant because the sample sizes were relatively large (greater than 200 in each condition; this study is reviewed in greater detail in Chapter 5). Similarly, Wampold and Brown (2005) found that in a naturalistic setting with more than 2,000 patients that the amount of change in psychotherapy was statistically dependent on their diagnosis, even though diagnosis accounts for less than 0.2 percent of the variability in outcomes. As sample sizes increase and other operations become more precise (e.g., more reliable instruments), the psychotherapy literature will be littered with significant results, many of which might reflect true effects very close to zero and some simply false positives (i.e., even if the null is true, 5 percent of studies will falsely reject the null).

Finally, because no study can rule out all threats to validity, no single study will provide an iron-clad refutation. Psychotherapy research, often involving the comparisons of two different treatments, illustrates nicely the ease with which results can be impugned. In a 1999 study, Tarrier et al. compared imaginal exposure (IE) to cognitive therapy (CT) and concluded, "A significantly greater number of patients receiving IE worsened over treatment" (p. 17) than in CT. However, Devilly and Foa (2001) claimed that Tarrier et al. delivered IE inappropriately:

> For example, although Tarrier et al. noted that the therapists guided the participants to speak in the present tense, was this integrated into the session effectively? Did the therapist note "hot spots" where appropriate and habituate the participants to these?
>
> (p. 115)

This is an adherence criticism (see Chapter 8) in the sense that the therapists delivering the treatment *may* not have been adhering to the treatment protocol—that is, the specific ingredients purported to be necessary were not being provided adequately. However, even when rated adherence to both treatments is sufficient, as it was in a comparison of behavioral marital therapy (BMT) and insight-oriented marital therapy (IOMT) that found that insight-oriented marital therapy had significantly fewer divorces after therapy (Snyder & Wills, 1991), an advocate for the inferior treatment (BMT) claimed that therapists in this condition did not sufficiently provide empathy and emotional nurturance and did not adequately foster hope, actions that were not specific to the treatment (Jacobson, 1991); that is, there was purportedly an inequivalence of the common factors. In another study that found that cognitive therapy was superior to relaxation therapy for panic disorder (Clark et al., 1994), it has been noted that the relaxation protocol was changed in critical ways so as not to overlap with cognitive therapy (an adherence issue) and the therapists, who delivered both treatments, had an allegiance to the superior treatment (allegiance effects) (Wampold, Imel, & Miller, 2009; see Chapter 5 for a review of allegiance effects).

The point here is that any single study will not provide definitive evidence about theory, but there is more to it than that. The manner in which studies are criticized reveals issues that relate to theory. Philosophers of science posit that auxiliary theories are needed to explain anomalous data or are even necessary to conduct research at all. In the examples discussed above, adherence and allegiance are auxiliaries that are invoked to help understand the results of psychotherapy trials. The reconstruction of science proposed by Lakatos makes these issues central to the progress of science.

According to Lakatos, focus on a theoretical edifice, solid and unchanging, which either survives attempts to falsify it or crumbles under a refutation, misrepresents how science works. Rather, theories are changed to accommodate new discoveries or unexpected results:

> It is a succession of theories and not one given theory which is apprised as scientific or pseudo-scientific. But the members of such series of theories are usually connected by a remarkable *continuity* which welds them into a *research programme*.
>
> (Lakatos, 1970, p. 132)

A programme has a *hard core*, which contains the essential tenets of the theory, as well as *auxiliary hypotheses* that are needed to conduct scientific research about the hard core and to interpret the results. Popper also recognized the existence of auxiliaries, which make theory testing difficult—was a falsification due to deficiencies of the hard core, because one of the auxiliaries was incorrect, or because something was learned and a new auxiliary is needed? However, according to Lakatos, who discussed auxiliaries in some detail, the auxiliary hypotheses can be modified to explain observations as long as the hard core remains untouched, thus providing a *protective belt* for the theory. As long as the changes to the auxiliary hypotheses result in better predictions or explanatory power, the program is termed *progressive*. On the other hand, if ad hoc amendments were needed to explain anomalies that do not result in novel predictions or increase explanatory power, the program is termed *degenerative*. Degenerative programs might apply auxiliaries inconsistently from one instance to another, accumulate so many auxiliaries that the theory becomes exceedingly complex, or utilize auxiliaries that themselves appear to be false.

According to Lakatos, a program of research should not be abandoned unless there is a progressive alternative. A theory, in the Lakotosian reconstruction, should be abandoned when "there exists a rival program that is powerful enough to account for all the facts of the former program and, importantly, possess sufficient generative power to anticipate novel facts, some of which have been corroborated" (Serlin & Lapsley, 1993, p. 205). As described by Larvor (1998), Popperian theories suffer refutation whereas "Lakatosian theories and programmes suffer abandonment . . . Our confidence in any dominant theory as a vehicle for a proof (i.e., justification) would be undermined by discoveries which either cast doubt on the dominant theory or which could not be expressed in it" (p. 34–35).

In this book, the Medical Model of psychotherapy is the received theory, as has been discussed in Chapter 1. As Lakatos' reconstruction demands, a rival programme must exist, and the Contextual Model provides such a rival. Both programmes are modified as research evidence is collected and presented, both programmes employ auxiliaries to conduct research and explain evidence, both programmes are supported by some individual studies that seem to "corroborate" the theory, and both programmes are weakened by some individual studies that seem to be contrary to predictions. Nevertheless, this volume presents evidence that suggests that the Contextual Model represents a progressive research programme and that the Medical Model shows signs of being degenerative. Before presenting predictions of the two programmes of research, a discussion of the type of evidence that is desirable or even admissible is presented.

Admissibility of Evidence: What Counts as Evidence?

There appears to be a general resistance to considering the scientific status of the Contextual Model, as exemplified by Baker et al.'s (2008) discussion of the science of clinical psychology:

> Research on nonspecific effects [i.e., the factors of the Contextual Model] provides little support for the current practices of psychology, however. Legitimate and important issues surround nonspecific effects, but the resolution of the debate about nonspecific effects has little potential to validate a science-based practice of clinical psychology. . . . It is important to note the marginal scientific status of those constructs.
>
> (p. 82)

Another criticism of the scientific validity of the Contextual Model is that the factors purported to be therapeutic cannot be shown to be causally related to outcomes of psychotherapy (Baker et al., 2008; DeRubeis et al., 2005; Siev, Huppert, & Chambless, 2009) because it is difficult or unethical to experimentally manipulate the variables. Randomized clinical trials (RCTs), according to this view, are given primacy, which ipso facto put a focus on the treatment method:

> Of all the aspects of psychotherapy that influence outcome, the treatment method is the only aspect in which psychotherapists can be trained, it is

the only aspect that can be manipulated in a clinical experiment [i.e., in an RCT] to test its worth, and, if proven valuable, it is the only aspect that can be disseminated to other psychotherapists.

(Chambless & Crits-Christoph, 2006, pp. 199–200)

Reconstructions of scientific progress typically are agnostic relative to what evidence is admissible, as all observations naturally come with baggage due to particular experimental arrangements (Lakatos, 1970; Latour, 1999; Larvor, 1998; Miller, 1994; Serlin & Lapsley, 1985, 1993). Many theories have been examined with naturalistic observations, including many in astronomy (e.g., planetary motion, big bang theory), economics (e.g., monetarism, common pool resources, new trade theory), biology (e.g., evolution), natural history (e.g., the extinction of the dinosaurs), and medicine (e.g., H. pylori and gastric ulcers, smoking and health). Indeed, a perusal of Nobel laureates will reveal that many used observational methods rather than experimental methods and few, if any, won Nobel Awards in physiology and medicine based on evidence produced by randomized clinical trials. From a causal standpoint, if a variable theoretically could be manipulated, it is appropriate to consider it as a causal factor, regardless of whether it is feasible or ethical to manipulate it (Holland, 1986, 1993; Rubin, 1986). As discussed earlier (as well as in subsequent chapters), RCTs are not free from controversy with regard to conclusions and have their own threats to validity. Consequently, there is no prioritizing of one particular research design over another, in terms of presentation of the evidence, although it is important to note the limitations of all studies, including RCTs, which have many.

There are some issues, however, that have to be addressed. There are thousands and thousands of studies on psychotherapy, with a proliferation of every kind, but especially clinical trials (see Chapters 4 and 5) and process variables such as the alliance (Chapter 7). As discussed above, each of these studies have some threat to their validity. Compounding that problem is that there is a rich history of selecting studies that support one theoretical position and either ignoring or impugning others. Therefore, the many studies investigating some research question have to be aggregated and summarized in a scientific way. Science has embraced meta-analysis as the quantitative means to aggregate studies (Hunt, 1997).

Effect Sizes in Meta-Analyses

Because meta-analyses are ubiquitous in psychology and these procedures are now taught regularly in methods classes, only the rudiments of the method are presented here, with a focus on the interpretation of effect sizes. An effect size is a standardized index that measures the strength of a relationship. In group designs, the effect size is the standardized difference between the means of the distributions for two groups. For example, take a comparison of the population of patients treated for a disorder with the population of untreated patients, where patients are randomly assigned to the two conditions (treatment, TX, and waitlist control, WLC). The sample effect size is given as $(M_{TX} - M_{WLC})/SD_{pooled}$, where M_{TX} is the mean of outcome measure after treatment for those patients in the treatment group, M_{WLC} is the mean of the outcome measure for those patients who did not receive treatment measured at the post-treatment time point (i.e., were on the waiting list), and SD_{pooled} is the pooled standard deviation of the two samples. Larger effects reflect greater treatment efficacy. The answer to the question "How big is big?" will be addressed below. The critical step in meta-analysis is to aggregate the effects from studies investigating the same hypothesis. If there have been ten studies that investigated the efficacy of the treatments for this disorder, then the effects from each study can be "averaged" to form an aggregate effect, providing an estimate of the treatment effect, which is more precise (i.e., has a smaller standard error of estimate) than the estimates provided by any single study. There is much statistical theory behind this process, including correcting for small sample bias, weighting studies by how precise each study is (more precise estimates, usually derived from larger samples, are weighted more heavily than less precise studies), estimating the error in estimation for effects for each study and for the aggregate effect, and creating confidence intervals for the effect (Cooper & Hedges, 1994; Cooper, Hedges, & Valentine, 2009; Hedges, 1981; Hedges & Olkin, 1985). It is customary now to conduct random effects meta-analyses, where effects (i.e., studies) are considered sampled from a population of studies (Raudenbush, 2009).

Studies of psychotherapy process often examine the correlation between some process variable and outcome; for example, the correlation of the alliance between the therapist and the client and outcome (see Chapter 7) or the correlation of therapist adherence or competence and outcome (see Chapter 8). These correlations can be aggregated across studies in a fashion similar to what is done for between group effects, creating an aggregate estimate of the population correlation coefficient as well as its standard error (Shadish & Haddock, 2009).

Hypotheses about the aggregate effect size, either d or r, are usually tested in meta-analyses. Typically, the null hypothesis tested is that the aggregate effect size is zero (in the continuing example, the treatment is not efficacious) versus the alternative that the effect is different from zero. As well, the heterogeneity of effects can be examined. If effects are heterogeneous, then there is more variability in the effects than is expected and it is important to examine what might have created the variability, usually accomplished by testing various moderators of the effects.

One of the advantages of effects sizes is that they provide different information than significance testing. For a given study, the effect may be very small but statistically significant, if the sample size is large, as discussed above. On the other hand, the effect might be large, but not statistically significant. To judge the size of an effect is somewhat tricky, but Table 3.1 is useful for this purpose.

Table 3.1 Effect Sizes

d	Cohen's Description	Proportion of Control Patients Less Than Mean of Treatment	r	R^2	NNT
1.0		0.84	.45	0.20	2
0.9		0.82	.41	0.17	3
0.8	Large	0.79	.37	0.14	3
0.7		0.76	.33	0.11	3
0.6		0.73	.29	0.08	4
0.5	Medium	0.69	.24	0.06	4
0.4		0.66	.20	0.04	5
0.3		0.62	.15	0.02	6
0.2	Small	0.58	.10	0.01	9
0.1		0.54	.05	<0.01	18
0.0		0.50	.00	0.00	∞

Note. d = between group effect size, Cohen's (1988) designation, proportion of success is the proportion of patients receiving treatment who would be better off than the average patient with the alternative, r = correlation coefficient, R^2 = Proportion of variance accounted for by factor, NNT = Number Needed to Treat.

The first column, labeled "d" is the effect size, as described above. Jacob Cohen, after reviewing results of studies in the social sciences, described a d of 0.8 as large, 0.5 as medium, and 0.2 as small (Cohen, 1988; see column 2), although many have criticized these descriptors as arbitrary. As will be discussed in Chapter 4, psychotherapy versus no treatment (e.g., waitlist control) produces an effect of approximately 0.8, which is a large effect, according to Cohen. The third column provides a common sense interpretation of effects based on overlapping normal distributions of the two groups (interpretation due to Glass, 1976). Suppose that a study found that a treatment was superior to no treatment with an effect size of 0.60. As shown in Figure 3.1, this can be interpreted as indicating that the average treated person will have a better outcome than 73 percent of those who are untreated. This interpretation is particularly appealing because it is a common sense interpretation; for example, it is understandable to a patient to say, on average, if you complete this treatment you will be better off than 73 percent of patients who do not get the treatment. Of course, if the treatment has no value at all (i.e., d = 0.00), then the average person receiving the treatment will be better off than 50 percent of untreated persons. The fourth column equates the effect size d with a correlation coefficient (Rosenthal, 1994), which allows a comparison of effects obtained from clinical trials (d) and effects from the correlation of process variables and outcome (r).[2]

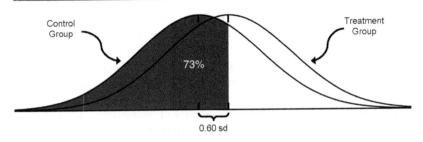

Figure 3.1 Interpreting effect sizes from overlapping distributions.

The next column gives the value of R^2, the proportion of variance in outcome explained by the factor being investigated.[3] Again, taking the example of a large effect of d = 0.80 implies that 14 percent of the variability in outcomes is associated with the factor. Consider an effect of .80 from an RCT comparing a treatment to a no-treatment control (e.g., a waitlist control); this effect implies that 14 percent of the variability in the outcome, say in depression scores, for the patients in the trial was associated with whether the patient received the treatment or not. There are a few issues that need discussion here. First, one has to be careful about implying that the factor is causal. Causality is a tricky concept and it is easier to ascribe causality in an experimental design where a variable is manipulated and the effects of this manipulation observed, as is the case in randomized clinical trials. However, it is vital to keep in mind that RCTs have threats to validity that make discussion of causality difficult. As well, the level at which causality is attributed is critical to making proper inferences. Consider an experiment where turning on a light switch is assigned to various time points—when the switch is turned on, light appeared. Is turning on a switch the cause of emission of photons? Clearly yes, but this is clearly not a very theoretically useful experiment. Causality is central to theories but terribly difficult to infer directly from studies, as will become clear through the presentation of the evidence in this volume. The second issue about variability accounted for by a factor is that it appears that even a large effect accounts for what might seem to be a relatively small percentage of the variability in outcome. If receiving psychotherapy accounts for 14 percent of the variability in outcomes relative to not receiving psychotherapy, then 86 percent of the variability in outcomes of patients is due to other factors—this might seem like psychotherapy is not really very effective. It is important to keep in mind that there are many other factors that contribute to the variability of outcomes of patients. Patients who are relatively more distressed before treatment will be relatively more distressed afterwards, regardless of the effectiveness of the treatment; initial distress accounts for about 50 percent of the variability in outcome. And then there are patient factors—some patients are more motivated, are ready for change, have economic resources and social support, and so forth (Bohart & Tallman, 1999; Prochaska & Norcross, 2002). Of course, there is also error variance attributable to measures, research operations, and other factors attributable to experimental arrangements. Even so, when compared to medical practices, 14 percent is quite impressive. Aspirin as a prophylaxis for heart attacks, established in an RCT that was halted because it was decided that it was unethical to withhold the aspirin from the placebo group, accounts for about one percent of the variability in outcomes, an order of magnitude smaller than psychotherapy. The superiority of antidepressants to placebos accounts for about three percent of the variability in outcomes. In terms of interpreting the evidence, the proportion of variability in outcome due to various factors will be compared to identify those factors important for the success of psychotherapy.

The final column in Table 3.1 converts effects into Number Needed to Treat (NNT) (Kraemer & Kupfer, 2006), which is defined as the number of patients who need to receive the treatment to achieve one additional success vis-à-vis the control condition. Returning to the example of an effect of 0.8 for a treatment in comparison to no treatment is equivalent to an NNT of three, which means that three patients need to receive psychotherapy to have one better outcome than they would have had receiving no treatment, or said another way, two of the three patients will not have a better outcome getting psychotherapy than they would have had without treatment. Again, this might be interpreted as an indictment of the effectiveness of psychotherapy until one compares this NNT to those of many medical practices. Keeping in mind that smaller NNTs indicate greater effectiveness, psychotherapy compares favorably to many commonly accepted medical practices, some of which are very expensive and have serious side effects, including most interventions in cardiology (e.g., b-blockers NNT = 40 vis-à-vis placebo), gastroenterology (e.g., proton pump inhibitors for bleeding peptic ulcers vis-à-vis placebo, NNT = 6), orthopedics (e.g., active treatment of whiplash versus treatment-as-usual, NNT = 5), respiratory disease (e.g., nicotine inhalers versus placebo on smoking cessation, NNT = 10), and primary care (e.g., influenza vaccine vis-à-vis placebo for the prevention of an episode of influenza, NNT = 12), among many others (see http://ktclearinghouse.ca/cebm/glossary/nnt/).

Extensions and Issues in Meta-Analyses

There are a number of advances in meta-analysis that further the understanding of psychotherapy as well as some issues, which will be briefly discussed here. As mentioned previously, it is customary to use random effects meta-analytic models, although this concept is often misunderstood. In random models, the studies included in the meta-analysis are treated as if they are randomly sampled from a population of studies investigating a particular effect, which introduces a variance term due to sampling studies as well as sampling participants within studies (Raudenbush, 2009). Suppose that there is a true population effect and many studies are designed to detect and estimate that effect. The estimates from the various studies will vary because of the random assignment of participants to conditions within the studies, as well as differences among the studies. If the variability of the effects of many studies is about what is expected due to statistical theory, then the effects are said to be homogenous. However, if the variability is greater than would be expected (i.e., a test of homogeneity leads to a rejection), then the effects are said to het-erogeneous. If effects are homogeneous, then confidence in the meta-analytic estimate of the true effect is increased. If the effects are heterogeneous, then there is between study variability that could be explained by some moderator, which would be some characteristic of studies. Often an index of heteroge-neity is given—for example, it might be that 30 percent of the variability of observed effects in a set of studies is due to between-study variability. Often we can account for the between-study variability with moderators and some-times the heterogeneity is unexplained. For example, as we shall see, stud-ies with better research designs produce larger psychotherapy effects than studies with poorer research designs. Tests of homogeneity can also be used to examine the relative efficacy of treatments, as discussed in Chapter 5 (see Wampold & Serlin, 2014).

One of the criticisms of meta-analysis is that it combines very different studies—combining "apples" and "oranges" if you will. This problem is dis-cussed in the context of absolute efficacy in Chapter 4, but at this point, it is simply noted that the differences among studies, in terms of some study level variable, such as quality of the design, can be examined by determining how they explain heterogeneity of effects.

Another issue that is consequential in psychotherapy outcome studies is that clinical trials typically involve multiple dependent measures. An effect size can be calculated for each outcome variable, but the outcome variables are *not* independent. This is a problem that was understood when meta-analysis was first applied to psychotherapy outcome studies but which has been largely ignored. If a study has eight dependent measures, then it is extremely problem-atic for that study to contribute eight effects to the meta-analysis, particularly if another study has only two or three effects. Over the years, various strategies have been used. First, the problem can be ignored and all effects are included in the meta-analysis—because of the problems with this, this strategy is rarely used any longer. Second, the effects can be averaged within studies, although this is usually done incorrectly. Although not stated in the meta-analysis, these averages are usually simply the means of the effects without taking into consid-eration that the outcome variables are correlated (see Gleser & Olkin, 2009), which significantly affects the standard error of the estimates (see Hoyt & Del Re, submitted). Wampold et al. (1997b) took into account the correlations among the dependent variables, using the methods presented by Gleser and Olkin, which produces a suitable estimate of the effect for the multiple outcome measures (see Hoyt & Del Re). A third way is to select only one variable from each study, a strategy that is often employed. This is problematic for several reasons, including a) it ignores the information from the other variables, creating a less precise estimate than could be obtained by using all the variables; and b) it focuses on one aspect of outcome to the exclusion of others. With regard to the latter, the one variable selected usually reflects symptoms targeted by the treatment (sometimes called disorder symptom specific measure, primary measure, or targeted measure), ignoring other important variables such as other symptoms, global measures of outcomes, quality of life, and so forth, which are important outcomes and affect the interpretation of the efficacy of the treatment (Bell, Marcus, & Goodlad, 2013; Laska, Gurman, & Wampold, 2014; Minami, Wampold, Serlin, Kircher, & Brown, 2007).

Conjectures of Medical Model and Contextual Model

One of the hallmarks of science is the notion that a theory T generates conjectures that can be examined. Conjectures are essentially predictions about what will be observed under certain conditions. In science, research creates the conditions and then it is determined whether the observations are consistent with the predictions. In the various reconstructions discussed previously, how conjectures lead to progress differs, but at the core of all reconstructions is the notion of theoretical specifications of what will be observed under what conditions. In the remainder of the chapter, predictions of the Medical Model and the Contextual Model are discussed. This discussion is approached through the lens of Lakatos' research programmes with the theoretical hard core and various auxiliaries. Many of the auxiliaries, however, only become apparent as various research evidence is examined in subsequent chapters.

Medical Model

The hard core of the Medical Model is that the specific ingredients that remediate particular deficits are what make psychotherapy work. David Barlow (2004) summarized this succinctly when he said that although potent psychotherapies all contain aspects that are common to all treatments, including "the therapeutic alliance, the induction of positive expectancy of change, and remoralization," they contain important "specific psychological procedures targeted at the psychopathology at hand" (p. 873). Certain conjectures flow from this theoretical proposition, as summarized in Table 3.2.

The first conjecture is that psychotherapy is effective because the specific ingredients are indeed effective. That is, psychotherapies should be more effective than no treatment, which is what is referred to as absolute efficacy (Chapter 4). Most advocates of a Medical Model recognize that the common factors are necessary for psychotherapy to be delivered and may be marginally beneficial by themselves, and, therefore, treatments with specific ingredients will be more effective than treatments without specific ingredients, although

Table 3.2 Conjectures of Medical Model and Contextual Model

Medical Model	Contextual Model
Absolute Efficacy (Chapter 4)	
1. Psychotherapy more effective than no treatment	1. Psychotherapy more effective than no treatment
2. Psychotherapy without specific ingredients will be less effective than psychotherapy with specific ingredients	2. Psychotherapy without specific ingredients will be less effective than psychotherapy with specific ingredients
3. Psychotherapy without specific ingredients more effective than no treatment	3. Psychotherapy without specific ingredients more effective than no treatment
Relative Efficacy (Chapter 5)	
1. Variability in efficacy of treatments (i.e., some treatments more effective than others)	1. Homogeneity of treatment effects: All treatments intended to be therapeutic will be equally effective
2. Tx A is more effective than Tx B for a particular disorder	
Therapist Effects (Chapter 6)	
1. Therapist effects are small, particularly when providing an evidence-based treatment and adhering to the model.	1. Therapist effects will be relatively large, especially in comparison to effects of specific ingredients
	2. Therapist differences will be due to relationship factors
General Effects (Chapter 7)	
1. Relationship factors will not be critical factors in psychotherapy outcome	1. Therapeutic alliance will be associated with outcome
	2. Other relationship factors (e.g., empathy, goal consensus and collaboration, real relationship) will be associated with outcome
	3. Expectations are important for outcomes
	4. Researcher allegiance, and particularly therapist allegiance, will be related to psychotherapy outcome
	5. Cultural adaptations will increase the effectiveness of treatments
Specific Effects (Chapter 8)	
1. Removing specific ingredient from a scientifically established treatment will attenuate the efficacy of the treatment; adding a component will augment efficacy	1. Removing specific ingredient from a scientifically established treatment will not attenuate the efficacy of the treatment; adding a component will not augment efficacy
2. A treatment T1 may be more efficacious than T2 for treating symptoms S1 but not for treating symptoms S2	2. Adherence and treatment specific competence will not be related to outcome
3. Adherence and treatment specific competence related to outcome	

treatments without specific ingredients might well be more effective than no treatment. In terms of the Contextual Model presented in Chapter 2, the Medical Model emphasizes the third pathway: specific ingredients.

The strongest conjectures that emanate from the Medical Model are in the area of relative efficacy, which addresses whether one treatment is more efficacious than another treatment. According to the Medical Model, ingredients of treatments that address a psychological deficit will be effective whereas treatments that contain ingredients that are scientifically inert—that is, do not remediate the deficit—will not be effective. The distinction between "scientific" ingredients and other ingredients goes back to the origins of behavior therapy, when Eysenck (1961) made a distinction between behavior therapy, based on scientifically based learning theory, and other types of therapy:

> Neurotic patients treated by means of psychotherapeutic procedures based on learning theory improve significantly more quickly than do patients treated by means of psychoanalytic or eclectic psychotherapy, or not treated by psychotherapy at all . . . It would appear advisable, therefore, to discard the psychoanalytic model, which both on the theoretical and practical plain fails to be useful in mediating verifiable predictions, and to adopt, provisionally, at least, the learning theory model, which, to date, appears to be much more promising theoretically and also with regard to application.
>
> (pp. 720–721)

Eysenck impugned psychoanalytic and eclectic therapy for being theoretically impoverished—in a sense unscientific. The important part of the logic here, which is fundamental to the Medical Model, is that the scientific status of the ingredients is related to the efficacy of the treatment. More recently, Baker et al. (2008) attempted to make the same distinction between scientific treatments and others:

> Scientific plausibility refers to the extent to which an intervention makes sense on substantive bases and whether there is formal evidence regarding its mechanisms. . . . However, the absence of a demonstrated or plausible *specific mechanism* of action, especially for a psychosocial intervention, leaves open the possibility that the intervention may merely be capitalizing on nonspecific credible ritual, or placebo effects.
>
> (emphasis added, p. 72)

As an example of a treatment with plausible specific mechanisms, consider prolonged exposure (PE) for post-traumatic stress disorder (PTSD) (Foa, Hembree, & Rothbaum, 2007), which is based on emotional processing theory (Foa & Kozak, 1986); the ingredients of PE (viz., exposure) activate a fear network, creating habituation that leads to extinguishing of the fear response. Scientific explanations for a disorder and ingredients endorsed by the science, such as is the case for PE according to Foa and colleagues, will lead to more effective treatments. In a sense, more potent ingredients imply more efficacious treatments.

Consequently, in terms of conjectures about relative efficacy, the Medical Model makes predictions at two levels. At the most general level, the Medical Model predicts that there will be variability in the effectiveness of treatments, with some—those with scientifically valid bases—more efficacious than others—those with less scientifically valid bases or no scientific bases at all. At the more specific level, a particular hypothesis about two particular treatments, say Tx A and Tx B, for a particular disorder, is made. For example, it might be hypothesized that PE is more effective than Eye-movement Desensitization and Reprocessing (EMDR) for PTSD, because PE contains scientific ingredients whereas many claim that EMDR does not (see Herbert et al., 2000; McNally, 1999). Medical Model adherents go one step further, suggesting a specificity in terms of symptoms targeted by specific ingredients: "A treatment T1 may be more efficacious than T2 for treating symptoms S1 but not for treating symptoms S2" (Hofmann & Lohr, 2010, p. 14).

A related conjecture about specific ingredients is derived from dismantling designs (Borkovec, 1990). In a dismantling design, a critical specific ingredient is removed from a treatment that has been proven to be efficacious. According to the Medical Model, removing the ingredient that is purportedly theoretically critical to the success of the treatment should attenuate the efficacy of the treatment. As well, adding a component with a scientific basis to an existing treatment should augment the efficacy of the treatment.

The Medical Model conjectures involve evidence produced by clinical trials, which involve random assignment of patients to various conditions in which treatments are delivered (or not delivered, which is the case for waiting list controls, for example). There are many methodological issues involved in designing RCTs, a few of which are discussed here as they relate to conjectures. To properly conduct an RCT, the treatment must be delivered properly so that the ingredients that are purported to be necessary to generate benefits are delivered adequately, as was alluded to earlier. That is, it is necessary for the validity of the study that the therapist adheres to the treatment protocol. Adherence, which is also referred to as *treatment integrity*, is defined as the "extent to which a therapist used interventions and approaches prescribed by the treatment manual, and avoided the use of interventions procedures proscribed by the manual" (Waltz, Addis, Koerner, & Jacobson, 1993, p. 620). In Lakatosian terms, adherence is an auxiliary, because it is necessary to conduct research and to make proper interpretations (see Bhar & Beck, 2009; Perepletchikova, 2009). As noted by Perepletchikova:

> Treatment integrity is integral to treatment outcome research methods, especially in conducting randomized controlled trials (RCT), where

precision and clarity are imperative (Kendall & Comer, in press). In order to draw valid inferences regarding the relationship between an intervention and the obtained results, it is necessary to establish and document that treatment was conducted as intended.

(p. 380)

Clearly, adherence is a reasonable auxiliary from a Medical Model perspective. However, as we noted adherence can be used to impugn the results of studies that are contradictory to one's point of view. Therefore, the adherence auxiliary and how it is applied must be examined carefully (see Chapter 8). Foremost, for adherence to be an explanatory auxiliary, the degree to which adherence is present (that is, in the treatment, the specific ingredients were delivered and avoided using proscribed ingredients) should be associated with outcome in clinical trials. Second, adherence should be assessed in clinical trials and attempts to impugn studies based on the adherence auxiliary should be applied consistently from one study to another and not simply when the result is contradictory to one's conjectures. A third aspect of adherence relates to therapist effects, which will be discussed as an auxiliary of the Contextual Model. Essentially therapist effects refer to variability among therapists in terms of outcomes—if therapist effects are present some therapists consistently will achieve better outcomes than other therapists, regardless of the characteristics of the patients. The Medical Model conjectures that therapist differences, if present, are due to the lack of adherence—when therapists provide evidence-based treatments with adherence to the protocol, therapist effects will be small or nonexistent (Crits-Christoph et al., 1991; Shafran et al., 2009).

A concept related to adherence is therapist treatment specific competence. Adherence refers to whether certain ingredients are delivered or not; treatment specific competence refers to how well the therapist delivers the ingredients. Competence has been defined as the "level of skill in delivering the treatment, [where] skill [is] the extent to which their therapists conducting interventions took the relevant aspects of the therapeutic context into account and responded to these contextual variables appropriately" (Waltz et al., 1993, p. 620). According to the Medical Model, ratings of competence should be associated with outcomes.

Contextual Model

Conjectures for the Contextual Model emanate from the three pathways of change discussed in Chapter 2. According to the Contextual Model, if a particular psychotherapeutic treatment contains the components of the three pathways, it will be effective. Of particular importance in terms of differentiating the Contextual Model from the Medical Model is the third pathway: specific ingredients. According to the Contextual Model, an effective treatment must have specific actions, an idea that goes back at least to Jerome Frank

(Frank, 1961). However, the power of the specific ingredients are that the patient is engaged in healing activities, necessary to create expectations, but also importantly leading to some desirable change (see Chapter 2). As opposed to the Medical Model, there is no assumption that the ingredient remediates a particular psychological deficit or even that the ingredient provides a scientifically "plausible" explanation for how it works; indeed, in this volume several treatments that contain what might seem to be bogus ingredients are shown to be effective. In Lakatosian terms, the hard core of the Contextual Model is that the effectiveness of the psychotherapy is unrelated to the scientific bases of the specific ingredients outlined by the treatment approach but works through the three pathways described in Chapter 2. It is worth reiterating that although in the Contextual Model the scientific bases of the specific ingredients are irrelevant to the effectiveness of the treatment, the model is scientific in that it is based on social science knowledge, but more importantly, produces conjectures that can be examined by observation, the hallmark of any reconstruction of science.

In terms of absolute efficacy, predictions of the Contextual Model are identical to those of the Medical Model, albeit for different reasons. According to the Contextual Model, treatments with a cogent rationale that is accepted by the client, administered by a therapist who believes in the treatment and who the client believes understands the client and has the expertise to help, and contain therapeutic actions that lead to some health-promoting change for clients will be effective. Moreover, treatment without specific ingredients, which are encountered in clinical trials as various kinds of controls and also are delivered by some therapists in practice, will be less effective than treatments with specific ingredients, as such treatments eliminate the third Contextual Model pathway. However, such treatments might well contain aspects of the first two pathways (the real relationship and expectations) and, therefore, will be more effective than no treatment.

A critical difference between conjectures for the Medical Model and the Contextual Model is found in in terms of relative efficacy. Whereas the Medical Model predicts that some treatments will be more effective than others, the Contextual Model predicts that treatments will be homogeneously effective. That is, all treatments will be equally effective, provided they contain the elements of the three pathways. As will be seen when the evidence is presented, "treatments" investigated in clinical trials are often not intended to be therapeutic and do not contain any cogent rationale and therapeutic actions rendering the third pathway null; as emphasized here, such treatments will not be as effective as treatment with the necessary components.

The Contextual Model predicts that there will be little evidence for the importance of any particular specific ingredient. Therefore, removing a critical specific ingredient from an established treatment will not attenuate the effectiveness of the treatment as long as the treatment remains cogent and there are sufficient specific ingredients remaining that provide the client an opportunity to make desirable changes. Similarly, adding a treatment component to an existing treatment will not augment treatment effectiveness.

A central component of the Contextual Model is the relationship between the therapist and the client. Some therapists are better able to form relationships with clients and more skillfully enact the components of therapy, and, consequently, some therapists will be more effective than other therapists. Moreover, therapist differences will not be due to adherence to a treatment protocol or the treatment specific competence but will be due to relationship factors.

The Contextual Model predicts that relationship factors will prominently account for much of the variability in outcomes. Related to the first pathway: real relationship, indicators of the real relationship and empathy will be associated with treatment outcomes. With regard to the second pathway: (i.e. expectations), the working alliance and goal consensus and collaboration will be associated with outcomes. As will be explored in Chapter 8, the working alliance is critical to many of the aspects that seem to make psychotherapy effective. As well, expectations created by therapy and the attributions made about the treatment will be important for the outcomes of psychotherapy.

In the Medical Model, the adherence auxiliary was necessary for conducting valid investigations and interpreting the observations made. In the Contextual Model, allegiance is an auxiliary that functions in a similar fashion as adherence. The prototypic randomized clinical trial in medicine is double blinded—neither the person administering the pill nor the patient receiving the pill are aware of whether the treatment has the purportedly active substance or is inert (i.e., a placebo). Such blinding is not possible in psychotherapy studies because the therapist is of course knowledgeable of what is contained in the treatment. Often—if not typically— researchers have an allegiance to one of the treatments being investigated. Researcher allegiance, which is often shown to increase the effects for that treatment (Luborsky et al., 1999; Munder, Brütsch, Leonhart, Gerger, & Barth, 2013; Wampold, 2001b), can be due to many factors, but one of particular importance for Contextual Model is the allegiance of the therapist. The Contextual Model places emphasis on the person of the therapist and predicts that therapy will be more effective when conducted by therapists who believe in the efficacy of the treatment being delivered.

As discussed in Chapter 2, expectations are only created if the patient accepts the explanation (Wampold & Budge, 2012; Wampold, Imel, Bhati, & Johnson Jennings, 2006). In the Contextual Model, it is conjectured that the explanations must be, to use Vygotskyian terms, in the zone of proximal development for a given patient—that is, the explanation and treatment must be compatible with the patient's cultural beliefs. According to this view, an evidence-based treatment will be more effective if it is adapted to the patient's cultural beliefs. This is contrary to the Medical Model, which stipulates that as long as the psychological deficit underlying a disorder, which is assumed to be culturally invariant, is addressed, the treatment will be effective.

The predictions of the two models are summarized in Table 3.2. These predictions are explored in more depth as the evidence for the predictions is presented in subsequent chapters.

Summary

In this chapter, the reconstruction of science perspective of Lakatos is adopted to examine the evidence for the Medical Model and the Contextual Model. Any reconstruction of science stipulates that theory must predict what will be observed under certain circumstances. According to Lakatos, a research programme is progressive provided observations are consistent with predictions and the auxiliaries needed to conduct research, interpret results, and explain anomalies that result can anticipate new evidence. On the other hand, a programme is degenerative if many *ad hoc* auxiliaries are needed to explain observations and the validity of the auxiliaries themselves are suspect. A programme is abandoned if there exists an alternate that can explain the evidence and anticipate novel facts.

In this volume, we rely on meta-analyses to aggregate the results of many studies. Meta-analyses avoid the problems of narrative reviews and are able to test many hypotheses generated by the Medical Model and the Contextual Model. The conjectures of the Medical Model and the Contextual Model, which were discussed in this chapter, predict very different outcomes of various psychotherapy investigations.

Notes

1. Lakatos used the spelling "programme" due to publication in the United Kingdom and reference to his reconstruction refers to "programmes," and, therefore, we utilize that spelling to refer to Lakatosian programmes, although the United States spelling is used as well.
2. Technically it is d and the point-biserial correlation that are being equated, but nevertheless the comparison of d and Pearson r is sufficient for our purposes. The formula for converting r to d or d to r is the following: $r^2 = d^2/(d^2 + 4)$.
3. The notation R^2 from regression is used here because it is commonly used. However, in the analysis of variance context this proportion would be labeled η^2. It should be noted that this is a sample value and is a biased estimate of the population value for the proportion of variance accounted for, which will be smaller than the sample value. When the distinction is important to the presentation it will be called to the attention of the reader.

Chapter 4

Absolute Efficacy

The Benefits of Psychotherapy Established by Meta-Analysis

It is now generally accepted that psychotherapy is efficacious, and slipping from memory is the "tendentious and adversarial" (Smith, Glass, & Miller, 1980, p. 7) debate about the benefits of psychotherapy that cast a pallor over the psychotherapy community from the early 1950s to the middle 1980s. On the one side were those who contended that psychotherapy was possibly harmful—that is, the rate of success of psychotherapy was less than or equal to the rate of spontaneous remission. The most notable advocates of this position were Hans J. Eysenck (1952, 1961, 1966) and Stanley Rachman (1971, 1977), both of whom were advocates of behavior therapy (as distinct from psychotherapy)[1] as a paragon of scientific activity. On the other side were defenders of traditional psychotherapy, such as Saul Rosenzweig (1954), Allen Bergin (1971; Bergin & Lambert, 1978), and Lester Luborsky (1954; Luborsky, Singer, & Luborsky, 1975), who contended that Eysenck's and Rachman's claims for the ineffectiveness of psychotherapy were flawed and that the evidence supported the benefits of psychotherapy. In 1977, the first meta-analysis of psychotherapy outcomes, conducted by Mary Lee Smith and Gene V. Glass (Smith & Glass, 1977), was published and changed the nature of the debate dramatically. Smith and Glass found that psychotherapy was remarkably beneficial and that the contentions of the various detractors were empirically unsupportable. In spite of criticisms of this particular meta-analysis, its sequel (viz., Smith et al., 1980), and meta-analysis as a method (e.g., Eysenck, 1978; Eysenck, 1984; Wilson & Rachman, 1983), the efficacy of psychotherapy now has been firmly established and is no longer a subject of debate. Interestingly, the estimate of the effect size produced in the early meta-analyses has turned out to be remarkably robust, as we shall see.

In the following we present the history of arguments for and against the efficacy of psychotherapy in two parts. The first section of this chapter we will discuss the research designs that are utilized to establish "absolute" efficacy (i.e., does a treatment work better than no treatment) and will summarize the period preceding meta-analysis in which the debate about the benefits of psychotherapy was particularly intemperate. Besides providing historical background, we will illustrate the problems inherent with heuristic reviews of the literature. The second section of the chapter will present the initial meta-analyses that were directed toward establishing efficacy, but will also include a) a review of more recent meta-analyses demonstrating the absolute efficacy of various psychotherapies for specific DSM disorders; b) studies that establish the effectiveness of psychotherapy in practice settings; and c) a review of evidence for the potential iatrogenic effects of specific psychotherapies.

Heuristic Reviews and Uncontrolled Studies: Inferential Chaos

Absolute efficacy refers to the effects of treatment vis-à-vis no treatment and is best addressed by a research design where treated patients are contrasted to untreated patients. At present, in the prototypical design to test for efficacy, patients meeting the study criteria (e.g., meeting diagnostic criteria for depression) would be randomly selected from a population and then randomly assigned to one of two groups: a treatment group and a no-treatment control group. The no treatment group often is a "wait-list control group," as the patients are promised the treatment at the conclusion of the study (assuming that the treatment proves to be efficacious). The waitlist control design examines the efficacy of the treatment as a whole (i.e., treatment package) and accordingly such designs are often referenced as *treatment package designs* (Kazdin, 1994). The logic of a treatment package design is that the only differences between the two groups (and by inference, the two populations) is that one has received the treatment and the other has not; consequently, any obtained difference is evidence that the treatment is efficacious. If the post-treatment scores of the treated sample are significantly superior to those of the waitlist control, the treatment is considered efficacious. The conclusions are typically derived from tests of statistical significance (e.g., ANOVA, ANCOVA, or more complex models such as multilevel modeling of longitudinal data).

However, the early history of psychotherapy did not have the benefit of controlled designs and was primarily distinguished by proponents' belief that the treatments of various psychodynamic and eclectic therapies were beneficial. Claims were "scientifically" justified by case studies and uncontrolled experiments, and proponents were free to justify their existence based on what now would be considered tenuous evidence, creating some interesting arguments, as mentioned in Chapter 1:

> Rivalry among theoretical orientations has a long and undistinguished history in psychotherapy, dating back to Freud. In the infancy of the field, therapy systems, like battling siblings, competed for attention and affection in a "dogma eat dogma" environment . . . Mutual antipathy and exchange of puerile insults between adherents of rival orientations were much the order of the day.
>
> (Norcross & Newman, 1992, p. 3)

Clearly, research was needed to examine the efficacy of psychotherapy so that claims could be made based on empirical evidence rather than the quality of one's rhetoric. In 1952, Eysenck sought to provide the evidence.

Eysenck (1952): The First Attempt to Review the Efficacy Literature

In 1952, Eysenck sought to "examine the evidence relating to the actual effects of psychotherapy, in an attempt to seek clarification on a point of fact" (p. 319) by reviewing 24 studies of psychodynamic and eclectic psychotherapy. The studies included in the review were uncontrolled (i.e., there were no published randomized clinical trials of psychotherapy at the time). Realizing that "in order to evaluate the effectiveness of any form of therapy, data from a control group of non-treated patients would be required" (p. 319), he used the spontaneous remission rate derived from two other studies, one of severe neurotics in state mental hospitals who received "in the main custodial care, and very little if any psychotherapy" (p. 319), and one based on disability claims due to psychoneurosis and treated by general practitioners. That is, the recovery rates derived from 24 studies were compared to the recovery rates derived from two separate studies. From his review, Eysenck made the following conclusion:

> Patients treated by means of psychoanalysis improve to the extent of 44 percent; patients treated eclectically improve to the extent of 64 percent; patients treated only custodially or by general practitioners improve to the extent of 72 percent. There thus appears to be an inverse correlation between recovery and psychotherapy; the more psychotherapy, the smaller the recovery rate. . . . [The data] fail to prove that psychotherapy, Freudian or otherwise, facilitates the recovery of neurotic patients.
>
> (Eysenck, 1952, p. 322)

Eysenck's findings were damning. This comprehensive and purportedly objective review of the literature had shown that psychotherapy was not effective and might even be harmful! The conclusions were widely cited and reported in the press, including a lengthy article in the *New York Times* entitled "Analysis of Psychoanalysis" (Hunt & Corman, November 11, 1962). However, Eysenck's conclusions were challenged by proponents of psychotherapy (e.g., Bergin, 1971; Bergin & Lambert, 1978; Luborsky, 1954; Rosenzweig, 1954). Although there were many problems with Eysenck's method, the most conspicuous and dangerous one was that the control group sample was quite different from the treated patients. Specifically, patients were not randomly assigned to the treatment and control groups (i.e., to the 24 treatment groups and the 2 control groups), creating numerous unknown differences between the treatment and the controls other than the presence or absence of treatment. Luborsky (1954) commented on this threat to validity:

I do not believe Eysenck has an adequate control group nor that comparisons of groups can be made within the experimental group. . . . To conclude as he does, Eysenck must assume patients do something they do not do: randomly self-select themselves to psychiatrists, general practitioners, and state hospitals.

(p. 129)

Clearly, trying to compare clients from one study with clients from another study creates unknown confounds. As we shall see, the determination of relative efficacy (see Chapter 5) suffers from similar attempts to make cross-study comparisons. Regardless, Eysenck was emboldened by his "success" in proving the failure of psychotherapy and as we shall see, published several subsequent reviews of the literature to bolster his original conclusion.

Eysenck's Sequels

Eysenck published two additional reviews that replicated his finding that psychodynamic and eclectic psychotherapy were inadequate, but supported the efficacy of behavior therapy (Eysenck, 1961; Eysenck, 1966). Rachman (1971) followed suit. As noted previously, here psychotherapy and behavioral interventions were not viewed as similar. Accordingly, the dispute of relative efficacy stems back all the way to early claims about the absolute efficacy of psychotherapy. In modern terms, this distinction does not apply. Psychotherapy is a broad term thought to include all types of interventions that rely on a conversation between a therapist and a patient who is seeking treatment for a mental health concern (see definition of psychotherapy in Chapter 2). Behavioral therapy, cognitive therapy, psychodynamic, and mindfulness-based stress reduction are all various forms of psychotherapy. Eysenck and colleagues divided the set of such treatments into two classes, those based on purported scientific principles that were presumably efficacious (viz., behavior therapy) and those that were not based on scientific principles, with the goal of showing the superiority of the former and the deficiencies of the latter.

Not to be deterred, the proponents of psychotherapy published their own reviews (Bergin, 1971; Luborsky et al., 1975; Meltzoff & Kornreich, 1970). Needless to say, the two sides came to very different conclusions. Eysenck and Rachman concluded that psychodynamic and eclectic psychotherapy were not efficacious, whereas Bergin, Meltzoff and Kornreich, and Luborsky concluded otherwise. How is it that these two sets of reviewers, having available essentially the same set of studies to review, can come to such different conclusions? The answer to this question will reveal the inadequacies of heuristic/qualitative reviews, which rely on subjective criteria for inclusion and non-meta-analytic methods for aggregation. The problems incurred by the two sides of this debate were discussed by Smith et al. (1980) and are illustrated in Figure 4.1, which contains the number of studies in each review, the number which were

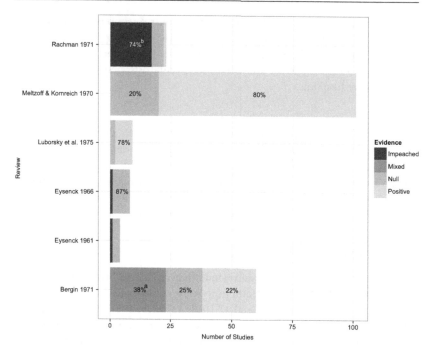

Figure 4.1 Review of non-meta-analytic psychotherapy clinical trial reviews.

[a] Fifteen studies were "in doubt," and eight not included in table for unknown reason.
[b] Seventeen studies were impeached (fifteen positive and two null results).

Additional notes: The grouping of "mixed" studies includes studies in which treated groups did not significantly differ from controls, in which controls were superior, in which treated groups did not exceed baseline. In both the Eysenck (1961/66) reviews, one study was disallowed (impeached) due to methodology (positive results). Treatments for children, psychotics, and behavioral treatments are excluded from the Rachman (1971) review. In Luborsky et al. (1975), the number impeached is unknown due to method of reporting and excluding studies based on low design quality. Behavioral treatments and treatments on psychotics were also excluded.

Adapted from *The benefits of psychotherapy*, by M. L. Smith, G. V. Glass, and T. I. Miller, 1980, Baltimore: The Johns Hopkins University Press.

impeached (disqualified due to inadequate study design), the number whose results were mixed (some results supporting the efficacy of psychotherapy and some not), the number which produced null results (no results favoring psychotherapy), and the number that were positive.

Several points related to the studies listed in Figure 4.1 need to be made. First, the figure only summarizes the controlled studies (i.e., psychotherapy versus control) that were reviewed. Comparisons to nonequivalent control groups persisted, with Eysenck (1961) sticking to a spontaneous remission rate of about two-thirds, whereas Bergin (1971) determined the rate to be about one-third, a figure that makes the benefits of psychotherapy more apparent. However, in either case, the comparisons were flawed because treatment and control subjects were not comparable.

The second point is that determining the effects of psychotherapy by counting the number of studies that are statistically significant is problematic, as was discussed in Chapter 2. Bergin (1971) for example, found that 37 percent of the controlled studies showed a positive result and concluded that "it now seems apparent that psychotherapy, as practiced over the past 40 years, has had an average effect that is modestly positive" (p. 263). What is a modest effect? And does the fact that 37 percent of studies were in a favorable direction establish that effect? Heuristic reviews lead to ambiguity and thus reviewers have great latitude in assigning verbal descriptions to the results.

The third and most important point is that the reviewers used different sets of studies on which to make their conclusions. For the most part, the reviewers did not indicate how studies were culled from the literature. Moreover, reviewers applied rules, often in inconsistent ways, to remove studies from their database due to flaws in design. In 1970, Meltzoff and Kornreich reviewed 101 studies, classifying studies as having either "adequate" or "questionable" designs (both designs are included in Figure 4.1). No studies were "impeached". On the other hand, Rachman (1971), publishing at nearly the same time, reviewed only 23 studies, 17 of which were "impeached." Interestingly, of the 17 studies impeached, 15 showed results supporting the effectiveness of psychotherapy! The judgments made by Rachman seem to be biased or, at least, arbitrary.[2] For example, studies were impeached because the dependent measures showed inconsistent effects (three measures showed positive outcomes whereas one did not, failure of positive results at termination to be maintained at follow-up, use of unpublished tests, and graphical presentation of the results).

The reviews of the controlled studies presented in Figure 4.1 present a tremendous dilemma for the scientific understanding of psychotherapy. Having available the same corpus of research studies, prominent researchers reached dramatically different conclusions. Moreover, the conclusions were consistent with the reviewers' preconceived positions—evidence at the service of a point of view rather than at the service of science (see Wampold, 2013). The reviews discussed here lacked a) systematic selection of studies from the literature; b) objective and scientifically based criteria for inclusion; c) coding of studies using objective rules and agreement among coders; and d) statistically appropriate means to aggregate the results of the studies. Thus, the reviews could be called heuristic, at best. The pre-meta-analytic reviews of the efficacy of psychotherapy demonstrate the inconsistencies that characterize such heuristic reviews.

In 1977, meta-analysis came to the rescue of psychotherapy, as will be shown in the next section.

Meta-Analyses of Treatment Package Designs: Order From Chaos

In the period following the heuristic reviews of psychotherapy research, Eysenck's indictment of psychotherapy cast a pallor over the field:

> Most academics [had] read little more than Eysenck's (1952, 1966) tendentious diatribes in which he claimed to prove that 75% of neurotics got better regardless of whether or not they were in therapy—a conclusion based on the interpretation of six controlled studies. The perception that research shows the inefficacy of psychotherapy has become part of the conventional wisdom even within the profession.
>
> (Smith & Glass, 1977, p. 752)

In 1977, Smith and Glass attempted to settle the efficacy issue using meta-analysis.

Smith and Glass (1977) and Smith, Glass, and Miller (1980)

The goal of the Smith and Glass (1977) meta-analysis was to aggregate the results of all studies that compared psychotherapy and counseling to a control group or to a different therapy to quantitatively estimate the size of the psychotherapy effect. They used various search strategies, which were well described, to locate 375 published and unpublished (i.e., dissertation or presentations) studies. No studies were excluded because of design flaws, but design characteristics, as well as many other features of the studies, were coded so that the relation between these features and effect size could be investigated.

For each dependent variable in each study, a sample effect size was calculated (the standardized mean difference or the difference between the mean of the control group and the mean of the treatment group divided by the standard deviation of the control group, denoted for now by d; see Chapter 3). As the statistical theory for meta-analysis of effect size measures was in its infancy, aggregation methods used by Smith and Glass consisted simply of taking the arithmetic average of each d to obtain an aggregate effect size.

The findings were clear. The 375 studies produced 833 effect size measures (more than two per study) and yielded an average d of .68. Interpretation of this effect can be made by consulting Table 3.1. This effect would a) be classified as between a medium and large effect in the social sciences, b) indicate that the average client receiving therapy would be better off than 75 percent of untreated clients, c) suggest that treatment accounts for about 10 percent of the variability in outcomes, and d) be equivalent to an NNT of 3 (i.e., three patients have to receive psychotherapy in order to have one better outcome than had the patients not received psychotherapy). Smith and Glass made a simple but important conclusion: "The results of research demonstrate the beneficial effects of counseling and psychotherapy" (p. 760). If this result were to stand up to various challenges, then it would show rather convincingly that the critics of psychotherapy were wrong.

In 1980, Smith et al. published a sequel to Smith and Glass (1977) with an expanded set of studies and a more sophisticated analyses. Again, an extensive search was made in order to find all published and unpublished controlled studies of counseling psychotherapy through 1977. In all, 475 studies were found, which produced 1766 effect sizes, calculated in the same manner as Smith and Glass. The aggregate effect size was .85, larger than that found previously. An effect size of .85 is a large effect in the social sciences and means that the average client receiving therapy would be better off than 80 percent of untreated clients (see Table 3.1).

There were many other findings in the Smith and Glass (1977) and the Smith, Glass, and Miller (1980) meta-analyses, but discussion of those conclusions will be presented as they relate to the various hypotheses tested in this volume.

Challenges to the Early Meta-Analyses

Not surprising, those who had sought to demonstrate that psychotherapy was not beneficial (e.g., Eysenck and Rachman) criticized the results of these meta-analyses (and subsequent meta-analyses) as well as meta-analysis in general (Eysenck, 1978; Eysenck, 1984; Rachman & Wilson, 1980; Wilson, 1982; Wilson & Rachman, 1983). These criticisms are briefly reviewed here.

One criticism is that meta-analysis aggregates studies that vary in quality, giving weight to poorly conceived and misleading results. Of course, as demonstrated in the heuristic reviews, the alternative is to have reviewers exclude studies that, in their judgment, are flawed, resulting in a systematic impeachment of studies that do not support preconceived positions. The strategy used by Smith and Glass (1977; Smith, Glass, & Miller, 1980) was to include all controlled studies regardless of quality, objectively rate the quality of the studies (i.e., with specific criteria and multiple raters), and determine if quality was related to outcome. Not all the results will be discussed here but, for example, consider internal validity of the study. The effect sizes for studies with low, medium, and high internal validity were 0.78, 0.78, and 0.88, respectively. Although the difference between the best designed studies (viz., high internal validity) and the poorer designed studies (viz., low and medium internal validity) was small (viz., .10), the conclusion was that the better designed studies produced larger effects and consequently excluding poorer studies would have increased the aggregate effect size, exactly opposite to what was contented by the critics! Essentially, the meta-analyst treats quality of the research design as an empirical question that can be answered with an analysis. Of course, if all studies are poor, the results of a meta-analysis may not be trusted, but then again so would the results of any other attempt to make sense of the same set of studies. The criticism and response involved here is an example of what

Lakatos described as a progressive research programme. A conjecture is made (psychotherapy is effective), observations are examined (the overall effect of psychotherapy is about 0.80) and found to be as predicted, criticisms of the conclusions are made (effect is due to poorly designed studies), and the theory anticipates the results of additional analyses addressing the criticism (better designed studies produce larger effects).

Another criticism of meta-analysis is that it is atheoretical, creating simply a fact or facts that accumulate unrelated to theoretical conjectures. But meta-analysis can be used, and is often used, to test theoretically derived conjectures. Certainly, primary studies and meta-analyses can be used atheoretically—for example, to determine whether Treatment A is efficacious. On the other hand, meta-analyses can be addressed to establish the validity of two competing theories, as is the case in this volume.

A third criticism is that meta-analyses aggregate "apples and oranges." For example, the meta-analyses discussed here lump together a wide variety of approaches to psychotherapy, and, therefore, the conclusion is a gross one. Unfortunately, when these early meta-analyses were conducted, tests of homogeneity of effect sizes had not been developed and, therefore, were not used to see whether "one size fits all." However, Smith and Glass (1977; Smith, Glass, & Miller, 1980) did segregate studies by treatment type to determine whether effect sizes differed by treatment; the results of this analysis are discussed in the context of relative efficacy (Chapter 5). While various "apples and oranges" arguments have been leveled against various meta-analyses, the veracity of the criticism could be empirically tested by conducting a between-group test of the "apples" and the "oranges." That is, are the effects produced by "apples" different that the effects produced by "oranges?" Similarly, narrative reviews suffer from the same problem in that they attempt to make sense of a variety of studies, yet lack an objective test of whether this phenomenon is operating in a given area.

A final criticism leveled at meta-analysis is around the criteria used for various ratings (e.g., of internal validity) and the criteria used for including or excluding studies. Eysenck (1984) and Rachman and Wilson (1980) contended that the conclusions of the Smith, Glass, and Miller (1980) meta-analysis were flawed because important behavioral studies were omitted. The meta-analytic response is that critics are invited to define inclusion/exclusion criteria differently and see if the conclusions are altered, an issue discussed in the next section.

Clearly, the meta-analytic response to most criticisms is that issues can and should be addressed empirically. One cannot help but think that most of the criticism of meta-analysis was generated by a distaste for the results. For the most part, the critics were reluctant to empirically test their alternative hypotheses. However, two meta-analyses reanalyzed the Smith and Glass (1977) and the Smith, Glass, and Miller (1980) data in order to challenge some of the conclusions (Andrews & Harvey, 1981; Landman & Dawes, 1982). These challenges are considered next.

The Smith et al. Results Stand up Under Scrutiny

A frequent criticism of the Smith and Glass (1977; Smith, Glass, & Miller, 1980) meta-analyses was that many of the studies analyzed involved clients who were not clinically distressed and were not seeking treatment for some disorder, problem, or complaint. Indeed, only 46 percent of the studies analyzed by Smith, Glass, and Miller involved "patients with neuroses, true phobias, depressions, and emotional-somatic disorders—the type of patients who usually seek psychotherapy" and only 22 percent "concerned patients who had entered treatment themselves or by referral" (Andrews & Harvey, 1981, p. 1204). This is an "apples and oranges" argument. It contends that the effects produced by studies with clinically representative samples would be different from the effects produced by the non-clinically representative studies.

Andrews and Harvey (1981) addressed this criticism by analyzing the 81 studies from the Smith, Glass, and Miller (1980) meta-analysis that involved clinically distressed subjects who had sought treatment for their disorder, problem, or complaint. The average of the 292 effects produced by the 81 studies was 0.72, an effect size similar to that produced by the two original meta-analyses, demonstrating that psychotherapy was beneficial for clinically distressed clients who sought treatment.

Landman and Dawes (1982) addressed several additional issues in Smith and Glass' (1977) meta-analysis. First, as discussed earlier, quality of the studies reviewed could impact the results of meta-analyses. The second issue was related to independence of observations (a problem alluded to in Chapter 3). Smith and Glass created dependent observations in many ways, but primarily by using multiple effect size measures derived from the multiple dependent measures in each study. Generally, dependent observations violate the assumptions of statistical tests, creating invalid conclusions. Whereas other violations of assumptions may have little effect on conclusions, non-independence can have drastic effects, as will be shown in Chapter 6 when therapist effects are discussed.

Landman and Dawes (1982) examined 65 studies randomly selected from the studies in Smith and Glass (1977), as well as 93 additional studies but restricted primary analyses to 42 "studies of uniformly high methodological quality" (p. 507). Additionally, the study was used as the unit of analysis, rather than the individual outcome measure, eliminating dependent observations. Based on these 42 studies, the average effect size was found to be 0.90, considerably larger than Smith and Glass' initial estimate of 0.68, which was reflected in the subtitle of Landman and Dawes' article: *Smith and Glass' Conclusions Stand Up Under Scrutiny*.

The impact of the Smith and Glass meta-analyses should not be underestimated. Until 1977, controversy reigned when it came to the issue of the benefits of psychotherapy. Many professionals as well as the lay public were lead to believe that psychotherapy was worthless. Although the initial Smith and Glass (1977) conclusion led to much criticism, it was heralded in the popular press under the headline "Consensus Is Reached: Psychotherapy Works" (Adams,

1979). Having withstood the challenges of the Andrews and Harvey (1981) and Landman and Dawes (1982) and other meta-analyses, the benefits of psychotherapy became accepted. Moreover, the meta-analysis method pioneered by Glass (1976) and used in the initial psychotherapy meta-analyses has been used in thousands of studies in education, psychology, and medicine (Hunt, 1997).

In the next section, the additional meta-analyses related to the efficacy of psychotherapy will be summarized.

Present Status of Absolute Efficacy: The Proliferation of Clinical Trials and Meta-Analyses

In the years since Smith and Glass's seminal contribution, the number of psychotherapy clinical trials and meta-analyses has exploded. A PubMed database search of the subject term "psychotherapy" (which is a generic PubMed term inclusive of different types of psychotherapies—i.e., psychodynamic, cognitive therapy, behavioral, etc.) and the publication type "clinical trial" reveals a rather shocking total of 12,511 hits with 619 in 2013 alone (see Figure 4.2).

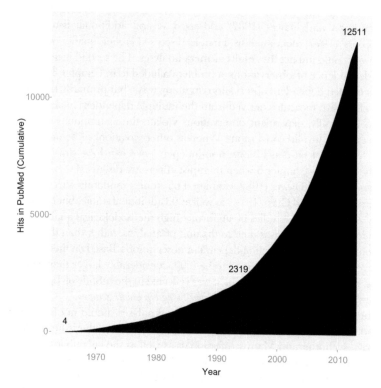

Figure 4.2 The number of psychotherapy clinical trials over time.

Not surprisingly, meta-analysis has become an increasingly used tool for making conclusions from this expanding set of clinical trials. A PubMed search of "psychotherapy" and publication type "meta-analysis" reveals a total of 703 hits for psychotherapy meta-analyses—51 in 2011 alone (see Figure 4.3). There are now more psychotherapy meta-analyses than there were clinical trials at the time of Smith and Glass's seminal reviews. As a result, it is no longer feasible to review the entire meta-analytic literature in psychotherapy in detail. Accordingly, we will summarize the findings of meta-analyses via published reviews of meta-analyses—as well as highlight several recent meta-analyses that are currently influential.

According to Lipsey and Wilson, by 1993, there were more than 40 meta-analyses of psychotherapy in general or of particular psychotherapies for particular problems. Generally, these meta-analyses showed that the treatment being studied was efficacious and provided evidence for the effectiveness of psychotherapy generally, as well as a variety of interventions broadly labeled as cognitive and behavioral in orientation. Although Lipsey and Wilson did not provide an aggregate effect size for psychotherapy, the effect sizes for meta-analyses that compared treatments to no-treatment controls for adults can be extracted from

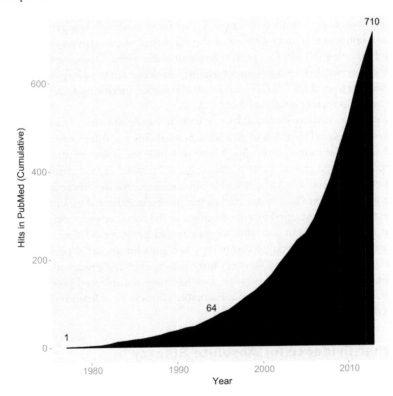

Figure 4.3 The number of psychotherapy meta-analyses over time.

their tabular results (see Lipsey & Wilson, 1993, Table 1, Section 1.1 Psychotherapy, General, p. 1183). The mean effect size for these 13 meta-analyses was .81, an effect remarkably comparable to that found earlier by Smith and Glass.

As noted by Lambert and Ogles (2004), recent psychotherapy meta-analyses have become fractured—perhaps reflecting the focus on developing specific empirically supported treatments for specific disorders. These meta-analyses focus on more limited questions regarding the effect of specific types of psychotherapy on specific sets of problems—typically DSM-IV diagnoses (e.g., CBT for panic disorder). Lambert and Ogles (2004) reviewed meta-analyses of treatments for depression (k = 19), anxiety (k = 28), as well as a group of miscellaneous treatments and disorders (k = 57). Across these classifications, the general conclusion is consistent with previous reviews. Interventions were consistently superior to waitlist and no-treatment controls and were comparable to medications for depression and anxiety. Similarly, Butler et al. (2006) reviewed 16 meta-analyses of CBT for various problems and disorders. Effect sizes were relatively consistent across disorders. There were positive effects of CBT across all problems tested (see also Westen & Bradley, 2005). The clinical trial literature for psychodynamic treatment is relatively small compared to CBT but has grown substantially in the last 20 years (i.e., there are no reviews of meta-analyses, but there are now several meta-analyses). Leichsenring et al. (2004) conducted a meta-analysis of the efficacy of short-term psychodynamic psychotherapy (STPP) for specific psychiatric disorders. Estimates of pre-post and differences between treatment waitlist/no treatment were large and similar to those reported for CBT. The relative efficacy of specific approaches will be discussed in further detail in Chapter 5.

From the various meta-analyses conducted over the years, the aggregate effect size related to absolute efficacy is remarkably consistent and appears to fall within the range .75 to .85. There was little variability in the effect size across this large group of meta-analyses that included diverse treatments and patients. A reasonable and defensible point estimate for the efficacy of psychotherapy would be .80, a value used in this book. As indicated in Table 3.1, this effect would be classified as a large effect in the social sciences, which means that the average client receiving therapy would be better off than 79 percent of untreated clients, that psychotherapy accounts for about 14 percent of the variance in outcomes, and for every three patients receiving psychotherapy, one patient will have a better outcome than had they not received psychotherapy. Simply stated, psychotherapy is remarkably efficacious, at least as determined by clinical trials.

Other Evidence for Absolute Efficacy

As it seems clear that psychotherapy is efficacious, research attention has focused on other more specific questions. Instead of testing the generic question about psychotherapy efficacy, researchers are focused on whether a particular treatment is efficacious. Of course, this is a critical question related to whether the treatment will be classified as evidence-based (i.e., as an empirically supported treatment, an evidence-based treatment, or as a psychological treatment with research support). In addition, because the goal of research in psychotherapy, broadly speaking, is to improve the quality of services, an important question to ask is whether psychotherapy works in practice. We now turn to these issues.

Empirically Supported Treatments, Evidence-Based Treatments, and Research-Supported Psychological Treatments

As noted elsewhere in this text, the Empirically Supported Treatments movement had a dramatic impact on how evidence for the effectiveness of specific psychotherapies was created, interpreted, and disseminated. This movement, and the subsequent variations (e.g., evidence-based treatments and research-supported psychological treatments) effectively changed the generic question "Does psychotherapy work?" to a more specific question about whether the evidence is sufficient to classify a specific treatment as an evidence-based treatment. Specifically, for a treatment to receive the status of "strong research support . . . well-designed studies conducted by independent investigators must converge to support a treatment's efficacy" (Chambless et al.,1998; SCP, 2007).

The focus on classifying treatments as supported by research has led to a proliferation of research on specific treatments. Based on the classification of the research evidence for the treatments for particular disorders as designated by the Society of Clinical Psychology (http://www.div12.org/PsychologicalTreatments/index.html, accessed 1/2013), Figure 4.4 illustrates the number of treatments in the various designations for each disorder. The size of each bubble indicates the number of treatments classified in each designation and the shading indicates the percentage of these treatments that are broadly cognitive-behavioral in approach. It is clear that treatments broadly labeled "CBT" represent the overwhelming majority of treatments reaching the status of "strong research support." However, a variety of other treatments are beginning to be more widely represented. Given the proliferation of psychotherapy clinical trials, it is likely that this number will continue to increase. However, for many disorders there are very few treatments (e.g. panic disorder, obsessive-compulsive disorder). There are also some treatments for which evidence appears to be lacking, controversial, or potentially harmful to patients— an issue we address later in this chapter.

Effectiveness of Psychotherapy in Clinical Settings

Treatment outcome research typically can be distinguished as either *efficacy* or *effectiveness* studies (Seligman, 1995). Efficacy refers to the benefits of psychotherapy that are derived from comparisons of the treatment and a no-treatment

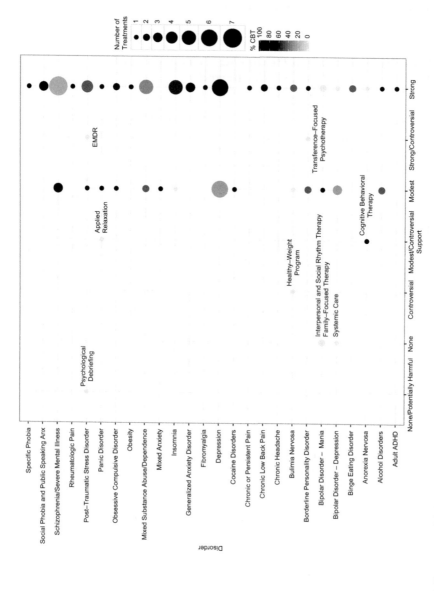

Figure 4.4 Proportional bubble plot illustrating the number of treatments and level of support for each treatment listed on Division 12's Empirically Supported Treatment Website.

control in the context of a well-controlled clinical trial (Westen, Novotny, & Thompson-Brenner, 2004; Westen, Novotny, & Thompson-Brenner, 2005). That is, if a treatment is found to be superior to a wait-list control group in a treatment package design, then the treatment is said to be efficacious. Effectiveness, on the other hand, refers to the benefits of psychotherapy that occur in community settings—and answers the question, "How effective is a treatment administered to clients in the 'real world'?" Many have contended that a clinical trial creates an artificial context that is not representative of how treatments are administered in the practice context, and, consequently, the establishment of the efficacy of psychotherapy does not ipso facto imply that the treatments are beneficial to clients in the community (Westen et al., 2004; Westen et al., 2005). It should be recognized that the distinction between the context of clinical trials and naturalistic setting is not always clear; for example, many clinical trials are conducted in settings that resemble naturalistic clinical settings (see Shadish, Matt, Navarro, & Phillips, 2000). For this reason, and because the terms *efficacy* and *effectiveness* are synonyms, we do not make a strict distinction between the terms. Nevertheless, the question about the effectiveness of psychotherapy in actual practice is a crucially important one, for theory, policy, as well as practice.

Researchers have utilized several methods to examine the effectiveness of psychotherapy in the community, including prominently a) examining the effects of psychotherapy "treatment package" studies that are investigated in more clinically relevant settings; b) benchmarking studies that compare estimates of treatment effectiveness obtained from naturalistic settings to effects derived from clinical trials; and c) clinical trials that compare an established treatment to treatment-as-usual (TAU; sometimes called usual care, or UC).

Clinical Representativeness

The delivery of treatments in clinical trials and in practice varies in many respects (Westen et al., 2004). In the prototypic clinical trial, treatment is given by select therapists who are given training and supervision to deliver a treatment guided by a manual. The patients typically are homogenous, selected by inclusion and exclusion criteria, which often rule out patients with co-morbidities (for depression, e.g., personality disorders, psychotic features, and substance use), dangerousness (e.g., suicidality), and use of psychotropic medications. They are typically recruited to participate in a clinical trial, often in a clinic associated with a university or medical institution.

The clinical representativeness strategy, which is the oldest method for testing the effectiveness of psychotherapy in practice settings, meta-analytically examines previously published studies to determine the extent to which factors that distinguish between the real world and the laboratory (e.g., setting, client recruitment method, random client assignment to treatment, use of treatment manual) moderate treatment effects. Interestingly, the first examination of clinical representativeness occurred in Smith and Glass' original meta-analyses

(Smith & Glass, 1977; Smith et al., 1980). Smith and Glass found that treatment setting influenced the effect of psychotherapy, as the treatment effect was largest in university settings (e.g., "psychology laboratory, therapy training center, or student mental health clinic") (p. 117, $d = 1.04$) and smallest in mental health centers ($d = 0.47$), although it was rare in this database for studies to be conducted in mental health centers. When patients were recruited through special advertisements for the study or when experimenters solicited participants, effects were larger ($d = 1.00$ and 0.92, respectively) than when patients were self-referred ($d = 0.71$). Smith et al. concluded that the "reliable differences in effects associated with the true-to-life methods and the laboratory methods of obtaining clients is evidence against the generalizability of results of laboratory-based therapies and argues for field-based evaluation to back up research conducted under artificial arrangements" (p. 122).

Although there have been attempts to conduct other clinical representativeness meta-analyses (e.g., Shapiro & Shapiro, 1982), they were methodologically problematic until Shadish and colleagues (Shadish et al., 1997; Shadish et al., 2000) systematically coded studies for clinical representativeness along a number of dimensions and examined these dimensions simultaneously (see Minami & Wampold, 2008). The dimensions included treatment setting, therapist characteristics, referral sources, use of manuals, adherence monitoring, additional training, client heterogeneity, and flexibility in length of treatment. Shadish et al. (2000), based on nearly 1,000 studies, concluded that an ideal, clinically representative psychotherapy would yield effect size estimates that would be similar to or slightly less than what is observed in clinical trials. Confidence in this conclusion is mitigated by the fact that most of these studies were not clinically representative (viz., only 56 contained treatments that met criteria for being "somewhat similar" to clinic therapy and only one met all criteria for clinic therapy) and consequently Shadish et al.'s conclusion is an extrapolation that must be taken as tentative.

Benchmarking

There is certainly evidence that psychotherapy can be helpful in clinical settings. For example, in a large sample (N > 10,700 patients) obtained from the National Health Service in the United Kingdom, Saxon and Barkham (2012) found that of those who initially were in the clinical range on the CORE-OM (a global measure of mental health), more than 61 percent recovered. However, how do we compare these effects to those observed in research settings? Benchmarking involves estimating the extent to which psychotherapy is effective in clinical trials and then comparing effects produced in naturalistic settings to what was found in clinical trials. More specifically, effect sizes are calculated from clinical trials to produce a benchmark against which the effects from naturalistic settings are compared. The naturalistic treatment might be treatment as usual TAU or it might be an evidence-based treatment that was transported and examined in a naturalistic setting.

An early benchmarking study assessed the effects of CBT transported to a community mental health center. In this study Wade, Treat, and Stuart (1998) compared the clinical outcomes of CBT administered to 110 clients seeking treatment for panic disorder with a benchmark derived from two clinical trials and found the effects to be "similar" (p. 237). Although this study indicated that an evidence-based treatment can be successfully transported to a naturalistic setting, it does not inform us about the effects of treatment in naturalistic settings as it is practiced, as there were "special" arrangements due to the fact that therapists received training in the use of the CBT manual and adherence to the protocol was assessed—procedures rarely seen in clinical settings. Merrill, Tolbert, and Wade (2003) replicated this study in the same clinic, but the conclusions were similarly uninformative about the effectiveness of psychotherapy as actually practiced.

Weersing and Weisz (2002) conducted the first study that benchmarked TAU against benchmarks derived clinical trials. They improved upon the previous studies by creating the benchmarks with a meta-analysis of published clinical trials of youth depression treatment. The benchmarks included effects for the controls (no treatment, waitlist, or "attention placebo") and treatment groups in clinical trials. They then compared the outcomes of 67 children who received treatment at six community mental health centers in the Los Angeles area to these two benchmarks. Three months into treatment, the progress of the children was nearly identical to the control benchmark and significantly poorer than the treatment benchmark. They concluded that there was little support for TAUs for youth depression.

One of the problems in benchmarking involves the hypothesis testing strategy. Typically the strategy is to reject the null hypothesis, but in benchmarking the goal is to say the effect produced in a naturalistic setting is "equivalent" to the benchmark; otherwise, the effect may be quite close to the benchmark, but if the sample size is large, which is desirable and common in many naturalistic studies (see e.g., Saxon & Barkham, 2012; Wampold & Brown, 2005), it is quite likely that there will be "statistically" significant differences from the benchmark. Minami and colleagues (Minami, Serlin, Wampold, Kircher, & Brown, 2008) developed a range null strategy, based on Serlin's good-enough method (Serlin & Lapsley, 1985, 1993), where it is determined whether an obtained effect is within a range of the benchmark. The range may be whatever the researcher believes is a clinical insignificant difference. Minami then used this strategy to benchmark treatment of depression in adults using naturalistic data collected in managed care (Minami, Wampold, Serlin, Kircher, & Brown, 2007). First, they created pretreatment to post-treatment benchmarks from a meta-analysis of clinical trials of evidence-based treatments for depression. There were three samples: intent-to-treat, completer, and natural history (i.e., effects for untreated patients in no-treatment controls). They found that focused measures, such as the Beck Depression Inventory or the Hamilton Rating Scale for depression, created larger effects than more global measures of psychological functioning. Specifically, when comparing against the treatment efficacy benchmarks, they considered effect size estimates 10 percent below the benchmarks—at most—were clinically equivalent. When comparing against the natural history benchmark (i.e., no-treatment control), clinical settings data needed to exceed it by at least $d = 0.2$. These criteria were selected to conduct conservative comparisons.

In the benchmark study (Minami, Wampold, et al., 2008), a large data set of patients (more than 5,700 in some analyses) was used. Patients completed the Outcome Questionnaire-30 (OQ-30; Ellsworth, Lambert, Johnson, 2006), a global measure of symptoms, social role functioning, and interpersonal relations, periodically during treatment—in this study the first and last observation was used. Because the OQ-30 is a global measure, the benchmarks corresponding to global measures were used. In this study, three clinical settings samples were benchmarked. The samples differed in degree of equivalence between the clinical settings data and the clinical trials based on client clinical characteristics. The first sample included all patients whether or not they had comorbid diagnoses (called the clinical sample) and that had distress comparable to distress levels in clinical trials. The second sample excluded patients with comorbidity or risk of suicide, making it similar to patients in clinical trials of depression (called the non-comorbid sample). The third sample included patients who had treatment intensity (12 to 20 sessions) similar to that of evidence-based treatments of depression. The first two samples were compared to the intent-to-treat benchmark and the third to the completer benchmark. Patients also were segregated by whether they were receiving concurrent medication. Effects for the naturalistic patients were based on their initial OQ-30 scores and their last observed OQ-30 score.

Results indicated that treatments effects observed in the naturalistic setting were equivalent to, and sometimes exceeded, the respective clinical trial benchmarks (see Figure 4.5). In all three comparisons, the samples met statistical criteria for clinical equivalence—that is, the outcomes attained by providers in a managed care environment were comparable to the outcomes attained in clinical trials and significantly above the benchmarks for natural history. Importantly, the average number of sessions in the clinical trials of depression was 16, whereas the average number of sessions in the naturalistic setting was less than 9, indicating that comparable effects were found with less treatment, suggesting that treatment as usual in naturalistic settings is effective (see Minami et al. 2009 for a replication of these results with clients at a university counseling center).

These benchmarking studies suggest that psychotherapy practiced in naturalistic settings is effective, although the evidence for youth settings suggests that this might not be the case. Of course, benchmarking has some severe limitations. In some ways, the benchmarking strategy is the inverse process used by

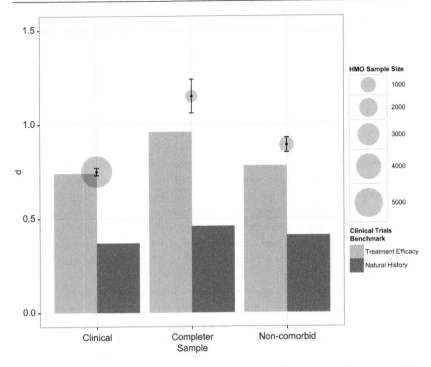

Figure 4.5 Benchmarked comparisons of naturalistic effect sizes and meta-analytic estimates from clinical trials. Each bar represents the treatment efficacy and natural history benchmark effect sizes that must be met to conclude treatment effects in the HMO surpassed or were comparable to clinical trial effects. The small point and standard error bars provide the observed effect size from the HMO for each sample calculation. The size of the grey point indicates the sample size.

Eysenck (1952, 1961, 1966), who created a benchmark from naturalistic settings to which he compared the results of the studies to assess whether psychotherapy effects in studies were as large as those in naturalistic settings. Of course, the sophistication of current benchmarking studies is superior to Eysenck's methods, but it is useful to keep in mind that the same criticism that was made of Eysenck's methods can be made of the benchmarking studies—patients are not randomly assigned to the naturalistic studies, treatment, and no treatment arms of a clinical trial.

Direct Comparisons of Established Treatments With TAU

The efficacy of TAU in naturalistic settings can be assessed by directly comparing a TAU and an established treatment that has been transported into a clinical setting. The outcomes of the established treatment are compared with the outcome of TAU in the same setting. Although this would seem to be a valid means to assess the TAU experimentally, there is much variability in how this is accomplished. The general strategy is illustrated with a study comparing an evidence-based treatment for panic disorder versus a TAU. Addis, Hatgis, Krasnow, Jacob, Bourne, and Mansfield (2004) randomly assigned volunteer therapists to deliver panic control therapy (Craske, Meadows, & Barlow, 1994) or to deliver their usual therapy. Patients were randomly assigned to the two treatment conditions. The therapists who delivered panic control therapy participated in a 2-day workshop on panic and panic control therapy and after conducting two trial cases using panic control therapy, they were further provided 30-minute phone consultations with the expert who provided the workshop as well as biweekly 1-hour group consultations with the principal investigator and the research team to "discuss cases and refine therapists' knowledge of [panic control therapy] and its underlying cognitive-behavioral principles" (p. 627). The panic control therapy sessions were audiotaped and were randomly checked for adherence based on a rating manual developed for panic control therapy.

The Addis et al. (2004) study has many commendable features, including randomization of therapists and patients to the two conditions ruling out threats due to therapist competence (but see Chapter 8). Nevertheless, the therapists providing panic control therapy received much that the TAU therapists did not—workshops by recognized experts, supervision, and consultation, providing an advantage to panic control therapy. However, the Addis et al. study is one of the best comparisons as other comparisons between an evidence-based treatment and TAU are deficient on a number of dimensions, including dose of treatment (EBTs often get more treatment), the nature of the TAU, allegiance effects due to the fact that the researcher was a developer of the EBT or an advocate of the EBT (see Chapter 5 for discussion of researcher allegiance), nonrandom assignment of therapists creating advantages for the EBT (e.g., the provider of the TAU may not be trained to deliver any treatment for the disorder), among others. Of these, the nature of the TAU is troublesome, because often the TAU does not provide *any* psychotherapy or provides questionable services (e.g., patients can present to their primary care physician, if they choose to, and receive any treatment that the physician may deliver or arrange).

There have been several meta-analyses of the comparison of evidenced-based treatment to TAU, all of which demonstrate the inadequacies of the comparisons. Weisz, Jensen-Doss, and Hawley (2006) meta-analyzed 32 randomized trials that directly compared EBTs with TAU for youth and concluded, "Our findings support the view that EBTs have generally outperformed TAU in direct, randomized comparisons" (p. 684). However, Weisz et al. recognized that fair comparisons of EBT and TAU should control for confounds related to patients, therapists, settings, and dose. Unfortunately, none of the 32 studies accomplished this goal! An example of a study with egregiously inadequate controls (viz., Kazdin, Esveldt-Dawson, French, & Unis, 1987) is the one that produced the largest effect size favoring EBP ($d = 1.12$). In this study, problem-solving skills training, the EBT, delivered more than twice the dose (45 minutes, 2–3 times/wk v. 20 minutes 2–3 times/wk) and the TAU was not a psychotherapeutic intervention by any definition ("The reason that the [dose was different was] to avoid in-depth discussion of affect-laden material likely to emerge in more protracted sessions . . . the therapist's task in these sessions was to engage the child in discussion of routine activities [and] there was no attempt to probe the child's feelings or clinical problems or to develop insight, self-acceptance, or related processes" p. 79). Clearly, the TAU in Kazdin et al. was distinctly disadvantaged and it is not surprising that the EBT elicited superior outcomes.

Spielmans, Gatlin, and McFall (2010) reanalyzed the studies used in Weisz et al. (2006) by modeling the confounds. When confounds were modeled one at a time, the advantage of the EBT was small and often not significant. Moreover, the more confounds modeled, the smaller the advantage became (see also Minami & Wampold, 2008).

There have been two meta-analyses of EBTs versus TAU for adults. In the first, Wampold et al. (2011) examined 14 studies that compared EBTs to TAU for depression and anxiety. Although overall effect favored EBT by a considerable margin ($d = 0.45$), when the TAU was actually a psychotherapy the advantage of the EBT was nonsignificant. Of the 14 studies, only 3 contained TAU that were clearly psychotherapy and none of those balanced training and supervision. Budge et al. (2013) examined 30 studies of EBT versus TAU for personality disorders, with similar results. The overall effect favored EBTs ($d = 0.40$), but only 7 of the 30 studies involved a TAU that was psychotherapy and those studies did not balance dose hours, supervision, and training as well. However, in this study, the EBT was significantly more effective than the TAU, even when the TAU was psychotherapy. These results suggest that special training and supervision for personality disorders might well be beneficial, although there was no direct test of this conjecture.

Conclusions About the Effectiveness of Psychotherapy in Practice

All three strategies used to examine the effectiveness of psychotherapy in naturalistic settings suffer from threats to their validity. However, the evidence suggests that psychotherapy practiced in a clinical settings is effective and probably as effective as psychotherapy tested in clinical trials and evidence-based treatment transported to clinical settings, although it may well be that therapists would benefit from training and supervision for the treatment of personality disorders.

While TAU studies provide good evidence that some psychotherapy can improve outcomes relative to minimal or no intervention, a case has also been made that the superiority of evidence-based treatments to TAU indicates that some treatments are superior to others. The evidence for the relative efficacy of treatments is reviewed in the next chapter (Chapter 5), but it should be noted that conclusions about relative efficacy need to emanate from trials that provide each treatment the opportunity to be successful. TAUs often do not involve psychotherapy at all and even when the TAU is a psychotherapy, the therapists delivering the TAU do not received the training, supervision, and consultation provided by the comparison evidence-based treatment.

Treatments That Harm?

After presenting the evidence that psychotherapy is efficacious, it may seem somewhat ironic to finish where we began—with assertions that psychotherapy can be harmful. In contrast to Eysenck's general claims cited earlier in the chapter, current debates regarding iatrogenic psychotherapy are more focused on specific treatments. This remains an important question, as the first ethical charge of a therapist is to "do no harm." For our purposes, the determination of whether some specific psychotherapies cause harm also is crucial to the distinction of the medical and contextual model. While we have little doubt that it is possible to construct or engage in practices that are harmful to patients (e.g., yelling, shaming, unethical behavior), the crucial question for the distinction of the Medical/Contextual Model is whether there is a class of psychotherapies that are consistent with the definition of traditional "bona-fide" psychotherapy, as defined in Chapter 2, that can be identified as harmful. If there are some psychotherapies that are harmful, while others are not, this is clear evidence that some specific approaches to psychotherapy are more effective than others and thus would be inconsistent with the Contextual Model.

Concerns about the likelihood of similar iatrogenic effects of psychological treatments have a long history in psychology, informed by reviews of the empirical literature dating back more than half a century (e.g., Bergin, 1963, 1971; Lambert, Bergin, & Collins, 1997). Interest in the evidence for harmful effects has grown in connection with the movement to identify empirically supported treatments, and recently Lilienfeld (2007) proposed an initial list of ten treatments for which certain types of empirical evidence supported a "probably harmful" designation and an additional two treatments more tentatively designated as "possibly harmful." (also see additional reviews citing evidence that specific therapeutic modalities are harmful; Mercer, 2002; Moos, 2005; Neimeyer, 2000; Rhule, 2005; Werch & Owen, 2002). But what is the basis for these claims?

Harm Defined

To investigate claims about the harmfulness of psychological treatments, it is necessary to distinguish between deterioration and harm. Deterioration for any person is established when scores at the end of treatment reflect poorer functioning on one or more outcome measures than at the beginning of treatment. Thus, a client who scores higher on a depression inventory at the end of treatment than before treatment has deteriorated. To characterize an outcome as harmful, however, it is necessary to show that this deterioration is in fact iatrogenic—that is, that the deterioration was caused by the treatment. Attribution of harm logically requires ruling out the plausible rival hypotheses for the observed deterioration. That is, one must ask whether the deterioration was caused by the treatment or by one or more factors unrelated to the treatment.

What other factors should be considered as explanations for deterioration? The most essential factor is *natural history*, which refers to changes in functioning that would have been observed in the absence of the treatment. Clients may deteriorate whether or not they received the treatment. Indeed, clients showing patterns of deterioration may nonetheless have benefited from the treatment, as in the case of a cancer patient whose life is extended by chemotherapy but who nonetheless gradually deteriorates over the course of treatment. Psychological functioning may also deteriorate because of a variety of causes external to the intervention, such as events in the client's life that are unrelated to treatment (e.g., deaths, unexpected relationship difficulties, loss of financial resources). *Measurement error*, a ubiquitous source of variance in scores on psychological measures, is another factor to consider when interpreting observed deterioration. Errors of measurement can create a false appearance of deterioration for some participants. To take an extreme example, if scores on a given measure are completely unreliable (i.e., $r_{XX} = 0$), then half of those tested will have poorer scores at Time 2 than at Time 1, regardless of their actual standing on the improvement of interest. Errors of measurement could account for apparent anomalies in studies with multiple outcome measures. For example, when a client improves on several outcome measures and deteriorates on another, this could indicate a meaningful divergence of outcomes for different symptoms or domains or it could simply reflect error of measurement.

Evidence of harm needs to go beyond simple claims of deterioration to show evidence of *treatment-induced deterioration*—decreased functioning following treatment that would not have been observed in the absence of treatment. Similar to research on beneficial effects of treatment, conclusions about treatment-induced harm are strongest when they are based on randomized experiments showing statistically significant differences between treated and untreated groups. As we will see, findings of this type are relatively rare and mostly apply to preventative interventions and/or those that would not be considered psychotherapy.

Unfortunately, authors writing on the subject of harmful treatments have not always relied on the stronger forms of evidence. Sometimes this reliance on less definitive evidence reflects the dearth of relevant empirical research but too often conclusions are based on selective interpretation of those studies that offer some support for the hypothesis of iatrogenic effects, while the results of other investigations that might support different conclusions are ignored, a problem that harkens back to the days of Eysenck. We now review the evidence relevant to purportedly harmful treatments to show how selective attention to the evidence may lead to overstated or even distorted conclusions about research findings. In the next section, we consider the evidence offered in support of claims about harmfulness of specific treatments.

Evidence for Harmful Effects

Many of the treatments listed as having "strong evidence for potential harm" are simply not psychotherapy. Clearly, "treatments" containing questionable practices can be found, a few of which are described here, but one should note that these treatments are not examples of psychotherapy, as we have defined it.

"Shock incarceration" or "Scared Straight" programs involve brief stints of incarceration with strict military-like discipline. These programs have been shown to increase delinquency rates significantly relative to control groups across seven randomized trials (Petrosino, Turpin-Petrosino, & Buehler, 2003). Based on this finding, it is reasonable to conclude that this type of intervention has unintended negative effects on targeted outcomes. Similar to shock incarceration, military-style boot camps emphasize discipline and obedience to authority. Lilienfeld (2007) noted that adolescent and adult offenders participating in "boot camp" interventions have rates of recidivism identical to those of untreated offenders (MacKenzie, Wilson, & Kider, 2001). In addition, sporadic media reports of deaths during boot camp interventions raise concerns about risks to participants from this type of intervention, particularly in the absence of documented benefits. While there are no clinical trials, various attachment therapies (rebirthing, holding therapy) have been classified as potentially harmful based on one or more reported deaths (e.g., one child was suffocated to death while wrapped in blankets during a rebirthing intervention; Lilienfeld, 2007). Many treatments, which have been cited as potentially harmful psychotherapies, are preventative programs that are offered to all comers who are potentially at risk, regardless of symptomology, or are programs mandated, usually due to some externalizing behavior that is problematic for families. Importantly, most of these treatments do not meet the definition of psychotherapy presented in Chapter 2, as the participants are not seeking treatment for a problem or complaint.

Psychological debriefing (PD) is a brief (3–4 hour) structured intervention intended to lessen adverse effects in those responding to trauma. A meta-analysis of randomized clinical trials found no evidence that PD recipients had fewer symptoms of PTSD at follow-up (Rose, Bisson, & Wessely, 2001). A later meta-analysis by van Emmerik, Kamphuis, Hulsbosch, and Emmelkamp (2002) suggested that treated participants were more likely than untreated controls to develop PTSD symptoms over a (usually) 6–12 month follow-up period. However, at the time of intervention debriefing participants reported that the intervention was helpful (McNally, Bryant, & Ehlers, 2003). Regardless, doubts about PDs long-term efficacy (and the possibility of long-term harm) raise serious questions about the advisability of PD as an intervention. Clearly, PD is not a psychotherapy, as it is an intervention that is provided to people who have been exposed to some traumatic event but have not developed symptoms and, more importantly, have not sought treatment for those problems, making this a prevention program.

Werch and Owen (2002) conducted a review of studies of alcohol and drug prevention programs (ADP) interventions for youth and college students (e.g., DARE), another prevention program. They found that of the 152 prevention studies (and 18 review articles) identified in this search, only 17 studies contained negative findings, defined as a significant difference between treated groups and controls for at least one alcohol- or drug-related outcome. As noted by the authors, this is a relatively small number of negative effects, which could well be due to Type I errors. Werch and Owen (2002) note that the 17 studies yielded 43 significant negative outcomes, but they do not document the total number of statistical significance tests conducted in these 17 studies nor the additional significance tests conducted in studies of ADP interventions that yielded no evidence of negative outcomes. Many of the studies reviewed had large sample sizes, so that the statistical power was relatively high to detect even small negative effects. For example, Ellickson, et al. (1993) followed about 4,000 students who participated in a similar prevention program over 6 years, looking at a variety of behaviors and attitudes relevant to substance use. In 324 significance tests, conducted over three assessment points, they found three statistically significant comparisons favoring the control group. One might reasonably wonder whether this trend in the data represents a true risk of treatment or a Type I error. Caution is certainly warranted in interpreting these findings, as is the case with any selective literature review.[3]

Following the death or loss of a loved one, some individuals seek one of various forms of grief counseling. Claims regarding the negative effects of grief counseling are subject of significant debate and have been featured in several news reports and in books targeted at the general public, as well as in scientific journals and policy papers (Hoyt & Larson, 2008; Larson & Hoyt, 2007). The claim that grief counseling is harmful is largely based on Neimeyer's (2000) summary of a dissertation project (Fortner, 1999) that included a meta-analysis of 23 RCTs of treatment-induced deterioration effects (TIDE) after grief therapy. Findings suggested 38 percent of clients were worse off following treatment than they would have been in the absence of treatment. Follow-up analyses of grief treatments for "normally bereaved" (versus traumatically bereaved) clients indicated even steeper TIDE rates approaching 50 percent of clients harmed. Fortner's dissertation provided no justification for the novel statistical technique that produced the TIDE findings but attributed the technique to an unpublished master's thesis conducted by Anderson (1988) and to a conference presentation, presumably based on this thesis research. A post hoc peer review by methodological experts (described in Larson & Hoyt, 2007) concluded that this analytic approach is not a valid index of harm and that there is no empirical or statistical basis for the claim that 50 percent (or any other percentage) of clients are harmed. In a more recent meta-analysis, grief counseling showed a modest positive effective at post-treatment that was not maintained at follow-up. However, this effect was substantially larger when treatment was proximal to the loss and among those with markedly difficult adaptions to their loss (Currier, Neimeyer, & Berman, 2008).

We now focus more directly on potentially harmful effects of treatments offered to symptomatic patients. Save one notable exception, the evidence for harm is quite thin. A series of techniques (e.g., hypnosis, suggestion) have purportedly been used to "recover" suppressed memories. The harmful effects of such interventions appear to center on the creation of inaccurate memories, not increases in post-treatment symptoms compared to controls. Loftus and Davis (2006) reviewed case reports and basic scientific research that suggested that memory- recovery therapies sometimes result in distorted or fabricated memories (e.g., Goldstein & Farmer, 1994). The potential importance of these findings should not be understated, as fabricated memories of abuse or trauma can have serious implications for patients' families as well as the patient. In the case of memory-recovery therapy, the evidence for potential harm has led to recommendations of caution in the use of suggestive techniques, as well as efforts to educate the public so that they can make informed choices about participating in these types of interventions (e.g., APA Office of Public Communications, 1995).

Teaching patients to relax via breathing, visualization, and biofeedback is a common treatment for anxiety. For example, applied relaxation is an evidence-based treatment for panic disorder (Öst, 1987) and is a component of many cognitive-behavioral treatments. Lilienfeld (2007) listed relaxation as a treatment that is "probably harmful to some individuals," noting that it may lead to an induction of panic attacks in "panic prone" patients. This claim was based on a series of case reports in the 1980s and 1990s. For example, Cohen, Barlow, and Blanchard (1985) reported on two cases where the patient experienced panic attacks during relaxation exercises. The first patient experienced the attack when the patient was told "relax her whole body, and then her face and forehead" and the second patient during a third biofeedback session (p. 97). In another study, Heide and Borcovec (1984) reported an increase in tension among 14 patients during an initial relaxation session. However, patients reported general improvements in anxiety symptoms post-treatment and patients were not assessed for panic disorder or panic attacks. Despite these early reports, there do not appear to be any clinical trials indicating the number, frequency, or intensity of panic attacks increase in patients who participate in relaxation conditions compared to controls.

Exposing patients to feared stimuli is a core ingredient of many cognitive behavioral treatments (e.g., prolonged exposure; Foa, Hembree, & Rothbaum, 2007) and has been listed as a common factor across many forms of psychotherapy (Garfield, 1995). Exposure-based interventions are listed as evidence-based treatments for a variety of anxiety disorders (PTSD, OCD, panic; SCP, 2007). Given this exalted status, it is not entirely surprising that Lilienfield (2007) did not list exposure as a potentially harmful treatment. Nevertheless, the evidence suggesting that patients can experience distress or symptom exacerbation as a result of exposure is decidedly more developed than the case reports suggesting relaxation induces panic. For example, Tarrier et al. (1999) found significantly more patients in an imaginal exposure (IE) condition experienced symptom worsening (as indicated by a numerical increase in PTSD symptoms from pre- to post-treatment) compared to those who received cognitive therapy. In response, Devilly and Foa (2001) noted that symptom worsening was not rigorously defined and the IE condition was less effective than previous trials, leading to questions about the integrity of IE in the Tarrier et al. trial.

Mohr (1995) asserted that a category of treatments he described as "expressive-experiential" (EE) may be harmful based on findings of two outcome studies (Beutler, Frank, Schieber, Calvert, & Gaines, 1984; Mohr et al., 1990). Beutler et al. (1984) randomly assigned psychiatric inpatients to three different short-term inpatient groups or to a no-treatment control group. Initial analysis based on post-intervention status showed no differences between the interventions: "All groups improved by the end of treatment" (p. 75). When outcomes were quantified as residualized change in symptoms, however, the results were negative (i.e., mean residualized scores less than zero) for the EE group, zero for the behavioral and no-treatment controls, and positive for the interpersonal process group. Although no significance tests for group differences in this analysis were reported, the authors noted that the residualized scores for the expressive-experiential group were "almost worse" (p. 74) than those for the control group, which implies that the differences were not significant. However, Beutler et al. (1984) interpreted the negative mean residualized change score for the EE group as indicative of deterioration for clients in this group. It should be noted that a negative residual in this analysis may or may not correspond with a negative pre-post difference score (the negative residual indicates only that the post-score was lower than predicted, based on the pre-score). The fact that the mean residualized change for this group was lower than that for the control group certainly merits attention, but if the two groups did not differ significantly, the basis for the conclusion that EE patients demonstrated a "systematic deterioration effect" (Mohr, 1995, p. 17) was unjustified.

In the second study (Mohr et al., 1990), three treatments for patients with depression were implemented: a) focused-expressive psychotherapy (a "gestalt-based, anger-arousing therapy" that was categorized as EE by Mohr, 1995, p. 17), b) cognitive therapy, and c) a supportive/self-directed intervention. There were no differences between treatments in the proportion of negative responders (p. 624). However, in support of the claim that EE treatments are potentially harmful, Mohr (1995) noted that the deterioration rates for the three groups appeared different, but did not refer to the lack of statistical significance for the differences among these proportions. Moreover, there were no significant differences among the treatments on mean scores, adjusted for pretest functioning. Finally, there was no control group to establish the natural history of the depression, and, therefore, it is not possible to interpret this as evidence of harm. Thus, the case for harmfulness of EE treatments (Mohr, 1995; see also Lilienfeld, 2007) relies on interpretation of selected non-significant findings from two studies. Moreover, these selected studies were considered in isolation from other rigorous clinical trials that have shown that treatments that might also be classified as EE therapies, such as Greenberg's emotion-focused therapy (EFT, formerly referred to as process-experiential therapy) (Ellison & Greenberg, 2007), are effective (e.g., Watson, Gordon, Stermac, Kalogerakos, & Steckly, 2003).

Dishion et al. (1999) discussed the evidence for iatrogenic effects for treating adolescents with behavior problems in group settings, based on the hypothesis that "deviancy training" (p. 755) among group members may accentuate rather than diminish conduct problems, including substance use, aggressive behavior, and delinquency. Dishion et al. (1999) summarized at length the findings of two intervention studies that suggested that the presence of harmful effects for group treatment for this population, (i.e., poorer outcomes relative to those for those receiving no treatment). Weiss et al. (2005) offered a careful review of the evidence presented by Dishion et al. (1999) and found several problematic practices among those claiming empirical support for iatrogenic effects of these treatments, including a) selective attention to findings from studies more favorable to the authors' preferred theory; b) selective attention to findings for one among many outcome measures within studies; c) reliance on marginally significant effects in tests of post hoc hypotheses; d) arbitrary attribution of apparent negative effects to one component of a complex treatment; e) inadequate attention to plausible alternative explanations for findings interpreted as supportive of the authors' preferred theory (Weiss et al., 2005). Weiss et al. (2005) also presented new meta-analytic evidence based on 66 studies and 115 separate treatment groups involving interventions focused on externalizing conduct problems in children and adolescents. Their analysis suggested that interventions involving a peer group component produced better (although not significantly better) outcomes than those without this component and that the peer group interventions were significantly less likely to produce negative effect sizes (in comparisons with no-treatment controls) than were interventions that did not involve peer groups. Their conclusion, based on this extensive review of published studies, was that there is "little support in the literature for iatrogenic effects [of peer group interventions for adolescent conduct disorders], deviancy training based or otherwise" (p. 1044).

Despite Weiss et al.'s findings to the contrary, Rhule (2005) featured the "deviancy training" hypothesis as a primary example of evidence for harm, and Lilienfeld (2007) included peer-group interventions for conduct disorder in his list of potentially harmful treatments (albeit in Level II, "treatments that possibly produce harm," rather than Level I, "treatments that probably produce harm"). Noting that Weiss et al.'s (2005) conclusions did not support Dishion et al.'s (1999) deviancy training account, Lilienfeld proposed that "the reasons for these marked discrepancies in study outcomes require clarification" (p. 62). On the other hand, Weiss and colleagues followed the recommended practice of casting a broad net in their search for relevant research studies and basing their conclusions on the preponderance of available evidence, whereas Dishion and colleagues used a selective strategy of focusing on studies and findings that supported their theoretical position. It is not surprising that these two approaches led to different conclusions, with preference given to the more systematic approach.

Summary of Findings on Treatments That Harm

In sum, claims about the iatrogenic effects of psychotherapy do not seem to be based on strong evidence. On close inspection, some studies cited as evidence for this phenomenon fail to provide clear evidence of negative outcomes, and those that do often offer little basis for attributing deterioration to the harmful effects of the intervention. While there appears to be evidence that some "behavioral" interventions—very broadly defined—can be harmful (e.g., re-birthing, CISD), these treatments are not psychotherapy, as defined in this volume or as is commonly understood to be the meaning of the term. Indeed, as we discuss in the conclusion of this volume, the question of harm raises important questions regarding the boundaries of what should be regarded as "psychotherapy." Every intervention that is applied via behavioral means should not automatically be considered an instance of psychotherapy. Many of the treatments listed by Lilienfeld do not meet this threshold. For example, critical incident stress debriefing, grief counseling for individuals with normal bereavement reactions, and Drug Abuse Resistance Education (DARE) programs are all preventative interventions that are offered to individuals regardless of symptomology and thus should not be considered traditional forms of psychotherapy. Attachment therapies and boot camps that include potentially dangerous physical interventions (e.g., sitting on the client to re-create birth, physical deprivation) more closely resemble forms of fraternity hazing than psychotherapy and may certainly be dangerous. Notably, the list of treatments identified by Lilienfeld is by no means exhaustive of the quackery that is offered to patients as a form of behavioral intervention (see final chapter for the boundaries of acceptable treatments performed by mental health professionals; Singer & Lalich, 1996). In regards to claims of harm directed against traditional forms of psychotherapy (e.g., experiential), conclusions are based on highly selective reviews of the literature, privileging negative findings (not always statistically significant) and ignoring the preponderance of the relevant research.

Conclusions

Approximately 40 years ago, there was controversy about whether psychotherapy produced outcomes that were better than the rate of spontaneous remission. Strikingly, it is difficult to find an example of an empirically tested psychotherapy offered to a treatment-seeking patient (i.e., a patient who has some problem or is in some distress and seeks treatment) that is not effective. While several treatments have been identified as potentially harmful, these treatments often are not psychotherapies at all, are offered to consumers that are neither in distress nor seeking treatment, or are based on very limited evidence. Before the use of meta-analysis, opponents and advocates of psychotherapy were able to review and find support for their respective positions. Although the first meta-analyses were controversial, the results of the original and subsequent meta-analyses have converged on the conclusion that psychotherapy is remarkably efficacious. The history of the investigations of psychotherapy efficacy establishes meta-analysis as an objective and useful way to aggregate studies addressing the same hypothesis.

Having established the efficacy of psychotherapy, we now focus on whether various psychotherapies are equally efficacious. Despite the expansive list of treatments that have demonstrated some efficacy, the proliferation of CBT-related treatments in lists of ESTs, and recent arguments that some psychotherapies may be harmful, evidence regarding the absolute efficacy of psychotherapy does not support either the Contextual Model or the Medical Model. If a particular treatment is found to be efficacious in treatment package designs that compare a treatment to a no-treatment condition, it is not possible to know whether the effects were due to the specific ingredients or the incidental factors of the treatment. That is, these designs are not sufficient to separate specific effects from general effects. Certainly, advocates of the treatment will claim that the benefits are due to the specific ingredient but the evidence cannot discriminate between the Medical Model and the Contextual Model of psychotherapy. Besides having immense practical importance, relative efficacy provides more specific evidence relative to the Contextual Model versus the Medical Model.

Notes

1. It is notable that the initial challenges to the effects of psychotherapy came from advocates of another form of "talk therapy." Essentially, early claims about the ineffectiveness of "psychotherapy" were driven by the behavioral criticisms of psychodynamic theory. Thus, at the time, even questions raised about absolute efficacy in psychotherapy were rooted in the relative efficacy of different treatment approaches. The tension between dynamic/non-behavioral and behavioral treatments stems the entire history of psychotherapy research and continues to this day. However, "psychotherapy" is now an omnibus term that is broadly applied to a class of treatments that are based in a conversation between and patient and therapist (i.e., behavioral treatment is now considered one *type* of many psychotherapies). Indeed, the PubMed subject heading "Psychotherapy" contains as sub-headings various psychotherapies including cognitive therapist, behavioral therapist, etc. In this chapter, we mostly ignore questions of the relative efficacy of different treatment and focus on the implications of the Eysenck findings, which—despite their original intention—resulted in a literature on the effects of psychotherapy in general.

2. Moreover, the criteria used by Rachman to impeach studies were different for psychotherapy and for behavior therapy, creating a further bias (see Smith, Glass, & Miller, 1980, Chapter 5).

3. The interpretation of selected negative effects is illustrated by subsequent reviewers, such as Rhule (2005) and Lilienfeld (2007), who relied on Werch and Owens' (2002) article to draw more pointed conclusions about harmful interventions than those offered by Werch and Owen. Rhule and Lilienfeld both asserted that Project DARE (Drug Abuse Resistance Education) is a potentially harmful treatment, citing Werch and Owen's (2002) review as evidence that DARE may actually lead to higher use of alcohol and perhaps other drugs. One problem with this proffered justification is that Werch and Owen found only a single study of DARE (Rosenbaum & Hanson, 1998) that showed evidence of any negative outcomes. As was often the case for studies reviewed by Werch and Owen, the negative effect was observed in only one (suburban schools) of several sub-populations examined on a number of different outcome variables. This effect disappeared for all outcomes except one when controlling for exposure to other drug-education programs.

   In contrast, West and O'Neal (2004) conducted a comprehensive meta-analysis focused specifically on DARE. The review included all studies that appeared in peer-reviewed journals that compared DARE to a control group and assessed variables related to alcohol, illicit drug, or tobacco use both prior to and following the intervention. Eleven studies were found that met these criteria (all published in 2002 or before and including Rosenbaum and Hanson, 1998). West and O'Neal found that the overall effect of DARE programs was near zero ($d = .023$, favoring DARE), suggesting that while it is not an effective preventative program, it is not harmful (i.e., does not increase the use of substances generally vis-à-vis comparisons across multiple studies). Only one of the 11 studies in the meta-analysis produced a negative effect ($d = -.117$, a very small effect). This meta-analysis reinforces the point that determination of harmful effects of a treatment should be made across the corpus of studies that evaluate the effectiveness of that treatment rather than on the basis of a single study selected from that corpus (especially if that study was selected specifically because it reported negative effects).

Chapter 5

Relative Efficacy
The Dodo Bird Still Gets It

In 1936, Rosenzweig suggested that common factors were responsible for the apparent efficacy of existing psychotherapies. The logical inference was that psychological treatments that contained the common factors would produce beneficial outcomes, and, consequently, all psychotherapies would be roughly equivalent in terms of their benefits. The uniform efficacy of psychotherapies was emphasized in the subtitle of Rosenzweig's article by reference to the Dodo bird's conclusion at the end of a race in *Alice in Wonderland*: "At last the Dodo said, '*Everybody* has won, and *all* must have prizes'" (p. 412). Evidence consistent with Rosenzweig's claim of uniform efficacy—commonly referred to as the Dodo bird effect—is typically considered empirical support for the conjecture that common factors are the efficacious aspect of psychotherapy. On the other hand, advocates of particular therapeutic approaches believe that some treatments (viz., those that contain "scientific" ingredients) are more efficacious than others.

In this chapter, the evidence related to the relative efficacy of various psychotherapies will be explored. First, predictions of the Contextual Model and the Medical Model will be discussed. Then, research design considerations for determining relative efficacy will be presented. Finally, the empirical evidence, which is predominated by meta-analyses, will be reviewed.[1]

Medical and Contextual Model Predictions

The predictions of the Medical Model and Contextual Model relative to the uniformity of psychotherapy efficacy are straightforward. There are two possible results. The first is that treatments vary in their efficacy. That is, some treatments will be found to be immensely efficacious, some moderately efficacious, and some not efficacious at all. Presumably, the relative differences in outcomes were due to the specific ingredients of some treatments that were more potent than the specific ingredients of other treatments. Thus, variability in outcomes for various treatments would provide evidence for the Medical Model of psychotherapy.

A second pattern of outcomes would be that all treatments produce about the same outcome. If the factors common to all therapies were responsible for the efficacy of psychotherapy, rather than specific ingredients, then the particular treatment delivered would be irrelevant and all treatments would produce equivalent outcomes. Of course, it could be argued that specific ingredients are indeed the causally important components but that all specific ingredients are equally potent—a logically permissible hypothesis but one that seems implausible.

It is worth reiterating the differential hypothesis here. Important evidence relative to the Medical/Contextual Model issue is produced by data about the relative efficacy of treatments. If specific ingredients are responsible for outcomes, variation in the relative efficacy of treatments is expected, whereas if the common aspects are responsible, homogeneity of effects (that is, general equivalence of treatments) is expected.

Research Methods for Establishing Relative Efficacy

Relative efficacy typically is investigated by comparing the outcomes of two treatments. However, as we shall see, there are inferential limitations of such designs. Many of the limitations can be addressed by meta-analytically aggregating the results of primary studies. In this section, research strategies for studying relative efficacy, in primary and meta-analytic contexts, will be presented.

Research Strategies for Studying Relative Efficacy in Primary Studies

The fundamental design for establishing relative efficacy is the comparative outcome strategy (Kazdin, 1994). In the comparative design, patients are randomly assigned to Treatment A and to Treatment B, the treatments are delivered, and post-tests are administered, rendering a design identical to the control-group design, except that two treatments are administered (rather than one treatment and a control group). Comparative designs typically contain some type of control group as well, such as a waitlist control group, so that it can be determined whether the treatments are superior to no treatment. However, the control group is not needed to answer the question, "Is Treatment A superior (or inferior) to Treatment B?"

There are two possible outcomes of comparative designs, both of which result in some ambiguity (see Wampold, 1997). One possible outcome is that the means of the outcome variables for the two treatments are not significantly different. Given the pervasive evidence for efficacy presented in Chapter 4, assume that both treatments were superior to a no-treatment control group. Thus, as administered and assessed, there appears to be no evidence that the two treatments differ. However, there is ambiguity around interpretation of this result. If both treatments were intended to be therapeutic and conform to the conditions of the Contextual Model, this result would be interpreted as support for the Contextual Model. However, it is difficult to rule out the possibility that the efficacy was due to the specific ingredients of the two treatments, where the specific ingredients have approximately equal potency. Moreover, it may be that one set of specific ingredients is more potent than the other but that the statistical power to detect this difference was low (Kazdin & Bass, 1989).

It would appear that a less ambiguous conclusion could be reached by the second possible outcome of a comparative design, namely that the study yielded a superior outcome for one of the treatments compared. Presumably, if Treatment A was found to be superior to Treatment B, then the specific ingredients constituting Treatment A are active—that is, these ingredients were responsible for the superiority of Treatment A. However, consider an example of such a finding that demonstrates ambiguity remains even when superiority of one treatment is found.

Snyder and Wills (1989) compared the efficacy of behavioral marital therapy (BMT) to insight-oriented marital therapy (IOMT). At post-test and 6-month follow-up, both BMT and IOMT were superior to no-treatment controls, but equivalent to each other. The authors recognized that the finding could not disentangle the common factor/specific ingredient explanations: "Although treatments in the present study were relatively uncontaminated from interventions specific to the alternative approach, each treatment used nonspecific interventions common to both" (p. 45). Four years after termination of treatment, an important difference between the treatments was found: 38 percent of the BMT couples were divorced whereas only 3 percent of the IOMT couples were divorced (Snyder, Wills, & Grady-Fletcher, 1991). This result would seem to provide evidence for the specific ingredients of IOMT, but Jacobson (1991), a proponent of BMT, argued otherwise: "It seems obvious that the IOMT therapists were relying heavily on the nonspecific clinically sensitive interventions allowed in the IOMT manual but not mentioned in the BMT manual. . . . To me, the . . . data suggest that *in this study* BMT was practiced with insufficient attention to nonspecifics" (p. 143). Jacobson argued that the playing field was not level because there was inequivalence in the potency of the aspects of treatment that were incidental to BMT and IOMT. Jacobson's critique also has specific application to the effects of "researcher allegiance" on relative efficacy—a research area that will be discussed later in this chapter.

There is another problem with interpretations of statistically significant differences between the outcomes of two treatments. As discussed in Chapter 3, statistical theory predicts that by chance some comparisons of treatments will produce statistically significant differences when there are no true differences (i.e., Type I errors). As noted in Chapter 4 (Figure 4.2), a large number of psychotherapy clinical trials are published each year. Given the large number of trials, we would expect some comparative studies to reveal differences between treatments (e.g., Butler, Fennell, Robson, & Gelder, 1991; Leichsenring et al., 2013; Snyder et al., 1991;Vos et al., 2012), but it may be that these studies represent the few that would occur by chance. This problem is exacerbated by the fact that differences are often found only for a few of the dependent variables in a study (e.g., one variable, divorce rate, in the Snyder et al. study).

The comparative treatment design is a valid experimental design to determine relative efficacy. Nevertheless, as is the case with any design, there are difficulties in making interpretations from a single comparative study, whether the results produce statistically significant differences or not. Meta-analysis can address many of the issues raised by the interpretation of primary studies and can be used to estimate a robust effect size for relative efficacy. We now address the various meta-analytic strategies for determining relative efficacy.

Meta-Analytic Methods for Determining Relative Efficacy

Meta-analyses can be used to examine the relative efficacy of treatments over many studies, thus testing the null hypothesis that treatments are uniformly effective versus the alternative that they vary in effectiveness. Meta-analysis provides a quantitative test of the hypotheses and avoids conclusions based on salient, but unrepresentative, studies. Qualitative reviews allow for the citation of studies that have shown the superiority of one treatment over another but, as discussed previously in this chapter and Chapter 4, each of these studies may be flawed (e.g., effects due to allegiance or lack of adherence) and the observed results may be Type I errors. In addition, studies that do not show differences may not receive adequate attention (see Ehlers et al., 2010; Persons & Silberschatz, 1998 for examples). This leaves questions about relative efficacy over the entire corpus of studies unanswered. Moreover, meta-analysis provides a quantitative index of the size of any treatment effect—if treatments are not equivalent in their effectiveness, then how different are they? Finally, meta-analysis can examine other hypotheses about relative effectiveness that cannot be answered easily by primary studies (e.g., do studies with researcher allegiance produce larger effects than studies without researcher allegiance?).

There are two primary meta-analytic means to examine relative efficacy. The first method reviews treatment package designs utilizing no-treatment control groups. According to this method, a) treatments examined in studies are classified into categories (e.g., cognitive behavioral therapy, CBT, dynamic, etc.); b) the effect size is computed for each treatment vis-à-vis the no-treatment control group; c) the effect sizes within a category are averaged (e.g., the mean effect size for CBT is calculated across the studies that contain CBT and a no-treatment control group); and d) the mean effect sizes for the categories are compared (e.g., CBT versus EMDR; see for example, Bisson et al., 2007).

Making inferences based on the meta-analysis of no-treatment control group designs is problematic because the studies of treatments in a given category may differ from the studies of treatments in other categories. For example, studies that compare CBT with a no-treatment control group may differ from studies that compare dynamic treatments with no treatment controls on such factors such as outcome variables used, severity of disorder treated, comorbidity of patients, treatment standardization, treatment length, and allegiance of the researcher. However, as we shall see, many claims about relative efficacy are made on the basis of meta-analytic comparisons of treatments to no-treatment control groups.

One way to deal with the confounding variables is to meta-analytically model their mediating and moderating effects. Shadish and Sweeney (1991) for example, found that setting, measurement reactivity, measurement specificity, measurement manipulability, and number of patients moderated the relationship of treatment and effect size and that treatment standardization, treatment implementation, and behavioral dependent variables mediated the relationship of treatment and effect size. However, modeling meta-analytic confounds post-hoc is extremely difficult, with the same problems encountered in primary research, such as leaving out important variables, misspecification of models, unreliability of measurements, or lack of statistical power.

A method that avoids most of the confounds that are created by comparing classes of treatments compared to controls is to test relative efficacy by aggregating only studies that directly compare two psychotherapies. For example, if one were interested in the relative efficacy of CBT and dynamic therapies, only those studies that directly compared these two types of treatments would be examined. This strategy avoids confounds due to aspects of the dependent variable, problem treated, setting, severity of the disorder, and other patient characteristics, as these factors would be comparable for each direct comparison due to random assignment (e.g., each direct comparison of CBT and a dynamic therapy would use the same outcome measures). Shadish et al. (1993) noted that direct comparisons "have rarely been reported in past meta-analyses, and their value for controlling confounds seems to be underappreciated" (p. 998). It should be noted that some confounds, such as skill of therapist and allegiance, remain in the direct comparison strategy. While the number of meta-analyses of direct comparisons in the area of psychotherapy outcomes has increased in recent years, as we shall see there are still many disorders for which direct comparisons studies are mostly unavailable. Further, researcher allegiance may be responsible for many observed differences between treatments because if allegiance is not well controlled in primary studies, then meta-analyses of such studies will be similarly confounded, although these confounds can be modeled, as discussed later in this chapter.

Meta-analysis of direct comparisons raises an issue that must be resolved. In order to properly test the Contextual Model hypothesis, it is important that the treatments compared are instances of psychotherapy, as stipulated by the

Contextual Model. That is, a) both treatments would need to appear to the patients to be efficacious and that the rationale would need to be cogent and acceptable; b) the therapists would have to have confidence in the treatment and believe, to some extent, that the treatment is legitimate (e.g., not a sham), c) the treatment would have to be delivered in a manner consistent with the rationale provided and contain actions that induce the patient to participate in therapeutic actions that reasonably address his or her problems; and d) the treatment would have to be delivered in a healing context. Studies often include treatments that are not intended to be therapeutic or are limited in some way and which, to any reasonably well-trained clinician, would not be legitimate. Such treatments are often called "alternative" treatments, placebo controls, or as we shall see, "supportive therapy" (Mohr et al., 2009; Wampold et al., 1997b; Westen, Novotny, & Thompson-Brenner, 2004). Westen et al. (2004) called such treatments "intent-to-fail" treatments because they were designed to be less effective than the treatments to which they were being compared. We refer to such treatments as pseudo-placebos (see Chapter 8 for a full discussion of these issues).

An example of a treatment that would not be intended to be therapeutic (and hence would not meet the Contextual Model test) was used by Foa, Rothbaum, Riggs, and Murdock (1991) to establish empirical support for Prolonged Exposure (a behavioral treatment for PTSD). The comparison treatment was supportive counseling (SC) and the patient sample included women diagnosed with PTSD who had recently (within the previous year) been raped. In the SC treatment a) clients were taught a general problem-solving technique (not individualized for the particular patient's problems); b) therapists responded indirectly and were unconditionally supportive; and c) clients "were immediately redirected to focus on current daily problems if discussions of the assault occurred" (p. 718). In all likelihood, this counseling would not be seen as viable by therapists because it contains no particular theoretical rationale or established principles of change, and, in the absence of other components, "few would accept deflecting women from discussing their recent rape in counseling as therapeutic" (Wampold, Mondin, Moody, & Ahn, 1997a, p. 227). Clearly, the SC treatment was not intended to be therapeutic, and therapists would not deliver the treatment with a sufficient sense of efficacy. Although proscribing discussion of the trauma in SC was intended to eliminate any exposure elements (e.g., covertly experiencing the trauma in a safe, supporting setting) so that it could be determined whether exposure to the trauma memory is an active ingredient in Prolonged Exposure, this "handcuffing" of therapists introduces numerous additional threats (Mohr et al., 2009). The resulting control treatment lost many of the elements purported by the Contextual Model that are needed to render a treatment effective, including therapists who believe the treatment is effective, a cogent rationale, agreement about the goals and tasks of therapy, therapeutic activity focused on patient's problems, and so forth. Examples of such "sham" treatments are extremely common in the literature and can be difficult to detect without closely reading method sections. For example, consider Gilboa-Schechtman et al. (2010) who compared PE to "psychodynamic treatment" for adolescents diagnosed with PTSD. In this study, PE was somewhat superior to psychodynamic treatment, and thus it might be logical to conclude that PE is more effective than a psychodynamic treatment for adolescent PTSD. However, a closer inspection of the research indicates that the psychodynamic treatment was not psychodynamic at all. The PD in this study was a pseudo-placebo control:

> [The PD treatment] consisted of 15 to 18 50-minute sessions. The initial sessions were primarily focused on building rapport and working alliance and on defining the central issue (two to three sessions). The remaining sessions were devoted to "working through" the central issue. Patients were encouraged to share their inner thoughts, daily difficulties, and free associations, while the therapist used selective listening and interpretation of themes related to the central issue. Therapists did not mention the traumatic event, and if the patient brought up details of the memory, they referred to the meaning of the event in the context of the central issue, without further encouragement to discuss the memory.
>
> (p. 1037)

The PE therapists attended a 5-day training workshop by the developer of PE and supervised by the first author, where the PD therapists received a 2-day training by a local psychodynamic supervisor, and PD therapists were proscribed from an action that would be common for most therapists (i.e., having the patient discuss the trauma) and which would certainly be central for most, if not all, psychodynamic therapists. To provide a fair test of the competing Medical and Contextual Models, the comparisons of treatments must involve treatments that are intended to be therapeutic.

In the following sections, we will review the evidence bearing on the question of relative efficacy. As allegiance is a crucial concept in the interpretation of trials comparing psychotherapies, we begin by introducing the concept and reviewing evidence for its effects. We then focus on the current evidence for relative efficacy claims, beginning again with a brief review of the chaos that was the treatment literature prior to the advent of meta-analysis, focusing on recent meta-analyses and key individual studies when appropriate.

Allegiance

Allegiance refers to the degree to which the therapist or researcher believes that the therapy is efficacious. One of the sacrosanct assumptions of clients is that their therapist believes in the effectiveness of the treatment being delivered. The client in a psychotherapy context expects that the therapist has an explanation for the client's disorder and the treatment strategy consistent with that explanation that will lead to improvement. This is the central mechanism of creating expectations for change, the second pathway of the Contextual Model. If the therapist does not believe the treatment is effective—that is, he or she believes it is a sham—then a basic element of psychotherapy, namely trust, is missing and would seem to undermine a basic tenet of psychotherapy practice. For the most part, practicing therapists choose the approach to psychotherapy that is compatible with their understanding and conceptualization of psychological distress and health, the process of change, and the nature of the client and his or her problem. Consequently, clients can rest assured that their therapist is committed to and believes in the therapy being delivered. Conceived in this way, more than a critical design issue, therapist allegiance is a basic common factor that should exist across therapies as they are typically delivered.

In the Contextual Model, trust that the therapist believes the treatment being delivered will lead to improvement is a critical component necessary for the efficacious delivery of a psychotherapeutic treatment. Although allegiance may be universal in practice settings, there is reason to believe that allegiance varies considerably in clinical trials of psychotherapy. Consider, for example, a clinical trial comparing cognitive-behavioral and interpersonal treatments for depression in which a crossed design was used. In such a design, each therapist would provide both of the treatments but may have allegiance to only one of the treatments. When proponents of a particular treatment conduct clinical trials, the therapists may be graduate students of the proponent or otherwise affiliated with the proponent's research laboratory and are often supervised by the proponent or the developer of that treatment. Consequently these therapists may have greater allegiance to the treatment affiliated with the laboratory than with the other treatment being delivered in the study, which is exaggerated when the therapists in the preferred condition are trained and supervised by the developer of the treatment or a nationally recognized expert, whereas the comparison treatment receives training and supervision from, say, a local clinician (as was the case for the adolescent dynamic treatment discussed earlier).[2] The effects of allegiance can be more pronounced when the therapists are affiliated with one treatment and are well aware they are providing another treatment for which it is desired by the researchers that the alternative treatment be found less effective than the preferred treatment—even more pronounced when the therapists are involved in the research (e.g., are coauthors). In randomized double-blinded placebo drug studies in medicine, allegiance effects are controlled because the clinicians administering the treatment do not know which treatment they are delivering; therapist blinding is impossible in psychotherapy studies because the therapist is always cognizant of the treatment being delivered. Therefore, in psychotherapy studies allegiance can be confounded with the treatment (i.e., some treatments use therapists with more allegiance than other treatments). Because allegiance varies, the effects of allegiance on outcome can be investigated.

Because therapist belief in the treatment is a critical component of the Contextual Model, it is predicted that allegiance will be related to outcome—the greater the allegiance of the therapist, the better the outcome. Proponents of the Medical Model might recognize that allegiance is consequential but would not consider allegiance to be central to treatment. The relative unimportance of allegiance in the Medical Model is demonstrated by the fact that allegiance has not historically been considered when control groups (placebos or alternative treatments) are designed. That is, clinical scientists seem to be unconcerned that therapists do not have allegiance to pseudo-placebo treatments, alternative treatments, or to theoretically coherent alternative treatments, thus making the assumption that allegiance effects are unimportant. However, the effect of allegiance to treatment provides a test of the Medical Model versus the Contextual Model: allegiance is a critical factor in the Contextual Model but relatively unimportant in the Medical Model. In the next sections, the research evidence related to allegiance will be presented.

Although primary studies do not assess individual therapists' allegiance to treatment, the allegiance of the therapists in outcome studies often can be inferred. As discussed above, if the researcher is a proponent of one of the treatments administered in the study and the researcher trains the therapists, then it can be inferred that the therapists have allegiance to that treatment. Similar to placebo effects, the effects of allegiance may be subtle and not detected by even the most well meaning researchers (hence the elusive pursuit of the double-blind psychotherapy clinical trial) and may include differences in recruitment strategies, the way treatments are described, etc. Before examining some studies and the meta-analyses of allegiance, an important distinction between researcher allegiance and therapist allegiance needs to be clear. A researcher may have an allegiance to treatment X, say, and design a study that carefully controls allegiance, say by using only therapists who have an allegiance to the treatments they are administering, with similar training and supervision provided by similarly qualified persons. However, researcher allegiance can be manifest in ways other than the therapists; it is not unsual to alter the comparison treatment in minor or major ways, often by removing a component of the treatment that might overlap with the preferred treatment (e.g., proscribing talking about the trauma in the session to rule out exposure). Such alterations often create treatments that are not delivered in a way they were originally designed.

Consider, for example, a study of CBT and applied relaxation (AR) (as well as a psychopharmacology condition) for the treatment of panic disorder conducted by Clark, Salkovskis, Hackmann, Middleton, Anastasiades, and Gelder (1994). The first author of the study (David M. Clark) is a leading proponent of cognitive therapy and a developer of the CBT being studied (along with the second author). The introduction of the article predominately discussed cognitive therapy and clearly identified AR as an established alternative that was selected in order to validate cognitive therapy. In the method section, two articles were cited as the basis for cognitive therapy and Clark authored both, while the alternative therapy was devised and advocated by another group of researchers. Additionally, the two therapists used in the study, and who provided both CBT and AR, were coauthors, one was a co-developer of the treatment and both were CBT advocates (viz., Salkovskis & Hackmann). Finally, the first author and proponent of cognitive therapy (Clark) served as the clinical supervisor for both treatments. The allegiance of the authors this study is unambiguous; moreover, the inference that the therapists were committed to the cognitive therapy and had less loyalty to AR is apparent, as well. This example demonstrates how researcher advocacy for a treatment translates into therapist allegiance. In this study however, there was another research operation that favored CBT, involving modifications of the standard AR procedure, as noted by Wampold, Imel, and Miller (2009):

> The second modification [of AR], more consequential, was that in Öst's development of [AR], exposure to anxiety-provoking stimuli was not introduced until after training in relaxation was completed (8 to 10 sessions), whereas in Clark et al.'s version, exposure was begun after four sessions—that is to say, Clark et al. exposed patients to the feared stimuli before they had learned to relax.
>
> (p. 148)

Although researcher allegiance can lead to multiple biases (e.g., recruitment, non-blind and biased evaluations, modifications of existing treatments, non-random data entry errors, etc.), it is clear that therapist allegiance in clinical trials is present when the researcher/treatment advocate trains and supervises the therapists and the therapists have loyalty to the researcher and the treatment approach. An issue is to determine the sources of researcher allegiance effects, should they exist.

Studies can be designed and undertaken that manage the impact of allegiance. A good example of a study that minimized allegiance effects is the National Institute of Mental Health (NIMH) Treatment of Depression Collaborative Research Program (NIMH TDCRP; Elkin, 1994). The authors of the study were not proponents of the two psychological treatments administered (viz., CBT and interpersonal psychotherapy, IPT) and the design of the study was developed through various committees of experts. The sites at which CBT and IPT were administered were selected from applications from groups using CBT and IPT. The treatments were delivered by therapists who had allegiance to the treatment they delivered and were trained and supervised by proponents of the respective treatments (more on this study later in the chapter).

While we might hope that investigators who design direct comparisons of psychotherapy are agnostic with respect to the effect of the treatments being investigated, the field has largely adjusted to the reality that psychotherapy science does not function in this way. Treatments most often are tested by the clinical scientists who developed them and are invested in establishing their efficacy and disseminating them to be widely used, not too different from efforts by pharmaceutical companies to have drugs approved for use (see Spielmans & Kirsch, in press)

Evidence Related to Allegiance

The effects of allegiance can be investigated by comparing results across studies. That is, comparisons of the size of effects obtained in studies where researcher allegiance to one of the treatments is present to the size of effects of studies where allegiance is not present. Examination of allegiance effects have been scattered throughout various meta-analyses of outcomes in psychotherapy.

The earliest attempt to identify allegiance effects appeared in Smith et al.'s (1980) meta-analysis. Recall from Chapter 4 that Smith et al. conducted an extensive search of all published and unpublished controlled studies of counseling and psychotherapy through 1977. In all, 475 studies were found, which produced an average effect size (treatment versus control) of 0.85, which is a large effect. Allegiance in each study in this meta-analysis was determined by the "direction of stated research hypotheses, favorable results of previous research uncritically accepted, rationalizations after failure to find significant effects for the favored treatment, and outright praise and promotion of a point of view" (p. 119). Often the alternative treatments against which the favored treatment was compared would "be treated with obvious disdain, and would not be given much opportunity for success" (p. 119). Unequivocal allegiance effects were detected. When compared to control groups, treatments for which the experimenter had allegiance produced an average effect size of 0.95, whereas treatments for which the experimenter had an allegiance against the treatment produced an effect size of 0.66. The difference between these two effect sizes (viz., an effect size of 0.29) is a rough estimate of allegiance effects. Shortly thereafter, Luborsky, Singer, and Luborsky (1975) noted, "It is natural to question whether or not . . . the therapeutic allegiance of the experimenter might . . . influence the results" (p. 1003).

A few years later, an interesting allegiance effect of a particular researcher appeared when Dush, Hirt, and Schroeder (1983) meta-analyzed studies that investigated self-statement modification (SSM). At the time, cognitive therapies were experiencing a wave of popularity. Three approaches predominated: Ellis's rational-emotive therapy, Beck's cognitive therapy, and Meichenbaum's SSM. Dush et al. retrieved 69 studies that compared SSM to a no-treatment control group or to a pseudo-placebo control group. The average of the effect sizes for SSM vis-à-vis no-treatment controls and pseudo-placebo controls were .74 and .53, respectively. These values are in accordance with treatment efficacy values found across meta-analyses (see Chapters 4 & 8). However, when studies were segregated based on whether the studies were authored or coauthored by Meichenbaum, dramatic differences in effect sizes emerged. The effect sizes produced by studies authored or coauthored by Meichenbaum were nearly twice as large as the other studies when comparisons were made to no-treatment controls and more than twice as large when comparisons were made to pseudo-placebo controls (see Figure 5.1). More telling is that the placebo controls appear to be markedly ineffective in those studies conducted by Meichenbaum, as the effect size using placebo controls and no-treatment controls produced almost identical effect sizes (i.e., placebo controls appeared to be essentially no-treatment controls). Using the difference between the Meichenbaum effect sizes and the other study effect sizes, allegiance effects in the range of .60 to .70 were obtained. These SSM studies show an allegiance effect for Meichenbaum, the developer and primary advocate for SSM treatments.

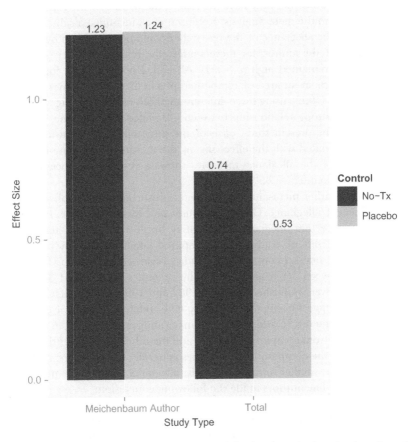

Figure 5.1 Effect sizes for self-statement modification by whether (co-) authored by Meichenbaum. Adapted from "Self-statement modification with adults: A meta-analysis," by D. M. Dush, M. L. Hirt, and H. Schroeder, 1983, *Psychological Bulletin, 94*, p. 414. Copyright by the American Psychological Association. Adapted with permission.

Another meta-analysis that found strong allegiance effects is Robinson, Berman, and Neimeyer's (1990) review of treatments for depression. Although Robinson et al. found differences in the efficacy of various treatments of depression, these differences were accounted for by differences in allegiance to the various treatments. In this meta-analysis, allegiance was rated on a 5-point scale, using the cues discussed previously (e.g., direction of hypotheses, degree of detail provided about treatments). The two raters used in this meta-analysis showed remarkable consistency in their ratings of allegiance (intraclass correlation of 0.95). The results indicated that the correlation between the allegiance ratings and the effects produced by the study was .58, which is remarkably large. That is, about one-third $[(0.58)^2 = 0.34]$ of the variability in effect sizes produced in the studies reviewed was due to the allegiance of the researcher. Because study outcomes may have influenced the writing of the introductions of the articles in the meta-analysis, Robinson et al. identified a subset of studies for which the allegiance of the researcher could be established by previous publications of the author; for these studies, the relation between allegiance and outcome remained high (r = .51). All told, Robinson et al. found large allegiance effects in an area of established psychotherapy outcomes research. Luborsky et al. (1999), using three different methods of determining allegiance, found a very strong relationship between allegiance and outcome, and concluded, "For the present study, each of the three allegiance measures is significantly associated with the effect size of the treatments compared, and the combination of the allegiance measures shows a very large association with treatment outcomes (r = .85!)" (p. 103).

Although earlier meta-analyses painted a disturbing picture of the pernicious effects of allegiance, Gaffan, Tsaousis, and Kemp-Wheeler (1995) produced evidence that allegiance effects may be decreasing over time. They examined two sets of studies that compared cognitive therapy and other therapies. The first set contained 28 studies reviewed in Dobson (1989) and published between 1976 and 1987. The second set contained 37 studies retrieved that were published between 1987 and 1994. For the first set, there was an advantage for cognitive therapy (CT) relative to control groups or alternate treatments. In addition, allegiance ratings were related to the effect sizes obtained from comparisons of CT and the other groups. For the second set of studies, the comparative effect sizes generally were smaller; indices of allegiance were smaller and, importantly, allegiance scores were not related to effect sizes. The authors made the following conclusion:

> The relationship is present in Dobson's set of studies partly because comparisons with large [effect sizes] favoring CT were associated with strong allegiance toward CT, especially before 1985, and partly because [effect size] and allegiance declined together from the late 1970s to the 1980s. By the 1990s, both these associations had disappeared.
>
> (p. 978)

To make sense of the various meta-analyses conducted on allegiance, Munder, Brütsch, Gerger, and Barth (2013) conducted a meta-analysis of 30 meta-analyses that have been conducted (a meta-meta-analysis, if you will), taking into account the fact that some studies were included in multiple meta-analyses. Across 30 meta-analytic studies, the overall correlation of allegiance and outcome was $r = .26$ (equivalent to $d = 0.54$, see Table 3.1, a moderate-sized effect). Interestingly, the allegiance of the meta-analysis researcher to the concept of the allegiance (allegiance to allegiance, if you will) made a marginal difference, but even if the meta-analytic researcher was not an advocate of allegiance (or even hostile to it), allegiance remained significantly correlated with outcome ($r = .17$, equivalent to $d = 0.35$). Allegiance effects were robust to all other moderators in this analysis.

A common criticism of the allegiance literature is that it is correlational. Thus, the association between allegiance and outcome may not be bias at all—the causality may actually be reversed such that researchers simply have allegiance to more effective treatments (Leykin & DeRubeis, 2009). Similarly, it is possible that the outcome of the study might influence the written report in a way that commends the superior treatment, creating the impression of allegiance (e.g., an editor could request a decrease in the length of a treatment description for an ineffective treatment). To test this criticism, Munder, Flückiger, Gerger, Wampold, and Barth (2012) conducted a meta-analysis that was restricted to treatments in which differences among them were thought to be minimal, namely trauma-focused psychotherapies for PTSD. In their meta-analysis there were no differences between direct comparisons of trauma-focused treatments, and thus allegiance effects could not be attributed to an allegiance to superior treatments or other artifacts. Nevertheless, allegiance ratings explained 12 percent of the variability in outcomes, suggesting that allegiance effects are not the result of true differences between treatments.

Munder, Gerger, Trelle, and Barth (2011) sought to examine the methodological factors of studies that were responsible for allegiance bias. Results of this meta-analysis suggested that design quality moderated the effect of allegiance on outcome such that when the quality of the research design was low, the allegiance effect was larger. Where there was allegiance to one of the treatments, but the design quality was high, the effect of allegiance was small. Moreover, the conceptual quality of the treatments, which focused on the theoretical credibility of the treatment, mediated the allegiance-outcome relationship. In sum, these findings confirm that one way in which researcher allegiance influences outcomes is through the design of the study. Munder et al. did not find evidence that therapist allegiance or training and supervision were related to allegiance effects.

In an attempt to directly address therapist (rather than researcher) allegiance, Falkenström, Markowitz, Jonker, Philips, and Holmqvist (2013) examined studies in which therapists provided both treatments being compared (i.e., in crossed designs). Most studies did not control for therapist allegiance. In studies that did not control for therapist allegiance, stronger researcher allegiance strongly predicted better outcomes for the preferred treatment, whereas when therapist allegiance was controlled in the study, researcher allegiance had no effect on outcome. This result suggests that therapist allegiance is an important factor in psychotherapy and explains, at least in these controlled studies, researcher allegiance effects. As well, Falkenström et al. found that CBT researchers controlled for therapist allegiance less than researchers of other theoretical orientations.

Conclusions Related to Allegiance

Meta-analyses that have investigated allegiance generally have found allegiance effects, with a few exceptions (e.g., Gaffan et al. 1995). The magnitude of allegiance effects ranged up to 0.65—a large effect compared to other sources of variability in response to psychotherapy outcome.

There are two conclusions about allegiance that are important. First, the Contextual Model predicts that allegiance, particularly therapist allegiance, would be an important factor in producing the benefits of psychotherapy. Although the evidence for researcher allegiance is fairly robust, the support for therapist allegiance is less so. Therapist allegiance is difficult to study. In naturalistic settings, for the most part, therapists provide the therapy that they believe in, so there is no natural variability in researcher allegiance. In clinical trials, therapist allegiance has never been manipulated directly but occurs only as a deficit in the design of the study, which brings up the second conclusion. When interpreting clinical trials, attention must always be paid to researcher allegiance, as well as therapist allegiance.

Evidence Related to Relative Efficacy

Pre-Meta-Analysis: Chaos Revisited

As has been mentioned several times, in 1936 Rosenzweig commented on the general equivalence of the various psychotherapeutic approaches. However, at the time, psychotherapy was predominantly psychodynamic. When behavior therapy came into existence, there was a concerted effort by advocates of this approach to show its superiority relative to (presumably psychodynamic) "psychotherapy." In 1961, when Eysenck reviewed studies on the efficacy of psychotherapy, he also addressed the relative efficacy issue. In previous chapters, it was noted that he came to the conclusion that there was no evidence to support the efficacy of psychotherapy. However, based on uncontrolled studies by Wolpe (1952a, 1952b, 1954, 1958), Phillips (1957), and Ellis (1957), Eysenck concluded that "neurotic patients treated by means of psychotherapeutic procedures based on *learning theory*, improve significantly more quickly than do patients treated by means of psychoanalytic or eclectic psychotherapy, or not treated by psychotherapy at all" (emphasis added, p. 720). Based on this evidence, Eysenck was quick to suggest that the specific ingredients of learning theory-based treatments were responsible for the superior outcomes:

> It would appear advisable, therefore, to discard the psychoanalytic model, which both on theoretical and practical plain fails to be useful in mediating verifiable predictions, and to adopt, provisionally at least, the learning theory model which, to date, appears to be much more promising theoretically and also with regard to application.
>
> (p. 721)

Interestingly, all three instances cited by Eysenck involved studies conducted by proponents of the method, which raises issues of allegiance. Moreover, each of these treatments involved dubious applications of learning theory.[3] Eysenck's claims are interesting because they represent an early attempt to show that a specific approach (viz., behavior therapy) is more scientifically defensible than other therapies and that the benefits of such therapies are due to the specific ingredients described in the theory.

About the same time Eysenck (1961) published his treatise on the superiority of learning-theory treatments, Meltzoff and Kornreich (1970) also reviewed the research on the relative efficacy of various types of psychotherapy. Essentially, they had available the same literature as did Eysenck, yet came to a very different conclusion:

> To summarize the present state of our knowledge, there is hardly any evidence that one traditional school of psychotherapy yields a better outcome than another. In fact, the question has hardly been put to a fair test. The whole issue remains at the level of polemic, professional public opinion, and whatever weight that can be brought to bear by authoritative presentation of illustrative cases. People may come out of different treatments with varied and identifiable philosophies of life or approaches to solving life's problems, but there is no current evidence that one traditional method is more successful than another in modifying psychopathology, alleviating symptoms, or improving general adjustment.
>
> (p. 200)

The early history of research summaries of relative efficacy mirrors that of absolute efficacy in that conclusions were idiosyncratic and influenced by the reviewers' preconceived notions.

In 1975, Luborsky, Singer, and Luborsky sought to conduct a comprehensive review of studies directly comparing different types of psychotherapy to address the relative efficacy question. Having realized the difficulty in locating and evaluating studies in past reviews, they commented that it was "not surprising that some previous reviewers have presented biased conclusions about the verdict of this research literature on the relative value of certain forms of psychotherapy" (p. 1000). Therefore, they systematically retrieved and evaluated studies. By reviewing only direct comparisons, they were able to rule out confounds mentioned earlier in this chapter. However, meta-analytic procedures were unavailable to Luborsky et al. and they had to resort to box scores (counting the number of significant results). Of 11 well-controlled studies comparing various traditional therapies (i.e., non-behavioral), only 4 contained any significant differences. Only client-centered therapy had a sufficient number of studies to examine relative efficacy of classes of traditional therapies; client-centered therapy was not significantly different from other traditional psychotherapies in four of five cases and the remaining one favored another traditional therapy. There were 19 studies that compared behavior therapy to psychotherapy and 13 found no differences. The remaining 6 favored behavior therapy, but five of the six received very low ratings for research quality. Luborsky et al. concluded, *"Most comparative studies of different forms of psychotherapy found insignificant differences in proportions of patients who improved by the end of psychotherapy"* (p. 1003) although "behavior therapy may be especially suited for treatment of circumscribed phobias" (p. 1004). Here we see a claim that has persisted in the psychotherapy literature to this day (even from staunch advocates of common factors theory, e.g., Frank & Frank, 1991)—namely that psychotherapies are generally equivalent, but that behavioral treatments (and now cognitive behavioral treatments) are clearly preferable for several anxiety disorders, including phobias, obsessive-compulsive disorder, and panic disorder. We will review the evidence regarding the relative efficacy of psychotherapies for these disorders later in this chapter.

Generally, we have seen that the early reviews of outcome research diverged in terms of their conclusions, with advocates of behavior therapy finding evidence that traditional psychotherapy was not efficacious, whereas behavior therapy was. On the other hand, other reviewers, having access to the same studies, came to the conclusions that traditional psychotherapy was just as efficacious. Toward the end of the pre-meta-analytic period, more rigorous reviews of controlled studies tended to find equivalence of outcomes for the various psychotherapies. As well, the best controlled and most rigorous comparative outcome study found few differences between traditional psychotherapy and behavior therapy (see Sloane, Staples, Cristol, Yorkston, & Whipple, 1975 for an early example of a well-controlled comparison of psychodynamic and behavioral treatment approaches). Nevertheless, the status of relative efficacy could not be examined critically until meta-analysis.

General Meta-Analyses: Order Restored

There are numerous meta-analyses that have addressed the question of relative efficacy, with each attempting to correct some problems of previous attempts and including current studies. We refer the reader to the first edition of this text for detailed information on early meta-analyses and focus mostly on meta-analyses published in the last 20 years.[4] Because the evidence continues to be debated in the psychotherapy research community (e.g., Crits-Christoph, 1997; Ehlers et al., 2010; Hofmann & Lohr, 2010; Howard, Krause, Saunders, & Kopta, 1997; Siev & Chambless, 2007; Wilson, 1982), the results of these meta-analyses will be presented in some detail, examining meta-analyses in specific diagnostic areas, criticisms, and prominent studies when useful.

Wampold et al. (1997b) sought to address primary methodological issues present in early meta-analyses by restricting the meta-analysis to studies that directly compared treatments and avoiding classification of treatments into therapy types. Classifying treatments into categories tests the hypothesis that there are no differences among therapy categories, whereas the Wampold et al. (1997b) meta-analysis tested the hypothesis that the difference among all comparisons of treatments is zero. Besides testing the more general Dodo bird conjecture, this strategy avoided several problems encountered by earlier meta-analyses that involved pairwise comparisons of treatment categories. First, in previous meta-analyses there were many pairwise comparisons of treatment categories that contain few or no studies (see Bisson et al. 2007 for a more recent example—indeed some pairwise comparisons are simply estimates from a single primary study). Second, classification of treatments is not as straight-forward as one would believe (see Baardseth et al., 2013). Third, comparison of treatment types eliminates from consideration all comparisons within treatment types, of which there are many and of which many were designed to test the efficacy of specific ingredients. Finally, and importantly, pairwise comparisons of treatment types obviates an omnibus test of the Dodo bird conjecture (are their any differences between all compared treatments?).

Wampold et al. (1997b) included all studies from 1970 to 1995 in six journals that typically publish psychotherapy outcomes research that directly compared two or more treatments intended to be therapeutic. Treatments were restricted to those that were intended to be therapeutic (i.e., bona fide), so that treatments that were intended as control groups (pseudo-placebos), or were not credible to therapists were excluded. This restriction is important because the Contextual Model of psychotherapy stipulates that the efficacy of a treatment depends on therapist and client believing that the treatment is intended to be therapeutic. A treatment was determined to be bona fide provided a) the therapist had at least a master's degree, developed a thera-peutic relationship with the client, and tailored the treatment to the client; b) the problem treated was representative of problems characteristic of cli-ents, although severity was not considered (i.e., the diagnosis did not have to meet DSM criteria); and c) the treatment satisfied two of the following four conditions: citation to an established treatment (e.g., a reference to Rog-ers, 1951a, client-centered therapy), a description of the treatment was pre-sented and contained reference to psychological mechanisms (e.g., operant conditioning), a manual was used to guide administration of the treatment, or the active ingredients of the treatment were specified and referenced. The retrieval strategy used resulted in 277 comparisons of psychotherapies that were intended to be therapeutic.

The primary focus of this meta-analysis was on the null hypothesis that the true differences among treatments intended to be therapeutic was zero. Two other hypotheses related to the Dodo bird conjecture were tested. Stiles et al. (1986) speculated that improving research methods, such as more sensitive outcome measures and manualized treatments, would detect true differences among treatments that had been obscured in the past. To test this hypothesis, Wampold et al. (1997b) determined whether more recent studies, which presumably used better research methods, produced larger differences than did older studies. The second hypothesis was related to classification of studies. If specific ingredients were causal to treatment efficacy, treatments within categories, such as cognitive-behavioral treatments, which contain similar ingredients, would produce relatively small differences, whereas treatments from different categories (cognitive behavioral and psychodynamic), which contain very different ingredients, would produce relatively large differences. Wampold et al. tested this hypothesis by relating treatment similarity to the size of treatment differences. If the Dodo bird conjecture is false (i.e., treatments differ in their efficacy), comparison of relatively dissimilar treatments would produce larger differences than comparisons of relatively similar treatments. On the other hand, if the Dodo bird conjecture is true, then treatment similarity would be irrelevant.

Avoiding classification of treatments into categories created a methodological problem. In previous meta-analyses of comparative outcomes studies, treatments were classified into categories and then one category was (arbitrarily) classified as primary so that the algebraic sign of the effect size could be determined. For example, in most meta-analyses a particular treatment is classified as primary so that a positive effect size indicated that a given treatment (e.g., cognitive therapy) is superior to an alternative. Wampold et al. (1997b), however, had to assign an algebraic sign to each comparison of treatments (i.e., for each primary study). There are two options, both of which were used. First, a positive sign could be assigned so that each comparison yielded a positive effect size. However, this strategy would overestimate the aggregated effect size; nevertheless, the aggregate of the positively signed effects provides an upper bound estimate for the difference in outcomes of bona fide treatments. The second option, which is to randomly assign the algebraic sign to the effect size for individual comparisons, creates a situation in which the aggregate effect size would be zero, as the "plus" and "minus" signed effects would cancel each other out. However, if there are true differences among treatments (i.e., the Dodo bird conjecture is false and specific ingredients are producing effects in some treatments), then comparisons should produce many large effects, creating thick tails in the distribution of effects whose signs have been randomly determined, as shown in Figure 5.2. On the other hand, if there are truly *no* differences among treatments (i.e., the

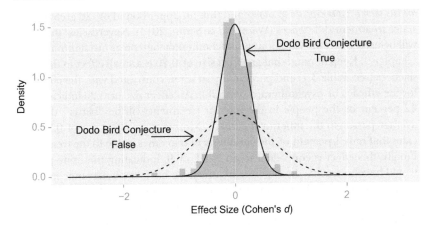

Figure 5.2 A distribution of effect sizes (with signs determined randomly) when the Dodo bird conjecture is true and when it is false. Histogram is of effect sizes from Wampold et al. meta-analysis. Adapted from "A meta-analysis of outcome studies comparing bona fide psychotherapies: Empirically, 'all must have prizes,'" by B. E. Wampold, G. W. Mondin, M. Moody, F. Stich, K. Benson, and H. Ahn, 1997b, *Psychological Bulletin, 122,* p. 206. Copyright 1997 by the American Psychological Association. Adapted with permission.

Dodo bird conjecture is true), then most of the effect sizes will be near zero and those further out in the tails of the distribution would amount to what would be expected by chance. Wampold et al.'s meta-analysis tested whether or not the effects were homogeneously distributed around zero, as would be expected if the Dodo bird conjecture were true, as illustrated by the actual distribution of effect sizes displayed in Figure 5.2. As it turns out, a statistical analysis of the method used in this meta-analysis revealed that the test used by Wampold et al. performs very well (i.e., has desired statistical properties); that it is unnecessary to randomly assign the "pluses" and "minuses" and that the expected value under the null hypothesis is known (Wampold & Serlin, 2014).

The evidence produced by the Wampold et al. (1997b) meta-analysis was consistent, in every respect, with the Dodo bird conjecture. First, the effects were homogeneously distributed about zero. That is, the preponderance of effects were near zero and the frequency of larger effects was consistent with what would be produced by chance, given the sampling distribution of effect sizes (see Figure 5.2). Second, even when positive signs were attached to each comparison, the aggregated effect size was roughly equal to .20,[5] which is a small effect (see Table 3.1 and below). It is important to note that even when the null hypothesis is true, there will be studies in the tails of the distribution due to random errors. Indeed, as discussed previously, an alpha set at .05 will yield 5 significant results for every 100 studies when there are absolutely no differences among treatments. It turns out that the absolute values of the effects *are less than what is expected by chance* and thus an upper bound of .20 greatly overstates treatment differences (Wampold & Serlin, 2014). Nevertheless this effect will be used when the variations in psychotherapy outcomes are summarized in Chapter 9. Keep in mind that an effect size of 0.20 is a small effect in the social sciences (see Table 3.1) and particularly so when contrasted with the effect size for the efficacy of psychotherapy (viz., .80). An effect size of 0.20 indicates that 42 percent of the people in the inferior treatment will be "better" than the average person in the superior treatment. Moreover, an effect size of 0.20 indicates that only 1 percent of the variability in outcomes is due to the treatments. Finally, this effect is equivalent to an NNT of 9, indicating that nine patients would have to receive the superior treatment to have one better outcome than if they had received the inferior treatment. The point here is that even the most liberal estimate of differences among treatments is very small.

Wampold et al. (1997b) found no evidence that the differences in outcome among treatments was related to either year in which the study was published or the similarity of the treatments. The lack of relation between year and effect size indicates that improving research methods are not increasingly detecting differences among treatments. It does not appear that comparisons of treatments that were quite different produce larger effects than comparisons of treatments that were similar to each other, a result consistent with the Dodo bird conjecture. The most comprehensive meta-analysis at the turn of the century (viz., Wampold et al., 1997b) produced evidence that was entirely consistent with the Dodo bird conjecture of uniform efficacy.

Meta-Analyses in Specific Areas

The possibility that there exists a subset of studies that show non-zero differences among treatments was discussed above. In particular, it may be that comparing the relative efficacy of specific treatments without respect to disorder is like comparing the efficacy of Tylenol and the antibiotic azithromycin without knowing if the patient has a minor common cold or a more serious bacterial infection. Despite the fact that the studies reviewed by Wampold et al. (1997b) involved treatments for a particular problem or disorder, the criticism suggests that analyses of particular disorders is needed. In the remainder of the chapter, meta-analyses and select primary studies are reviewed that test relative efficacy for particular disorders, including a) depression, b) PTSD and other anxiety disorders, and c) substance use disorders. Of course there are many other disorders that could be examined, but the debate about the importance of specific ingredients is most heated, and most researched, in these areas. Moreover, review of these meta-analyses will demonstrate issues related to a) confounding due to variables such as allegiance, b) lack of direct comparisons, and c) classification and multiple comparisons. As we will see, many claims have been made that one treatment, typically specific cognitive-behavioral treatments, is superior to all other, or some other, treatment.

Depression

Research on psychotherapy for depression is perhaps the most developed of all the major psychiatric disorders. In a recent meta-analysis described later in this section, Barth et al. (2013) presented a useful visualization of the currently published direct comparisons of different classes of psychotherapy for depression (see Figure 5.3). The size of the "node" represents the number of patients enrolled in direct comparison trials of that category and the width of the line between categories of treatments represents the number of times the categories have been directly compared. As can be seen, CBT is by far the most tested treatment, which is not surprising because it has been the established therapy for depression since 1979.

It is also clear from this figure that the majority of comparisons are to wait-list controls. The most common comparisons that involve some intervention include "usual care" and "supportive therapy," which are both treatment conditions that do not typically meet the definition of a bona fide psychotherapy utilized in this book. Thus, the question is, in a fair test between cognitive therapy and another bona fide therapy for depression, delivered by advocates of the respective therapies (i.e., controlling allegiance), would cognitive therapy be superior?

Before turning to meta-analyses, we return to the seminal NIMH Treatment of Depression Collaborative Research Program (NIMH TDCRP; Elkin, 1994). It was the first attempt in psychotherapy to conduct the analog of the collaborative clinical trial used in medical studies and deserves full consideration as it has inspired a generation of psychotherapy clinical trials.

The NIMH TDCRP compared four treatments for depression: CBT, interpersonal psychotherapy (IPT), an antidepressant medication (viz., imipramine) plus clinical management, and pill-placebo plus clinical management. The contrast between CBT and IPT provided a good test of the relative efficacy of CBT, the standard psychotherapy for depression at the time, to another treatment. CBT was conducted according to the manual generally used for this treatment (Beck, Rush, Shaw, & Emery, 1979) and thus represents the prototypic cognitive therapy for depression. IPT, which is based on assisting the client to gain understanding of his or her interpersonal problems and to develop adaptive strategies for relating to others, was conducted according to the manual developed by Klerman, Weissman, Rounsaville, and Chevron (1984). IPT, originally developed as a control intervention for drug trials, is a derivative of dynamic therapy and in various meta-analyses might be classified as a "verbal therapy," "dynamic therapy," or "other psychotherapy," depending on the type of classification scheme used, although recently IPT is sometimes considered a distinct category. The specific ingredients of the two therapies were distinctive and readily discriminated (Hill, O'Grady, & Elkin, 1992).

The treatments were delivered at three sites (hence the classification as a *collaborative* study), thereby decreasing the possibility that the results were due to

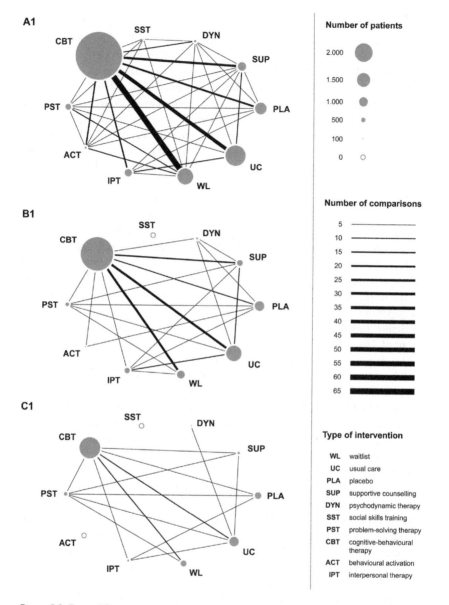

Figure 5.3 From "Comparative efficacy of seven psychotherapeutic interventions for patients with depression: A network meta-analysis," by J. Barth, T. Munder, H. Gerger, E. Nuesch, and S. Trelle, 2013, *PLoS Med, 10(5)*, p. 12. Copyright Barth et al.

idiosyncrasies of a particular site. The therapists, eight in CBT and ten in IPT, were experienced in their respective treatments, resulting in a design in which therapists are nested within treatments (see Chapter 6). Moreover, therapists were trained and supervised by experts in the respective treatments. Finally, therapists adhered to the respective treatments. Given these therapist design aspects, it would appear that allegiance effects were well controlled.

The results for three overlapping samples of clients are considered here. Of 239 clients who entered treatment, 204 received an "adequate dose" of treatment (defined as staying in treatment for at least 3.5 weeks) and 84 clients the complete treatment (e.g., "completers"). The relatively large number of clients provided good estimates of the relative efficacy of CBT and IPT. All clients met diagnostic criteria for a current episode of major depressive disorder. Outcome relative to depression was assessed with four measures: the Hamilton Rating Scale for Depression, the Global Assessment Scale, the Beck Depression Inventory, and the Hopkins Symptom Checklist-90 Total Score.

The results of this prototypic trial were quite clear. Despite the large samples (i.e., sufficient power to detect an effect should it be present), none of the differences between the treatments approached significance for any of the samples. Examining the effect sizes for this study can make a poignant point about relative efficacy. The aggregate effect size for the completers favored IPT by 0.13 standard deviation units; for individual variables the effect sizes ranged in magnitude from 0.02 to 0.29 (see Figure 5.4). These effect sizes translated into small and non-significant differences in recovery rates favoring IPT, a difference that was eliminated if therapist effects are taken into account (Kim, Wampold, & Bolt, 2006). In Chapter 6 it will be shown that although the effects due to relative efficacy are small, they are inflated by therapist differences—that is, true treatment differences are even smaller than they appear.

Although there were criticisms of the NIMH TDCRP (e.g., Elkin et al., 1989; Elkin, Gibbons, Shea, & Shaw, 1996; Jacobson & Hollon, 1996a, b; Klein, 1996), it is among the most comprehensive clinical trials ever conducted and one that provided a fair and valid test of relative efficacy of a cognitive therapy and a verbal, dynamic therapy for depression.

Of course, any individual study can be flawed, thus we turn our focus to meta-analyses of treatments for depression. In general, when controlling for allegiance, meta-analyses of depression treatment are consistent with the TDCRP, revealing no differences among treatments. Dobson (1989) found evidence for the superiority of cognitive therapy vis-à-vis other treatments. However, this study relied on the Beck Depression Inventory (BDI; Beck, Ward, Mendelson, & Erbaugh, 1961), a measure that consistently favors a cognitive approach[6] and did not control for researcher allegiance. Robinson, Berman, and Neimeyer (1990) analyzed 58 controlled studies that compared treatments Robinson et al. classified as a) cognitive, b) behavioral, c) cognitive behavioral, or d) general verbal therapy. The latter category was a collection of

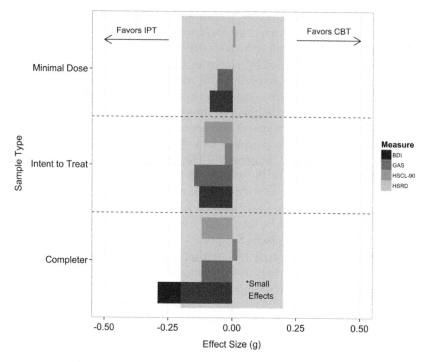

Figure 5.4 Comparison of cognitive-behavioral treatment and interpersonal psychotherapy for depression—NIMH Treatment of Depression Collaborative Research Program.

Note. HRSD, Hamilton Rating Scale for Depression; GAS, Global Assessment Scale; BDI, Beck Depression Inventory; HSCL-90 Hopkins Symptom Checklist-90 Total Scores; IPT, Interpersonal Therapy; CBT, Cognitive Behavioral Therapy.

Adapted from "National institute of mental health treatment of depression collaborative research program: General effectiveness of treatments," by I. Elkin, T. Shea, J. T. Watkins, S. D. Imber, S. M. Sotsky, J. F. Collins, . . . M. B. Parloff, 1989, *Archives of General Psychiatry, 46,* p. 975.

psychodynamic, client-centered, and interpersonal therapies. When allegiance was controlled, differences between treatments disappeared.

In an update of the Dobson meta-analysis, Gaffan, Tsaousis, and Kemp-Wheeler (1995) reanalyzed the studies reviewed by Dobson (1989) and 35 additional studies published before 1995. All studies compared cognitive therapy for depression to another treatment. Generally, these comparisons yielded small effects (magnitudes in the range of 0.03 to 0.34) and non-significant differences (only one of the six effect sizes was statistically significant).

The one statistically significant comparison was between cognitive therapy and "other psychotherapies" and needs further scrutiny. The superiority of specific treatments over those classified as "other" will appear again in meta-analyses of depression and treatments for other disorders. As an initial example, consider some of the 12 comparison therapies classified as "other psychotherapies." One psychotherapy was pastoral counseling, which was described as follows:

> Each session [included] approximately 75% of the time spent in nondirective listening and 25% of the time spent in discussing bible verses or religious themes that might relate to the patients' concerns. Parallel to the CBT treatments, homework was assigned. In the [pastoral counseling], however, this consisted of merely making a list of concerns to be discussed in the subsequent session.
>
> (Propst, Ostrom, Watkins, Dean, & Mashburn, 1992, p. 96)

One of the essential features of the Contextual Model is that treatments are intended to be therapeutic and that they be based on psychological principles, as stipulated in the definition of psychotherapy given in Chapter 2. The above treatment is not based on psychological principles and would not be considered a treatment intended to be therapeutic. Another treatment in this class was supportive, self-directed therapy, which was provided over the telephone by non-experts, and involved bibliotherapy and therapists' comments were restricted to "reflection of feelings, clarifications, and information seeking" (Beutler & Clarkin, 1990, p. 335). This therapy does not fit the definition of psychotherapy used in this book because there were no face-to-face interactions, the therapists were not trained, and the treatment was not based on psychological principles.[7] A third therapy classified as "other psychotherapy" was an exercise group. The point here is simple: it is meaningless to claim that the cognitive therapy is a superior form of psychotherapy by showing that it is superior to pastoral counseling, supportive, self directive therapy, exercise, or other treatments that plainly are not psychotherapy. Care must be exercised here because, as a general rule in this book, deleting studies from a meta-analysis because they don't support a position is discouraged. Nevertheless, comparisons of treatments intended to be therapeutic (e.g., cognitive therapy) to treatments that are not intended to be therapeutic and do not fit the definition of psychotherapy, particularly when the study is conducted by advocates of the former, cannot be used to test the relative efficacy of psychotherapies.

A meta-analysis of cognitive therapy for depression by Gloaguen, Cottraux, Cucherat, and Blackburn (1998) is noteworthy because it used the state-of-the-art meta-analytic procedures developed by Hedges and Olkin (1985, see also Chapter 3). Gloaguen et al. reviewed all controlled clinical trials published from 1977 to 1996 that involved comparisons of cognitive therapy for the treatment of depression to other types of treatments for depression. All 48 studies met the inclusion criteria and used the BDI to standardize the comparisons, and to avoid non-independent effect sizes, evaluation of outcome was restricted to this measure of depression. Moreover, effect sizes were computed from direct comparisons, eliminating many confounds. Effect sizes were adjusted for bias, aggregation was accomplished by weighting by the inverse of the estimated variance, and homogeneity of effect sizes was determined (see Hedges and Olkin, 1985; see Chapter 3). When compared to behavior therapies, the aggregate effect size was 0.05, which was not statistically significant. The 13 effect sizes derived from these comparison were homogenous, indicating a consistency that provides confidence in the conclusion that cognitive and behavior therapies of depression are equally effective, as there do not appear to be any moderating influences. However, cognitive therapy did appear to be superior to the class of "other therapies" (aggregate effect size for the 22 such comparisons was 0.24, which was significantly different from zero, $p < 0.01$) but still small (see Chapter 3, Table 3.1). However, the effect sizes were heterogeneous, indicating that there was a moderating variable or variables affecting the results.

Similar to Gaffan et al., the "other therapies" in the Gloaguen et al. (1998) meta-analysis contained therapies that were not intended to be therapeutic (e.g., supportive counseling, phone counseling) as well as therapies that were intended to be therapeutic. Wampold, Minami, Baskin, and Tierney (2002) hypothesized that the heterogeneity of the CT/"other therapies" contrast was due to the fact that "other therapies" contained treatments intended to be therapeutic (i.e., bona fide therapies) and those not intended to be therapeutic (i.e., not bona fide). They predicted that when CT was compared to bona fide "other" therapies, the effect size would be zero, consistent with the Dodo bird conjecture. Indeed, when CT was compared to bona fide "verbal therapies," the null hypothesis that the effect size was zero could not be rejected; when an outlier was eliminated, the aggregate effect size for this comparison was negligible (viz., 0.03). As expected, CT was superior to treatments that were not bona fide (i.e., were essentially control groups). The results of the Gloagen et al. results and the Wampold et al. reanalysis demonstrate that psychotherapies for depression that are intended to be therapeutic are uniformly efficacious.

The general pattern of no differences between cognitive behavioral and "other therapies" has been replicated in subsequent meta-analyses (Cuijpers, van Straten, Andersson, & van Oppen, 2008a; Cuijpers, van Straten, Warmerdam, & Andersson, 2008b; Spielmans, Pasek, & McFall, 2007). However, in an update of the CBT vs. "other therapies" debate, Tolin (2010) conducted a meta-analysis of 26 studies that compared CT to other bona fide therapies. He reported that in general CBT was superior to psychodynamic therapy ($d = 0.28$), although not interpersonal or supportive therapies, at post-treatment and at follow-up. They also found that CBT was only superior to other therapies for depression on targeted measures, although the effect size was small ($d = 0.21$).

The Tolin (2010) depression result brings up an important issue about classes of variables. Typically clinical trials, particularly trials of focused treatments, such as CBT, emphasize effects on symptom-specific measures, often called targeted variables. However, these trials also have an array of non-targeted measures, such as measures of related symptoms (e.g., depression measures for an anxiety study), quality of life measures, and so forth. Meta-analyses that focus exclusively on targeted symptoms, as we have alluded to earlier, advantage focused treatments. Clients rarely come to psychotherapy simply to remove the symptoms of a specific disorder. Some treatments, such as psychodynamic treatments, conceptualize therapeutic change more broadly:

> The goals of psychodynamic therapy include, but extend beyond, alleviation of acute symptoms. Psychological health is not merely the absence of symptoms; it is the positive presence of inner capacities and resources that allow people to live life with a greater sense of freedom and possibility.
>
> (Shedler, 2010, p. 105)

A propos of this concern, Baardseth et al. (2013) examined the depression studies in Tolin (2010) to estimate the effect for non-targeted variables and found that CBT was not superior to other treatments for depression on non-targeted variables ($d = .03$).

Finally, two recent meta-analyses used standard as well as "network" meta-analytic techniques to examine relative efficacy. Network meta-analysis is a relatively new statistical approach that relies on Bayesian methods to simulate the direct comparison of treatments that were not actually compared in the same study, potentially offering more powerful tests of the extant literature (see Del Re et al., 2013 for potential problems with this approach). Essentially, if a CBT is tested directly against Acceptance and Commitment Therapy (ACT) and Interpersonal Therapy (IPT) is compared with a CBT, that information can be used to simulate a direct comparison of ACT and Interpersonal Therapy. Braun, Gregor, and Tran (2013) examined the outcomes of 53 studies (3,965 patients) that directly compared two or more bona fide psychotherapies for major depressive disorder. Barth et al. (2013) conducted a larger meta-analysis that included 198 studies, including 15,118 patients that included both bona fide and non-bona fide treatments, waitlists, and usual care comparisons. Across both analytic approaches, results were broadly consistent with prior work on the comparative efficacy of bona fide psychotherapies for depression: generally no differences among treatments were detected. However, there were several specific treatment effects that warrant further examination.

Using the network meta-analytic approach, Barth et al. (2013) found a small but significant difference between interpersonal therapy and supportive therapy (there were no significant differences among these two treatments in the standard meta-analysis). In addition, Braun, Gregor, and Tran (2013) conducted 31 separate meta-analyses of direct comparisons of a given treatment category to all other categories (using standard meta-analytic procedures) across patient reported outcomes, clinician reported outcomes, and clinically significant change. There were four small but significant effects suggesting supportive therapy was less effective than other therapies (out of eight meta-analyses involving supportive therapy). However, when meta-analyses were restricted to pairs of treatments with at least five direct comparisons, there were no differences among treatments.

At first glance, these meta-analyses are consistent with the now all well-established finding that active or bona fide treatments are generally equivalent, while interventions designed as controls—supportive therapy being the most common example—are generally less effective. However, the Braun et al. analysis was purportedly restricted to only treatments that were bona fide—that is, the supportive therapies supposedly met the criteria laid out in Wampold et al. (1997b). In addition there was no effect of researcher allegiance on any effects observed in the Barth et al. meta-analysis. Upon closer inspection, it appears that some of the treatments might meet the *letter* of the bona fide criteria (citation to an established approach), but most were clearly intended to be controls. Many of the treatment descriptions were no more than two sentences (e.g., Milgrom et al., 2005) and some actually included the word control in the treatment name (i.e., "High-demand Control," McNamara & Horan, 1986). Moreover, most of the studies were designed by researchers interested in evaluating the treatment compared to the "supportive therapy," creating little variability in allegiance. Given this lack of variability, it is not surprising that allegiance did not account for variability in effects. Indeed, supportive therapies had dubious theoretical rationales that are presented to clients and almost all had no therapeutic actions, other than empathic responding, and thus were pseudo-placebos—lacking some of the elements proposed in the Contextual Model. What is quite remarkable from a theoretical perspective is that these treatments were almost as effective as treatments that are designed to be therapeutic and are tested by advocates of these treatments.

Given all of the evidence related to various treatments, it appears that the most appropriate conclusion remains that no psychotherapy consistently outperforms any other bona fide psychotherapy in the treatment of depression. The meta-analyses reviewed above indicate that generally cognitive therapies do not produce statistically different outcomes from other therapies, although in some cases the null results appeared only after allegiance was controlled. The most perspicuous difference appears to be between cognitive therapy and verbal or "other" therapies, although as was pointed out, the therapies often contain treatments that do not fit the definition of psychotherapy (e.g., are not intended to be therapeutic or are clearly not psychotherapies at all). However, the therapies that are intended to be therapeutic appear to be equally efficacious as cognitive therapy, the generally accepted standard. Indeed, the Society of Clinical Psychology lists psychological treatments that have strong or modest research support, using the criteria for empirically supported treatments (see Chapter 4), which now include Behavior Therapy/Behavioral Activation (strong research support), Cognitive Therapy (strong research support), Cognitive Behavioral Analysis System of Psychotherapy (strong research support), Interpersonal Therapy (strong research support), Problem-Solving Therapy (strong research support), Self-Management/Self-Control Therapy (strong research support), Acceptance and Commitment Therapy (modest research support), Behavioral Couple Therapy (modest research support), Emotionally-Focused Therapy (modest research support), Rational Emotive Behavioral Therapy (modest research support), Reminiscence/Life Review Therapy (modest research support), Self-System Therapy (modest research support), and Short-Term Psychodynamic Therapy (modest research support) (see http://www.div12.org/PsychologicalTreatments/disorders/depression_main.php). Clearly, many treatments with a variety of therapeutic ingredients are efficacious for the treatment of depression.

PTSD and Other Anxiety Disorders

Since the demonstration that fear reactions in animals and humans could be induced experimentally (see Chapter 1), behavioral therapists have contented that various techniques imbedded in the classical conditioning paradigm would be effective in the treatment of anxiety disorders. The most perspicuous therapeutic ingredient thought to lead to the reduction of anxiety is exposure to the feared stimulus. Although there are many variations of exposure techniques, exposure is a central component of behavioral treatments of anxiety disorders (e.g., obsessive compulsive disorder, panic disorder, social anxiety, PTSD).[8] However, cognitive treatments also have been developed and tested; these treatments are based on the notion that the cognitive appraisal of the feared stimuli is critical and that altering such appraisals is therapeutic. Cognitive-behavioral treatments combine techniques for altering cognitions with some behavioral techniques. Not surprisingly, outcome studies in this area have focused primarily on behavioral, cognitive, and cognitive-behavioral techniques = hypotheses regarding the relative efficacy of various CBTs in comparison to non-cognitive/non-behavioral treatments have only been tested more recently.

Because behavioral and cognitive perspectives rely on distinct theoretical models, evidence on the relative efficacy of outcomes will be informative about specific effects. Moreover, claims for the superiority of cognitive-behavioral treatments for specific anxiety disorders are perhaps the most persistent and frequent claim made in the area of specificity. Even those who concede that differences between treatments for most disorders are likely small maintain that cognitive-behavioral treatments are superior to alternatives for many anxiety disorders (Frank & Frank, 1991; Lilienfield, 2007). Thus, the relative efficacy of treatments for specific anxiety disorders appear to be central to the durability of the Medical Model in psychotherapy and should be examined in detail.

The standard view in the treatment of PTSD with psychotherapy is that specific trauma-focused treatments that contain repeated exposure to the traumatic memories and related circumstances (i.e., some form of in vivo and/or imaginal exposure) are required to achieve the best results (National Collaborating Centre for Mental Health, 2005; Surgeon General, 1999). While the vast majority of treatments developed and tested for PTSD include some focus on traumatic experience, debates regarding the relative efficacy of these treatments still mirror the literature in the area of depression. Specifically, there is generally little evidence to suggest that any specific bona fide treatment is more effective than any other treatment. Differences between treatments only emerge when there is a comparison of specific treatments to the "other" category that we have described above—a category that typically contains a mix of treatments, some of which are bona fide and some that are not.

Cognitive therapies and exposure therapies often contain overlapping elements. For example, if in cognitive therapy, clients discuss the feared stimulus, then the clients are experiencing an imaginal representation of the event, which could be interpreted as imaginal exposure. To address this limitation, Tarrier et al. (1999) designed a clinical trial examining treatments for chronic post-traumatic stress disorder. Recognizing that cognitive therapy and exposure typically are confounded, Tarrier compared CT without any discussion of the trauma to an exposure treatment. Subjects were stratified on trauma category and randomly assigned to cognitive therapy without any exposure (CT) or imaginal exposure (IE). In this study, CT was "aimed to be emotion focused and to elicit patients' beliefs about the meaning of the event and the attributions patients made following it, taking into account their previous belief system, then to identify maladaptive cognitions and patterns of emotions and to modify these" (p. 14). Discussion of the trauma itself was avoided in order to distinguish the treatment from exposure. IE was "trauma focused and aimed to produce habituation of emotional response by instructing the patient to describe the event as if it was happening in the present tense while visualizing it" (p. 15). This study found that the patients' assessment of the credibility of the treatment and therapists' ratings of the motivation of the patients did not differ between the two treatments. Although patients generally improved from pre-test to post-test, the important result from a relative efficacy perspective is that there were no significant differences between the two treatments on any of the seven outcome measures. The results of this study failed to support that exposure was a necessary specific ingredient for improvement in the area of post-traumatic stress disorder. This study suggests that perhaps the specific ingredients of PTSD treatments are not the major factor in producing benefits, and we now turn to reviews of the PTSD literature.

In an early PTSD meta-analysis, Sherman (1998) examined all controlled studies of treatments of PTSD. The predominant treatments were behavioral and cognitive-behavioral but also included psychodynamic, hypnotherapy, the Koach program, anger management, eye movement desensitization and reprocessing (EMDR), adventure-based activities, psychodrama, and the Coatsville PTSD program. Effect sizes were calculated from treatment versus control contrasts and were derived from aggregating over the dependent variables in the individual studies and by aggregating within classes of dependent variables (viz., intrusion, avoidance, hyperarousal, anxiety, and depression). When one outlier, with an unrealistic effect size of 8.40, was eliminated, the remaining effect sizes derived from aggregating over all dependent variables within a study were found to be homogenous. The only target variable that showed heterogeneity was hyperarousal, a difference the authors attributed to the variety of methods used to assess this construct.

Bradley, Greene, Russ, Dutra, and Westen (2005), Bisson and Andrew (2009), and Bisson et al., (2007) found similar effect sizes for a variety of treatments including CBT, exposure plus cognitive therapy, and EMDR. However, supportive therapy controls produced smaller effects and "other therapies" did not different from waitlist or usual care. Note however, that all of the above findings are based on the comparison of effect sizes across studies, rather than on direct comparison of treatments in the same study, which is necessary to make more valid conclusions.

Several PTSD meta-analyses have used the direct comparison method, producing some contradictory findings. Davidson and Parker (2001) found no differences between direct comparisons of EMDR and exposure based treatments but the number of comparisons were few (see also Seidler & Wagner, 2006). Similarly, Bradley et al. (2005) found little evidence of differences among treatments in direct comparisons but noted that the number of treatments in specific categories was not sufficient to make strong conclusions. Both Bisson and Andrew (2009) and Bisson et al. (2007) generally found no differences between comparisons of different treatments but that a variety of treatments (e.g., trauma-focused CBT, EMDR) were superior to "other therapies" as well as stress management.

As noted in earlier sections of this chapter, the focus on direct comparisons of treatment categories limits direct tests of relative efficacy when the number of treatments compared is small (as is the case in PTSD and other anxiety disorders generally, see below). In 2008, Benish, Imel, and Wampold conducted a meta-analysis modeled on Wampold et al. (1997b) that only included bona fide interventions that were directly compared in the same study. The meta-analysis included 15 studies comparing bona fide treatments (17 direct comparisons; 958 patients), which included treatments as diverse as prolonged exposure, dynamic therapies, EMDR, present-centered therapy (PCT; see below for further detail), and CBT (with and without exposure), among others. Similar to Wampold et al. (1997b), the authors avoided treatment categorization and examined homogeneity around zero as a test of the null hypothesis that all treatments were equally efficacious. Consistent with Wampold et al. (1997b), effects were indeed homogenously distributed about zero, suggesting no differences between treatments that were directly compared. While the results and methods of this study have been harshly criticized by leading PTSD treatment researchers as only including "effective" treatments (Ehlers et al., 2010) in their meta-analysis, these critiques are based on a flawed understanding of how treatments are classified as bona fide or not (see Wampold et al., 2010). In addition, results are broadly consistent with more recent meta-analyses that indicate there is no difference between direct comparisons of exposure-based treatments and other active treatments (e.g., Powers et al., 2010).

There appears to be little evidence to suggest that one treatment for PTSD is superior to any other. However, there is additional evidence that creates a severe challenge to the Medical Model as applied to PTSD. As discussed above, one of the challenges to research in PTSD is to design treatments that do not contain particular therapeutic ingredients. As discussed above, Foa et al. (1991) developed a supportive counseling treatment that contained no exposure and no cognitive components, which was intended to be a control group for PE and which was clearly not a bona fide treatment. However, Schnurr et al. (2007) developed a treatment called Present-Centered Therapy (PCT; see also Frost, Laska, & Wampold, 2014) that would "provide a credible therapeutic alternative to control for nonspecific therapeutic factors so that observed effects of prolonged exposure could be attributed to its specific effects beyond the benefits of good therapy" (p. 823). However, as opposed to Foa et al, Schnurr et al. included therapeutic ingredients, including psychoeducation regarding the impact of trauma on the client's current life, a focus on altering present maladaptive relational patterns/behaviors, and the use of problem-solving strategies. PCT, however, remained a treatment without exposure (clients were redirected to solving current problems if they mentioned the trauma) or any actions that could be construed as cognitive restructuring or alteration of attributions about the trauma. That is, PCT purposefully did not contain the ingredients that were considered scientific (exposure, a processing of the trauma, or cognitive restructuring of any kind) but had a cogent rationale and therapeutic actions. Various manuals for PCT were developed, therapists were trained to deliver the treatment, and it took on the trappings of a legitimate treatment. Importantly, when PCT was compared to the most scientific evidence-based treatments in five clinical trials, a meta-analysis demonstrated that PCT was as effective as the evidence-based treatment to which it was compared for targeted and non-targeted variables (Frost et al., 2014). Indeed, the Society of Clinical Psychology now considers PCT as a psychological treatment for PTSD with strong research support (see http://www.div12.org/PsychologicalTreatments/disorders/ptsd_main.php). The case of PCT is a disturbing finding for the Medical Model, which considers some particular ingredients necessary for the treatment of PTSD.

There is more disturbing evidence imbedded in treatments for PTSD. All of the meta-analyses discussed above that have examined the efficacy of EMDR have found it to be comparable to the best treatments for PTSD (see Seidler & Wagner, 2006). However, EMDR is based on questionable ingredients from a scientific perspective. It has been labeled as pseudoscience (e.g., Herbert et al., 2000) and compared to Mesmerism (McNally, 1999) by Medical Model adherents. Clinical scientists have been annoyed by unjustified claims of efficacy and efficiency and the way it is publicized and disseminated (see also Davidson & Parker, 2001; Rosen, 1999). Herbert et al. (2000) asserted that "the promotion of EMDR provides a good illustration of pseudoscience in general and of how pseudoscience is marketed to mental health clinicians, some of whom may be relatively unfamiliar with the published research on EMDR" (p. 955). Yet this purportedly pseudoscientific treatment is as effective as the "scientific" evidence-based treatments for PTSD.[9]

The evidence from PTSD clinical trials creates multiple issues from a Medical Model perspective, but is entirely consistent with the Contextual Model. It appears that treatments with a variety of ingredients are equally effective, including CBT without exposure, PCT, and EMDR.

We now turn to other anxiety disorders. A number of meta-analyses in the 1990s addressed the relative efficacy of cognitive and behavioral treatments of anxiety, as well as some other treatments (Abramowitz, 1996, 1997; Chambless & Gillis, 1993; Clum, Clum, & Surls, 1993; Mattick, Andrews, Hadzi-Pavlovic, & Christensen, 1990; Sherman, 1998; Taylor, 1996; van Balkom et al., 1994). Although claims that cognitive and behavioral treatments are superior to alternatives are pervasive, this research has not escaped the threats to validity that are apparent in the larger psychotherapy literature.

Before reviewing the results of the various meta-analyses, several limitations should be noted. First, many of the outcome studies of the early anxiety studies were uncontrolled (i.e., did not contain a control group), thus the effect sizes typically were calculated by comparing the post-test to the pre-test [i.e, (post-test mean—pre-test mean/standard deviation)]. Such effect sizes are inflated by regression toward the mean, as clients are selected because they are distressed (i.e., they score high on anxiety measures) and will tend to score closer to the mean on the post-test, in the absence of treatment (see Campbell & Kenny, 1999, for an excellent discussion of regression artifacts). More troublesome, however, is that only a minority of the meta-analyses examined direct comparisons of various treatments (e.g., Abramowitz, 1997; Clum et al., 1993; Ougrin, 2011), leaving the conclusions of the other meta-analyses suspect because of confounds. Moreover, none of the meta-analyses using indirect comparisons attempted to model allegiance. Another problem is that early meta-analyses did not take advantage of the statistical theory underlying the effect size statistics; no tests of homogeneity were conducted and tests of average effect sizes and differences among treatments were not based on the sampling distributions of the statistics. Consequently, results from these meta-analyses must be interpreted cautiously. Finally, it should be noted that primary studies of various treatments, particularly those that directly compare two bona fide psychological treatments, are sparse. For example, the Abramowitz meta-analysis (1997) examined direct comparisons of psychological treatment for obsessive-compulsive disorders, but was based on only six comparisons derived from five studies

The most recent meta-analyses for both panic and OCD found exposure-based treatments had large effects vs. waitlist and pseudo-placebos for behavioral and cognitive treatments but did not include meta-analyses of direct comparisons of bona fide treatments (Rosa-Alcázar, Sánchez-Meca, Gómez-Conesa, & Marín-Martínez, 2008; Sánchez-Meca, Rosa-Alcázar, Marín-Martínez, & Gómez-Conesa, 2010).

The authors also reported that exposure-based treatments had superior response to active controls and waitlists compared to effects from non-exposure-based treatments. However, there were only 3 (of 24) studies that compared non-exposure-based treatments to a control in OCD (Rosa-Alcázar et al.) and 13 (of 65) in the panic meta-analysis (Sánchez-Meca et al.). Note, however, one of the panic treatments categorized as "non-exposure based" that had a very small negative effect vs. control ($d = -0.01$) was exposure and systematic desensitization (Mavissakalian & Michelson, 1986). When this treatment is categorized as exposure, type of treatment (exposure vs. non-exposure) was not a moderator of treatment effects in either case (waitlist or active control).[10] Regardless, none of these tests of treatment effects were derived from direct comparisons of treatments in the same study and, therefore, the effect of between-study differences is unknown.[11]

Ougrin (2011) conducted a meta-analysis of direct comparisons of behavioral and cognitive approaches to treatment for specific anxiety disorders, including, OCD (five studies), panic (seven studies), PTSD (five studies), and social phobia (three studies). There were no significant differences for any disorder except social phobia, where cognitive therapy was superior to behavioral treatment, a finding which was based entirely on a meta-analysis of three studies where exposure-based treatments did very poorly relative to cognitive therapy (Clark et al. 2003; Clark et al. 2006). In Clark et al. 2006, the exposure protocol was labeled "self-exposure" wherein the patient received instructions from a therapist, but the therapist did not have an engaged relationship with the patient and did not assist with the exposure protocols, raising questions about whether this intervention meets the definition of psychotherapy. It clearly does not contain the therapeutic elements of the Contextual Model. Finally, in each Clark et al. study, behavioral experiments were included in the cognitive therapy while cognitive interventions were not allowed in the exposure-based interventions (see Siev & Chambless, 2007; Siev, Huppert, & Chambless, 2009; Wampold, Imel, & Miller, 2009, for a similar discussion in treatment of generalized anxiety disorder). Despite the general pattern of a lack of differences between behavioral and cognitive treatments for anxiety disorders, relative efficacy conclusions are limited by the relative similarity of these treatments in which many cognitive treatments include behavioral components and many of the behavioral treatments include cognitive interventions.

Some recent individual trials comparing CBT to other treatments have provided some limited evidence that CBT may be more effective for some anxiety disorders. Leichsenring et al. (2013) randomly assigned 495 patients diagnosed with social anxiety disorder to up to 25 sessions of manualized CBT or psychodynamic treatment. Both treatments were superior to waitlist with large pre-treatment to post-treatment effect sizes ($d = 1.32$ for CBT and $d = 1.02$ for psychodynamic treatment). Although between-group effect sizes were small (treatment condition accounted for 1–3 percent of variance in outcomes) remission rates were significantly higher for CBT (36 percent) than psychodynamic treatment (26 percent). Response rates did not differ significantly between treatments. Interestingly, differences between treatments were smaller than differences between therapists, which accounted for between 5–7 percent of variability in outcomes (see Chapter 6). Two final limitations were the manualized psychodynamic therapy was only recently developed and tested for the first time in this trial and that the analyses of therapist adherence indicated that CBT therapists used more dynamic interventions than dynamic therapists used CBT interventions. This final point raises the question that some of the advantage of CBT may have been due to this increased technical flexibility (see Clark, 2013; Leichsenring, Salzer, & Leibing, 2013 for more details on the debate).

IPT has performed poorly in comparison to CBT in two smaller trials, one for panic (n = 91; Vos, Huibers, Diels, & Arntz, 2012) and the other for social anxiety disorder (n = 117; Stangier et al., 2011). However, the literature for specific anxiety disorders remains immature relative to research on depression and other disorders. Thus, to make firm conclusions we must await additional trials.

A larger point in the comparison of CBTs to other treatments is related to what is meant by "CBT." Tolin (2010) found that CBT was superior to other treatments for anxiety (d = .43, a moderate-sized effect), a result that is often cited to support the superiority of CBT for anxiety disorders. A more careful reading of this result is informative however. This effect was based on only four studies, two of which were published before 1972, and was restricted to disorder-specific symptoms only. It is also curious that Tolin retrieved only four direct comparisons of CBT to a non-CBT bona fide treatment for anxiety disorders when Benish et al. (2008) in their meta-analysis of PTSD found at least ten such comparisons. The answer appears to be that Tolin defined CBT quite broadly such that it included EMDR, as none of the EMDR comparisons with CBT were included in his analysis. This brings up the issue of classification. To Ehlers et al. (2010), EMDR is not CBT, whereas for Tolin it was. Sometimes Stress Inoculation is a CBT, sometimes not; sometimes PCT is a classified as CBT, sometimes not (see Baardseth et al., 2013; Wampold et al., 2010). To make inferences about a class of treatments, such as CBT, the taxon has to be clearly defined and should be invariant from one investigation to another (Baardseth et al., 2013). To address this issue, Baardseth et al. classified a treatment for anxiety as CBT based on a survey of members of the Association for Behavioral and Cognitive Therapies who specialized in anxiety disorders. Using this consensual definition of CBT, Baardseth et al. were able to locate 13 studies that directly compared CBT to a bona fide non-CBT treatment for anxiety disorders. Neither the effect for targeted nor non-targeted variables (d = 0.13 and d = − 0.03, respectively) was statistically significant. Here a comprehensive meta-analysis investigating the superiority of CBT for anxiety disorders failed to provide evidence that CBT was especially efficacious.

In sum, the preponderance of meta-analytic evidence suggests there are not substantial differences in efficacy between bona fide psychotherapies for anxiety disorders. What evidence does exist is pulled from single trials or meta-analyses of three or four studies that are often driven by one or a few studies with very large effects in which allegiance is particularly troublesome. Evidence that suggests exposure is a necessary ingredient is based on comparisons across studies and is not found in direct comparisons of treatments with and without exposure. Thus, despite the persistent claims from prominent advocates the relative efficacy of CBT and other active treatment interventions for these specific anxiety disorders is for the most part untested. The tests of this conjecture, when made, fail to support that claim. For sure, CBT works. However, strong claims regarding the relative superiority of CBT over alternative psychotherapies are based on very limited number of clinical trials.

Substance Abuse

Substance abuse is the number one public health problem in the United States (Schneider Institute for Health Policy, 2001). Although there are as many potential substance-use disorders as there are specific drugs, alcohol remains the most problematically used substance and perhaps the most researched. As a result we focus on the treatment of alcohol-use disorders (AUD) in order to examine the relative efficacy of specific treatments. The treatment of AUD is among the most controversial and hotly debated topics in mental health (Marlatt, 1983, 1985; Pendery, Maltzman, & West, 1982; Sobell & Sobell, 1976, 1984a, b; Sobell, Sobell, & Christelman, 1972). New treatments are offered as scientific breakthroughs, improvements upon the flawed technology or theory of the past and a source of hope for clients who continue to struggle with substance abuse and dependence (White, 1998). For example, consider Marlatt's prediction regarding the use of relapse-prevention treatment as compared to Alcoholics Anonymous (AA):

> Learning precise prevention skills and related cognitive strategies would seem to offer more help to the client than relying on vague constructs like willpower or attempting to adhere to the advice embedded in various prophetic slogans such as, "You are only one drink away from a drunk."
> (Marlatt, 1985, p. 51)

Accordingly, it would appear that if differences were present in certain disorders, they would likely be present in the treatment of alcohol use. However, primary studies, qualitative reviews, and meta-analytic reviews have not provided clear answers regarding the superiority of a particular treatment over any other.

Although a number of treatment alternatives are available (Miller et al., 1998), the psychosocial treatments for alcohol-use disorders that remain of primary interest to researchers include behavioral and cognitive-behavioral treatments, which include behavioral self-control training, relapse prevention/skills training, and motivational interviewing, as well as 12-step facilitation based programs (Emmelkamp, 2004; Marlatt & Gordon, 1985; Nowinski, Baker, & Carroll, 1992; White, 1998). However, the proliferation of scientific research has done little to clarify the ambiguity of the previous two centuries of alcohol treatment. Tension between competing models of treatment has continued into the modern era of addiction research, reaching a crescendo in the 1970s and 1980s with the controlled drinking debate (Marlatt, 1983, 1985; Pendery et al., 1982; Sobell et al., 1972; Sobell & Sobell, 1976, 1984a, b). Specifically, behaviorally oriented researchers began to question the assumption that the only acceptable goal of alcohol-dependence treatment was total abstinence (Davies, 1962; Mills, Sobell, & Schaefer, 1971; Sobell et al., 1972; Sobell & Sobell, 1973). Advocates of controlled drinking were accused of scientific fraud and critiques of their research were published in *Science* (Pendery et al., 1982) and the *New York Times* (Boffey, 1982), appeared on "60 Minutes," and were ultimately the subject of a congressional investigation (Marlatt, 1983).

The Pendery et al. critique of controlled-drinking interventions involved detailed interviews and case reviews of patients originally involved in the controlled-drinking arm of the Sobell and Sobell (1973) trial. Pendery's findings demonstrated that the controlled-drinking treatment, in the absolute sense (i.e., how much did patients improve), did quite poorly (e.g., a number of patients died and a majority relapsed). This finding led to the fallacious conclusion by many that controlled drinking was an ineffective and possibly unethical treatment goal (Marlatt, 1983). However, the Pendery study failed to include an analysis of the comparison condition (abstinence-based treatment), which was also quite ineffective in the long term (e.g., a greater number of patients who received abstinence-based treatment died then those who received controlled-drinking treatment). Thus the most justifiable conclusion from the controlled-drinking debate is that there are no treatments that are particularly effective for severely dependent clients (Marlatt, 1983; Sobell & Sobell, 1984a). However, the acrimony of the debate suggested that a core assumption of the treatment of alcohol-use disorders (i.e., the disease concept of alcoholism and the corollary of abstinence as the only viable treatment goal) was in question.

The most well-known study comparing treatments for alcohol abuse is Project MATCH (1997), perhaps the largest study directly comparing bona fide psychotherapies ever conducted (n ≈ 1200 patients). In this study, patients were randomly assigned to one of three treatment modalities: a) Twelve-Step Facilitation (TSF), b) cognitive-behavioral therapy (CBT), and c) motivational interviewing (MI). TSF (Nowinski et al., 1992) was developed for use in Project MATCH and consisted of individual meetings with a counselor trained in aiding the patient in the recovery process. The content of the session was designed to mirror and reinforce the philosophy and strategies offered in AA. Thus, individuals who participated in TSF were expected to both attend the facilitation sessions and regularly attend 12-step meetings. Despite the fact that these three treatments had very different theoretical bases, there were essentially no differences among the treatments. However, we turn to meta-analyses to examine relative efficacy more fully.

The meta-analytic literature of AUD treatment is broadly limited by the same methodological problems present in other disorders noted above (e.g., categorization of treatments, limited numbers of comparisons for specific categories, lack of modern meta-analytic methods—tallies of significant p-values, use of "other" category that contained both bona fide and non-bona fide interventions; see Imel et al., 2008 for a review). Accordingly it is not surprising that some researchers suggest that certain treatments are more clearly supported by scientific evidence (e.g., Miller et al., 1998/2002), while others suggest that there is little evidence to indicate any specific treatment is superior to any other (Berglund et al., 2003).

To address these limitations, Imel, Wampold, Miller, and Fleming (2008) conducted a meta-analysis similar to Wampold et al. (1997b) and Benish et al. (2008) wherein they included all clinical trials for alcohol-use disorders that directly compared at least two bona fide psychotherapies. They avoided classification of treatments into categories and tested treatment differences by examining the heterogeneity in treatment effects around zero. Thirty studies (47 effects, and 3,503 patients) met inclusion criteria. There was no evidence for treatment effects for alcohol-use measures or in a restricted set of studies that included measures of abstinence. That is to say, when directly compared, very different treatments for AUD are equally effective.

Criticisms of Meta-Analytic Conclusion of Uniform Efficacy

A number of issues have been raised with regard to the general meta-analytic finding that psychotherapies intended to be therapeutic produce equivalent outcomes. These issues will be addressed briefly here.

An ironic criticism of the meta-analytic findings was that the "indiscriminate distribution of prizes . . . is absurd" (Rachman & Wilson, 1980, p. 167). The irony lies in the fact that such a claim would be made by the camp that was critical of the advocates of traditional psychotherapy who were convinced of its effectiveness and were unwilling to consider the empirical evidence contrary to their opinion:

> An emotional feeling of considerable intensity has grown up in this field which makes many people regard the very questioning of its [psychotherapy's] effectiveness as an attack on psychotherapy; as Teuber and Powers (1953) point out; "To some of the counselors, the whole control group idea . . . seemed slightly blasphemous, as if we were attempting a statistical test of the efficacy of prayer . . ."

(Eysenck, 1961, p. 697)

Yet, when the empirical evidence supports a contrary position, the conclusion is labeled "absurd" and some return to overall Eysenckian skepticism of the meta-analytic endeavor. Barlow (2010) similarly criticized meta-analysis as a viable means to assess relative efficacy:

> Methods used are retrospective re-analyses of other work using meta-analytic procedures . . . these procedures are notoriously subject to distortion with just the slightest tweaks (see Dieckmann, Malle, & Bodner, 2009) . . . Is there any clinician out there who really believes that you can use exactly the same procedure with, say, someone with chronic schizophrenia, specific phobia, bipolar disorder, or OCD as long as it's a "bona fide" treatment that both patient and therapist believe in? So client-centered therapy would work as well for cognitive deficits in schizophrenia as would cognitive remediation therapy, and as well with OCD as ERP? The fundamental reason this argument has never gained traction is because it just plain doesn't make sense no matter how the clinical trials are reinterpreted.
>
> (pp. 15–16)

Here, Barlow extends the uniform efficacy argument to ridiculous lengths (i.e., that the Dodo bird conjecture holds that therapists should use the *exact* same procedures no matter the client or presenting concern) and implies the superiority of certain treatments is simply obvious. The theoretical proposition of uniformity in treatment efficacy has never implied that a clinician ignore the disorder and simply provide exactly the same treatment to everyone. To be included in the meta-analyses, the treatments must be intended to be therapeutic for the disorder. What is found is that a wide variety of treatments for particular disorders are equally effective.

Moreover, it is common to question the clinical expertise of the meta-analyst: "All too often, the people who conduct these [meta-] analyses know more about the quantitative aspects of their task than about the substantive issues that need to be addressed" (Chambless & Hollon, 1998, p. 14). This last statement could just as well have been made by a psychoanalyst in 1960 with regard to the behaviorally oriented clinical scientists who used control group designs! Are advocates of specific pharmacotherapies the only researchers with valid critiques of the pharmacotherapy literature? It is unscientific to discount evidence because it cannot be brought into accord with one's underlying model, in this case the Medical Model of psychotherapy. Indeed, the spirit of science relies on the ongoing dialectic of criticism and response, as noted by Popper (1962),

> "How can we hope to detect and eliminate error?" . . . By criticizing the theories or guesses of others . . . So my answer to the question "How do you know? What is the source or basis of your assertion?" . . . would be:

"I do not know: my assertion was merely a guess. Never mind the source, or the sources, from which it may spring—there are many possible sources, and I may not be aware of half of them . . . But if you are interested in the problem which I tried to solve by my tentative assertion, you may help me by criticizing it as severely as your can . . .".

(pp. 26–27)

Another criticism of meta-analytic results is that the Dodo bird conjecture cannot be true because there are counter examples—that is, there exist studies that have found differences between treatments (Chambless & Hollon, 1998; Crits-Christoph, 1997). However, it is expected that a small proportion of studies will find a significant difference when the true difference between therapies is zero because the probability of a Type I error (falsely rejecting the null hypothesis of no differences) is typically set at 5 percent. Wampold et al. (1997b) showed that the tails of the distribution of effect sizes for comparisons were consistent with a true effect size of zero—that is, the number of studies showing a significant difference for one treatment was exactly what would be expected by considering sampling error (see Figure 5.2). Of course, the sampling error rate is exacerbated if counter examples are selected on the basis of statistical significance on one or a few of many outcome measures. Crits-Christoph (1997) was able to locate 15 studies contained in the Wampold et al. (1997b) meta-analysis that compared cognitive-behavioral treatment to a non-cognitive-behavioral treatment and for which one variable showed the superiority of the cognitive-behavioral treatment. Although there were numerous problems with the studies selected (e.g., the comparison group was not intended to be therapeutic), the primary issue is that culling through a database to find instances of results in this case 15 variables from a set of more than 3,000 that confirm one's notion will surely lead to confirmation of that notion.

The implications drawn from reviewed meta-analyses have been discounted by some because they represent the current state of outcomes research but perhaps do not reflect the true state of relative efficacy or the future state of outcome research (Howard et al., 1997; Stiles et al., 1986). As noted by Wampold et al. (1997a):

We would cherish the day that a treatment is developed that is dramatically more effective than the ones we use today. But until that day comes, the existing data suggest that whatever differences in treatment efficacy exist, they appear to be extremely small, at best.

(p. 230)

In any case, until data are presented to the contrary, the scientific stance is to retain the null hypothesis, which in this case is that there are no differences in efficacy among treatments.

A number of alternative hypotheses for the uniform efficacy result have been offered. For example, Crits-Christoph (1997) commented that including follow-up assessments in the Wampold et al. (1997b) meta-analysis attenuated differences because clients in the less efficacious treatment would seek other treatment for their disorder. Another alternative hypothesis is that differences will only be apparent for severe disorders: "With mild conditions, the nonspecific effects of treatments . . . are likely to be powerful enough in themselves to affect . . . outcomes leaving little room for the specific factors to play much of a role" (Crits-Christoph, 1997). These and several other alternative hypotheses could be true but must be put to an empirical test in order to establish that some treatments are superior to other treatments (Wampold et al., 1997a). It should be noted that Wampold et al. (1997a) reanalyzed their data and showed that when treatment outcomes was measured at termination only and disorders were limited to those that were severe (viz., DSM-IV disorders), the uniform efficacy result persisted.

Others have blamed the diagnostic system for the equivalence of outcomes. The argument is that DSM disorders are categories that contain multiple etiological pathways and that treatments specific to the pathways are needed (Follette & Houts, 1996). For example, cognitive-behavioral treatment would be indicated for those who depression is caused by irrational cognitions or social skill training would be indicated for those who depression is caused by loneliness resulting from a social skill deficit that limits social relations. This conjecture, if true, would provide strong evidence for specific ingredients and would definitely support the Medical Model. However, as will be shown in Chapter 8, there is little evidence that the predictions of an interactive effect of treatment and etiological pathway exist.

Others have argued that the primary studies synthesized in meta-analysis are flawed, due to problems with randomization, attrition, interactions with unknown causal variables, choice of outcome measures, and limited external validity (Howard, Krause, & Orlinsky, 1986; Howard et al., 1997) and that consequently meta-analyses are flawed as well. Howard et al. (1997) noted that meta-analysis "inherits all of the problems of these kinds of comparative experiments" (p. 224), which is true, to a certain extent but does not invalidate the conclusion for the following reasons. If the outcomes research conducted in psychotherapy is so flawed that the results transmit no information, then they should be abandoned altogether and decisions should not be based on results produced by such designs. But, of course, no one seriously is recommending that such designs are totally invalid, only that there are threats to validity. Meta-analysis is advantageous because it can be used to determine whether results of such studies are consistently drawing the same conclusion (i.e., converge on a common estimation), in which case confidence is increased. This is exactly the case with uniform efficacy. There are flaws with all comparative studies and making strong statements, either for practice or theory, from an individual study is risky. However, when 277 comparisons are homogeneously distributed about zero, as was the case in the Wampold et al. (1997b) meta-analysis and replicated in subsequent disorder-specific meta-analyses, then it must be understood that the corpus of comparisons are consistent with a uniform efficacy conjecture, a conclusion that can be made with confidence.

Conclusions

Rosenzweig (1936) speculated, "All methods of therapy when competently used are equally successful" (p. 413). In the 1970s and 1980s, the evidence from initial meta-analyses were consistent with Rosenzweig's conjecture. In the next 30 years, exemplary studies and methodologically sound meta-analyses unfailingly produced evidence that demonstrated that there were small, if not zero, differences among treatments. This result generalized to the subpopulations of treatments for depression and anxiety, two areas where behaviorally oriented treatments are thought to be particularly appropriate and superior to alternatives. Claims that specific cognitive-behavioral therapies are more effective than bona fide comparisons are common but overblown and in need of additional testing. The Dodo bird conjecture has survived many tests and must be considered "true" until such time as sufficient evidence for its rejection is produced.

The lack of differences among a variety of treatments casts doubt on the hypothesis that specific ingredients are responsible for the benefits of psychotherapy. One would expect that if specific ingredients were indeed remedial, then some of these ingredients would be relatively more beneficial than others. Uniform efficacy of treatments represents the first evidence that the Medical Model cannot explain the empirical findings in psychotherapy research.

Notes

1. In the first edition, a number of early reviews and primary studies were reviewed. Due to the expansion of the clinical trial literature in the last 15 years, we have removed much of these early citations. Save for a few classic references (e.g., Elkin et al. 1989; Smith & Glass, 1977) the current review focuses on more recent primary studies and meta-analyses. Readers interested in these early studies should consult the first edition.
2. Ellis' (1957) study was probably the most egregious as Ellis, who developed and promoted rational therapy, was the sole therapist for all treatments and was the evaluator of therapeutic change.
3. The reciprocal inhibition mechanisms proposed by Wolpe have been found to be flawed (see Kirsch, 1985). Phillips claimed that all behavior, pathological and normal, is the result of "assertions" made about oneself and relations with others, a claim that appears to be far afield from extant learning theories of the time. Although Ellis proposed no learning theory basis for his rational treatment, Eysenck commented that developing a learning theory explanation for it "would not be impossible" (Eysenck, 1961, p. 719).
4. Early meta-analyses conducted to date have produced generally consistent results. While early meta-analyses (viz., Smith & Glass, 1977; Smith et al., 1980) that did not rely on reviewing primary studies that directly compared psychotherapies found

some differences in efficacy among various classes of treatments, when confounds were statistically modeled, these differences were negligible. Early meta-analysis of direct comparisons among classes of treatments (viz., Shapiro & Shapiro, 1982) produced a few differences but not more than expected by chance. Moreover, the one result that might have supported specific ingredients (viz., the superiority of cognitive treatments to systematic desensitization) was later shown to be nonexistent and most likely due to allegiance (see Berman et al., 1985).

5. Grissom (1996) meta-meta-analyzed 32 meta-analyses that compared various psychotherapies, assigned positive signs to the differences, and calculated an effect size difference of 0.23, replicating the upper bound found by Wampold et al. (1997b).

6. The bias of the Beck Depression Inventory (BDI) is suggested by an examination of the items, many of which refer to cognitions. However, empirical evidence is provided by the Shapiro et al., (1994) study of cognitive-behavioral and psychodynamic-interpersonal therapy. Of the eight outcome measures, the F values for six of the differences were less than 1.00, indicating that there were absolute no differences between the treatments. The BDI, however, produced a large effect in favor of the cognitive-behavioral treatment. Further evidence for the cognitive bias of the BDI is revealed in a meta-analysis that found that changes in cognitive style fostered by psychotherapy are related to decreases in depression as measured by the BDI but not by other measures of depression (Oei & Free, 1995).

7. Interestingly, for some types of patients, supportive, self-directed therapy was the most efficacious treatment.

8. While in the Diagnostic and Statistical Manual of Mental Disorders, Fifth Edition, post-traumatic stress disorder (PTSD) is no longer formally labeled an anxiety disorder, many of the treatments for both PTSD and other anxiety disorders often include exposure-based mechanisms. While we separate the discussion of PTSD and anxiety disorders generally, we have paired these discussions as many of the theoretical issues are similar.

9. Critics of eye movement desensitization and reprocessing (EMDR) generally account for its effectiveness by noting that it is essentially an exposure-based treatment. Essentially, EMDR is pseudoscience not because it doesn't work or because it doesn't contain any therapeutic ingredients but rather because clients are given a misleading rationale about why the treatment works and asked to engage in specific actions that are unnecessary (see Chapter 8).

10. This result is based on effect sizes reported in the corrigendum to Sánchez-Meca et al. (2010) with variances calculated from n's reported in the appendix. After re-categorizing the effect from Mavissakalian and Michelson (1986), we separated effects into those from active controls and waitlist comparisons. Type of treatment (exposure-based vs. non-exposure-based) was not a moderator of effect size in either case, $d_{exp} = 0.32$, 95% CI [−0.01–0.64] for active controls, and $d_{exp} = 0.59$, 95% CI[−0.1,1.27] for waitlist controls. Also note that while the authors reported that publication bias was not a threat to the results, they did report evidence for publication bias on panic measures in a footnote on p. 42, suggesting fewer small effects than expected among published studies with small sample sizes, creating a potential upward bias on the aggregate effect of treatment.

11. Abramowitz (1997) conducted the first meta-analysis for obsessive-compulsive disorder that reviewed direct comparisons among exposure and response prevention, cognitive therapy, and components of exposure and response prevention (i.e., either exposure alone or response prevention alone). Exposure-response prevention was also compared to relaxation, but relaxation in these studies was used as a control group and did not meet the definition of psychotherapy used in this book. No differences among any pair of treatments were found.

Chapter 6

Therapist Effects
An Ignored but Critical Factor

The qualities of the therapist that lead to beneficial outcomes have been of interest to psychotherapy researchers and clinicians since the origins of the field. It seems intuitive that some characteristics or actions of therapists would be more desirable than others and that, consequently, some therapists would be more effective with clients than others. In this regard, therapists are similar to other professionals, as some lawyers win more cases than others, some artists create more memorable and creative sculptures than others, and some teachers facilitate greater student achievement than others.

Despite an interest in therapist effects, there has been a tendency to ignore therapists as a therapeutic factor. Almost 50 years ago, Donald Kiesler (1966) noted:

> The Uniformity Assumption still abounds in much psychotherapy research. Patients are still assigned to "psychotherapy" as if it were a uniform homogeneous treatment, and to psychotherapy with different therapists as if therapist differences were irrelevant . . . If psychotherapy research is to advance, it must first begin to identify and measure these therapist variables so relevant to eventual outcome (personality characteristics, technique factors, relationship variables, role expectancies, and the like).
>
> (pp. 112–113)

To understand the many ways that therapists influence psychotherapy process and outcome, Beutler et al. (2004) created a taxonomy of therapist variables. Aspects related to the therapists were classified along two dimensions: a) objective versus subjective, and b) cross-situation traits versus therapy-specific states, thereby yielding four types of therapist variables. Many of the therapy-specific states are discussed in other chapters, including *therapist interventions*, which relate to adherence and specific effects (Chapter 8); *therapeutic relationships*, which relate to the working alliance and other relationship aspects (Chapter 7); and therapeutic *orientation*, which relates to relative efficacy (Chapter 5). The cross-situational traits for therapists are aspects of the therapist that are relatively constant across the various clients treated by the therapist, including demographics (e.g., age, gender, and ethnicity of the therapist) and characteristics of the therapists, including personality, coping style, emotional well-being, values, beliefs, and cultural features.

Beutler et al. (2004) reviewed the research to identify therapist variables in the four classes that were related to psychotherapy outcome. The preponderance of the evidence was related to therapy-specific variables and was consistent with the evidence reviewed in earlier chapters. For the most part, Beutler et al. concluded that none of the variables examined were clearly related to therapist effectiveness and that research focused on therapist variables had been decreasing up to the time the chapter was written (i.e., up to 2003). Although examining therapist variables is interesting and informative, it puts the cart before the horse. Before a search of variables that are related to therapist effectiveness, it must be established that indeed the therapists providing the treatment make a difference in outcomes. If therapists are uniformly effective, then there is no need to find the characteristics and actions of effective therapists because there will be none. This chapter is focused on whether the therapist makes a difference at all, and if so, how much?

A central issue for differentiating the Medical Model and the Contextual Model is to estimate the degree to which the therapist affects the outcome of therapy—stated as a question, "Is the particular therapist important?" The Medical Model posits that the specific ingredients are critical to the outcome of therapy and, therefore, whether the ingredient is received by the client is more important that who delivers the ingredient. On the other hand, in the Contextual Model, the therapist is critical because it is recognized that how the treatment is delivered is critical to the success of therapy. Furthermore, the Contextual Model proposes that the actions of effective therapists will be unrelated to specific ingredients (e.g., adherence to a protocol) but rather to what we think of as common factors: empathy, understanding, ability to form an alliance across a range of patients, and so forth. Medical Model proponents clearly recognize that some therapists will be more competent than others in delivering a specific treatment:

> *Competence* [refers] to the level of skill shown by the therapist in delivering the treatment. [Skill is] the extent to which the therapists conducting the intervention took the relevant aspects of the therapeutic context into account and responded to these contextual variables appropriately. Relevant aspects of the context include, but are by no means limited to, (a) client variables such as degree of impairment; (b) the particular problems manifested by a given client; (c) the client's life situation and stress; (d) and factors such as stage in therapy, degree of improvement already achieved, and appropriate sensitivity to the timing of interventions within a therapy session.
>
> (Waltz, Addis, Koerner, & Jacobson, 1993, p. 620)

Competence, as defined in this way, typically is assessed by raters who are expert therapists themselves or trained by experts (see Chapter 8). However, the characteristics of therapy measured by these expert raters may be irrelevant to outcome. Indeed, researchers are hard-pressed to find correlations between measures of competence and outcome, as was the case in the NIMH Treatment of Depression Collaborative Research Program, and confirmed in a meta-analysis (e.g., Shaw et al., 1999; see also Webb et al. 2010 and Chapter 8).

The important issue for the Medical versus Contextual Model debate addressed here, however, is not how competence is measured or whether it is related to outcome, but whether there is much variability among therapists with regard to outcomes at all. In clinical trials comparing treatments intended to be therapeutic, therapists are screened, trained, supervised, and expected to reach an adequate level of competence before delivering the treatment. Nevertheless, the Medical Model supposition that some ingredients are better than others, combined with minimization of therapist differences in clinical trials, suggests that the variability among treatments should be greater than variability among therapists. Essentially, the treatment a patient receives (Treatment A vs. Treatment B) should be more important than who delivers the treatment, especially if the therapist adheres to the treatment protocol. This is an important question that will guide the remainder of this chapter.

In this chapter, competence is defined by outcome. Simply put, more competent therapists produce better outcomes than less competent therapists. Of course, it is productive to identify those characteristics that differentiate more competent from less competent therapists, yet surprisingly little research has been directed toward this goal (see Anderson, Ogles, Patterson, Lambert, & Vermeersch, 2009; Baldwin, Wampold, & Imel, 2007; Blatt, Sanislow, Zuroff, & Pilkonis, 1996 for examples of this type of research). When competence is defined by outcome, variability in outcomes due to therapists reflects differences in competence. The Contextual Model predicts that variability among therapists will be relatively large, especially in comparison to variability among treatments. A competent therapist will achieve commendable outcomes regardless of the treatment provided.

To summarize, the two models have divergent hypotheses:

Medical Model: **Variability of Treatments > Variability of Therapists**
Contextual Model: **Variability of Therapists > Variability of Treatments**

The first section of this chapter will discuss design issues relative to assessing therapist effects. The second section will then examine studies that produce evidence about the size of therapist effects.

Design Issues

Consideration of therapists in any study of psychotherapy is critical to proper conclusions about the efficacy of treatments. Ignoring therapists in the design of psychotherapy studies can lead to erroneous conclusions, as will be shown in this chapter. Understanding the nature of therapist effects in psychotherapy studies is vital. In this section, two alternatives for assigning therapists to treatments, nested and crossed designs, will be presented.

Nested Design

In the nested experimental design, therapists are randomly assigned to treatments, as shown in Figure 6.1. That is, each therapist delivers one and only one treatment. Although nested designs are well discussed in most experimental design texts (e.g., Kirk, 1995), the design is presented in some detail here.

Let m be the number of subjects randomly assigned to each therapist, k be the number of therapists assigned to each treatment, and p be the number of treatments. Thus there are mk subjects in each treatment and mkp subjects total. When a nested design is used, historically the therapist factor is ignored (Crits-Christoph & Mintz, 1991; Wampold & Serlin, 2000); however, as will be discussed below, ignoring the therapist factor to leads to increased Type I errors and overestimation of treatment effects (Wampold & Serlin, 2000). While acknowledgement of therapist effects in primary RCT articles is becoming more common in large-scale studies published in quality journals (e.g., Ball et al., 2007; Leichsenring et al., 2013), many trials are too small to adequately estimate therapist differences in outcomes (e.g., Taylor et al., 2003). Thus, while authors may test for therapist differences, such effects are unlikely to be detected, due to lack of power. In such cases, therapists should still be explicitly included in statistical models even if statistical significance is not found, because the deleterious consequences are there nonetheless.

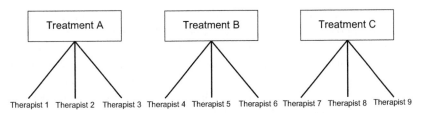

Figure 6.1 Therapists nested within treatments.

Before examining the design further, it should be noted that therapists should be considered a random factor (Crits-Christoph & Mintz, 1991; Wampold & Serlin, 2000):

> In this model, the researchers are interested in making conclusions about the specific treatments chosen to be studied, and consequently treatment should be considered a fixed effect. On the other hand, rarely is the researcher interested in the particular [therapists] used in the study. The issue is whether [therapists] in general differ in the outcomes they produce. Therefore, [therapists] should be treated as a random factor so that conclusions can be made about [therapists] in general. Ideally, [therapists] would be randomly selected from the population of [therapists] and then assigned to the treatments. In practice, [therapists] who have chosen a treatment or have an affinity to a treatment often are used to deliver that treatment, a condition that mirrors the real world situation in which [therapists] are free to deliver their preferred treatment chosen from a set of professionally accepted treatments. In the latter case, the [therapists] are not randomly assigned to treatments, and the conclusions need to be restricted to "[therapists] who have an affinity to treatment X" rather than to [therapists] in general.
>
> (Wampold & Serlin, 2000, p. 427)

In the nested model, if therapists vary in their effectiveness, clients assigned to some therapists will have better outcomes than clients assigned to other therapists, regardless of client variables (recall that patients are randomly assigned to therapists in the nested design). The variability of therapists, as we will see, contributes to apparent treatment differences, which if ignored, will make differences between treatments appear larger than they really are.

Statistically, differences among therapists are expressed as a ratio of the variability due to the therapists to the total variability among patients, which produces an intraclass correlation coefficient (ICC). That is, the ICC is the proportion of variability in outcomes due to which therapist the patient was assigned. The ICC indexes the degree to which outcomes of two patients being treated by the same therapist are more similar than the outcomes of two patients treated by two different therapists (Kenny & Judd, 1986; Kirk, 1995; Wampold & Serlin, 2000). The larger the ICC, the greater the variability among therapists, indicating that some therapists will consistently achieve better outcomes with their patients than will other therapists. It is important to note that observations (i.e., patient outcomes) in such designs are not independent (i.e., they depend on the therapist), violating a major assumption of statistical tests used in RCTs if therapists are ignored.

The correct analysis of the nested design requires the therapist be considered a random factor in the analysis (Serlin, Wampold, & Levin, 2003; Wampold &

Table 6.1 Source Tables for Nested and Incorrect Designs

$\widehat{\omega}^2 = .1, \widehat{\rho_I} = .3, m = 4, p = 2, k = 5)$

Source	SS	df	MS	F	Effect Size
		Nested Design (Correct Analysis)			
Treatment	9.064	1	9.064	3.339	$\widehat{\omega}^2 = .100$
Therapists	21.714	8	2.714	2.714	$\widehat{\rho_I} = .30$
WCell	30.000	30	1.000		
Total	60.778	39			
		Design Ignoring Nested Therapist Factor (Incorrect Analysis)			
Treatment	9.064	1	9.064	6.660	$\widehat{\omega}^2 = .124$
Error	51.714	38	1.361		
Total	60.778	39			

Note. Reprinted from "The consequences of ignoring a nested factor on measures of effect size in analysis of variance designs," by B. E. Wampold and R. C. Serlin, 2000, *Psychological Methods, 5,* p. 428. Copyright 2000 by the American Psychological Association. Reprinted with permission.

Serlin, 2000). The expected value for the mean squares for treatments contains a term that includes the variance due to therapists; that is, variability of therapists contributes to the observed differences between treatments. Thus the proper F is calculated as the ratio of the mean squares for treatment and the mean squares for therapists. The correct and incorrect analysis (i.e., ignoring the therapist effect) is shown for a hypothetical example in Table 6.1. When the correct analysis is conducted using the correct denominator, the F value and degrees of freedom for the treatment effect are considerably less than the respective values for the incorrect analysis.

When the nested factor is ignored, the assumption that the observations are independent is violated because some therapists are more effective than others. The consequences of ignoring the fact that observations are not independent have been derived and disseminated to the research community (Barcikowski, 1981; Kenny & Judd, 1986; Kirk, 1995; Walsh, 1947; Wampold & Serlin, 2000) but have been for the most part ignored. Unfortunately, the incorrect analysis yields an F which is liberal, in that the probability of Type I error will be larger than its nominal value, and thus the null hypothesis will be rejected more frequently than expected when there are no true treatment differences. Based on a Monte Carlo study, Wampold and Serlin derived the error rates for rejecting the null hypotheses when there are no true treatment differences between treatments, for different therapist effects, and clients/therapist ratios; these error rates are found in Figure 6.2. Consider a comparison between two treatments, with four therapists per treatment ($k = 4$), each seeing five clients ($m = 5$), where therapists account for 10 percent of the variance in outcomes; 15 percent of

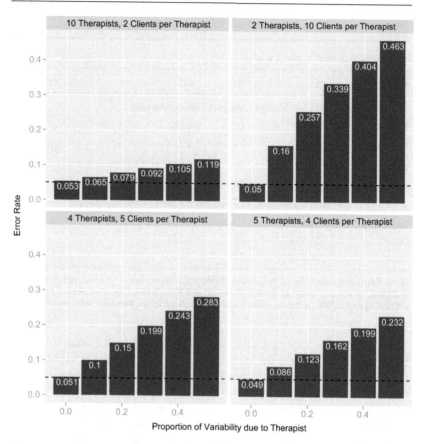

Figure 6.2 Error rates when nested therapist factor is ignored (nominal error rate is .05, two treatments). Adapted from "The consequences of ignoring a nested factor on measures of effect size in analysis of variance designs," by B. E. Wampold and R. C. Serlin, 2000, *Psychological Methods, 5,* p. 429. Copyright 2000 by the American Psychological Association. Adapted with permission.

such comparisons will result in rejection of the null hypotheses when *there is no true difference between the treatments.* It is disturbing to find that such a high percentage of studies like these would have concluded that one treatment was more effective than another treatment when absolutely no differences existed. Given the relatively few studies that show treatment differences (see Figure 5.2) and the fact that therapist effects typically are ignored, one has to wonder how many of the observed treatment differences are ignoring therapist effects.

The important determination in this chapter is the estimation of therapist effects. In the appropriate analysis of the nested design, the proportion of variance attributable to therapists (within treatments) can be estimated. Let ρ_I be the population intraclass correlation coefficient for therapists with the interpretation that it represents the population proportion of variance accounted for by therapists within treatments. The estimator of this number can be calculated easily (see Wampold & Serlin, 2000). In the example shown in Table 6.1, $\widehat{\rho}_I$ was equal to 0.30, indicating that the estimate of the proportion of the variance accounted for by therapists was 30 percent.

Discriminating between the Medical and Contextual Models of psychotherapy has relied largely on the determination of effect sizes for various critical questions. In Chapter 5, estimates of the effect size for the direct comparisons of two treatments were calculated. However, these estimates do not take into account therapist variability, resulting in an overestimation of effect sizes. Wampold and Serlin (2000) derived the degree to which failure to take into account dependence of observations affects the size of proportion of variance measures. As can be seen in Table 6.1, the correct estimate for the proportion of variability due to treatments $\widehat{\omega}^2$ was .100, whereas the when therapist effects were ignored researchers would have reported .124, indicating that ignoring therapist variance inflates the size of the estimates of treatment effects.[1] Figure 6.3 shows the degree to which treatment effects are inflated in various instances. Take the case where there are absolutely no treatment effects (i.e., in the first panel in Figure 6.3, $\widehat{\omega}^2 = 0$), when there are two therapists per treatment (i.e., $k = 2$), ten subjects per therapist (i.e., $m = 10$), and therapists account for 30 percent of the variance in outcomes (i.e., $\widehat{\rho}_I = .30$); the expected value of the incorrect estimate is 0.067. *That is, in this case, researchers would conclude that nearly 7 percent of the variability in outcomes was due to treatments, when in fact absolutely none of the variance was due to treatments (i.e., treatments are equally efficacious).* Later in the chapter, the consequences for ignoring the therapist factor in psychotherapy will be modeled.

The nested design has been presented in some detail in order to establish that ignoring the therapist factor results in grossly liberal tests of treatment differences and an overestimation of treatment effects. The bottom line is simple: *use the appropriate analysis when therapists are nested within treatments.* Not only does it provide the correct conclusion, but it provides an estimate of therapist effects, which is extremely important information, as will be seen later in this chapter. When the incorrect analysis is conducted, the detrimental effects of ignoring therapist variance are increased even further when few therapists are used (see Figures 6.2 and 6.3).

Crossed Design

In the crossed design, therapists deliver each of the treatments being studied, as illustrated in Figure 6.4. As in the case of the nested design, therapists are considered a random factor because the researcher wishes to make conclusions about therapists in general rather than the specific therapists being studied.

Suppose that there are k therapists (randomly selected from a population of therapists) and p treatments; n subjects are assigned to each of the kp combinations of therapists and treatments. This factorial design is often called a mixed model,

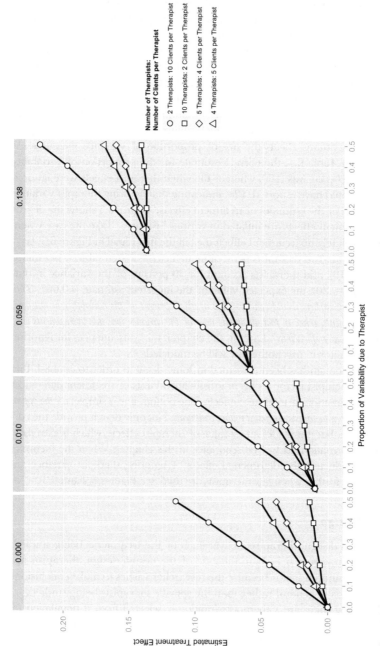

Number of Therapists:
Number of Clients per Therapist

○ 2 Therapists: 10 Clients per Therapist
□ 10 Therapists: 2 Clients per Therapist
◇ 5 Therapists: 4 Clients per Therapist
△ 4 Therapists: 5 Clients per Therapist

Figure 6.3 Incorrect estimates of the population proportion of variance accounted for by treatments. Adapted from "The consequences of ignoring a nested factor on measures of effect size in analysis of variance designs," by B. E. Wampold and R. C. Serlin, 2000, *Psychological Methods, 5*, p. 430. Copyright 2000 by the American Psychological Association. Adapted with permission.

	Tx A	Tx B	Tx B
Therapist 1	n subjects	n subjects	n subjects
Therapist 2	n subjects	n subjects	n subjects
Therapist 3	n subjects	n subjects	n subjects
Therapist 4	n subjects	n subjects	n subjects

Figure 6.4 Therapists and treatments crossed.

due to the inclusion of a fixed and a random factor. Details of this design are found in standard textbooks (see e.g., Hays, 1988; Kirk, 1995; Wampold & Drew, 1990).

The analysis of the mixed model is similar to the nested design in that the expectation of the mean squares for treatments contains a term other than the error and treatment terms. In this context, the expected mean squares contain a term involving the variance due to the interaction. If some therapists produce better outcomes with one therapy and other therapists produce better outcomes with another therapy, the interaction effects will be large. The proper F ratio is determined with the mean squares interaction as the denominator rather than the mean squares error. Consequently, ignoring therapists in the design (and consequently ignoring the interaction) will result in an overly liberal test of treatment effects and an overestimation of the size of treatment effects, similar to the consequences of ignoring therapist effects in the nested design. Although the reader is spared a detailed discussion of the crossed design (but see Hays, 1988; Kirk, 1995; Wampold & Drew, 1990), the bottom line is the same as in the nested design: *use the appropriate analysis when therapists are crossed with treatments.* Not only does it provide the correct conclusion, but it provides an estimate of therapist effects.

Relative Advantages of the Nested and Crossed Design

One of the distinct advantages of the nested design is that one can compare treatments administered by therapists who are skilled in and have allegiance to each of the therapies being compared. Because allegiance is so important to successful outcome (see Chapter 5), the nested design permits a comparison of treatments conducted by therapists who have allegiance to those treatments, provided of course that researchers appropriately balance the allegiance of the therapists. A good example of a nested design is the NIMH Treatment of Depression Collaborative Research Program, which used ten therapists in the interpersonal therapy (IPT) and the pharmacotherapy conditions and eight in the cognitive-behavioral (CBT) condition. Skill and allegiance were controlled in the following way:

> All [therapists] had to meet specific background and experience criteria: at least two years of full-time clinical work following completion of professional training (ie, following the Ph.D. and clinical internship for clinical

psychologists and following the MD and psychiatric residency for psychiatrists); treatment of at least ten depressed patients; and a special interest in and commitment to the therapeutic approach in which they were trained. In addition, IPT therapists had to have previous training in a psychodynamic oriented framework, CB therapists were to have had some cognitive and/or behavioral background, and the past training of pharmacotherapists had to include a considerable emphasis on psychotropic drug treatment. . . . *Thus, the treatment conditions being compared in this study are, in actuality, "packages" of particular therapeutic approaches and the therapists who both choose to and are chosen to administer them.*

(emphasis added, Elkin, Parloff, Hadley, & Autry, 1985, p. 308)

The disadvantage of the nested design as used in psychotherapy research is that different therapists administer the treatments. Thus, technically therapists and treatments are confounded. It may be that the therapists delivering one of the treatments are generally more skilled than the therapists delivering the other treatment. However, the conclusion is that, if properly analyzed, Treatment A, given by therapists with adequate training in and with sufficient allegiance to Treatment A, produces better outcomes than Treatment B, given by therapists with adequate training in and with sufficient allegiance to Treatment B (see Serlin et al., 2003; Wampold & Serlin, 2000).

In the crossed design, the general characteristics of the therapist are equivalent across treatments, but care must be taken to ensure that the training, skill, and allegiance are balanced. For example, in a study comparing behavior therapy (BT) and cognitive-behavioral therapy (CBT), Butler, Fennell, Robson, and Gelder (1991) used clinical psychologists who had originally been trained in BT but who had received special training in CBT from the Center for Cognitive Therapy in Philadelphia. Although the psychologists initially may have had allegiance to BT, their special training would certainly increase their skill, if not their allegiance, to CBT. However, a comparison of cognitive therapy (CT) and applied relaxation (AR) conducted by Clark et al. (1994) demonstrates the problems with a crossed design. In this study, which was discussed in Chapter 5, two of the authors, who clearly were proponents of CT and skilled in its delivery, also administered both CT and AR. Moreover, these two therapists were supervised by the first author, who had developed the CT used in the study. In this study, treatment was confounded with allegiance, and, therefore, it is not possible to determine whether the observed superiority of CT was due to the efficacy of CT or to the allegiance and skill of the therapists. As noted previously (Chapter 5), allegiance in crossed designs is often ignored, especially in CBT studies, with deleterious effects (Falkenström, Markowitz, Jonker, Philips, & Holmqvist, 2013).

Both of the methods for assigning therapists to treatments contain potential confounds, and, therefore, the researcher must be cognizant of the threats and minimize threats to validity. Clearly, ignoring the variability of therapists, whether in a nested or a crossed design, produces a liberal F test and overestimates treatment effects. Unfortunately, in a review of 140 comparative studies, Crits-Christoph and Mintz (1991) found that not a single study correctly analyzed the treatment effect by conducting the appropriate nested or crossed analysis. This is particularly problematic as the size of therapist effects may not be predictable without direct examination (discussed further in the following). For example, in a recent reanalysis of 20 clinical trials (495 effects), Baldwin et al. (2011) found that ICCs varied widely across measures and studies, meaning the impact of therapist differences on tests of treatment effects could vary from negligible to dramatic. Thus, it remains crucial for researchers to model therapist effects in clinical trial data. The failure to do so may result in the overestimation of treatment effects in clinical trials.

The Size of Therapist Effects

Although Crits-Christoph and Mintz (1991) could not find studies that correctly tested treatment differences properly taking variability among therapists into account, there have been a number of attempts to estimate the size of therapist effects by reanalyzing data from the primary studies. In this section, we provide examples of several of these attempts but also focus on comprehensive meta-analyses that provided a summary of this literature (Baldwin & Imel, 2013; Crits-Christoph & Mintz, 1991). We describe the importance of therapist effects by comparing the relative amount of variance in outcomes explained by therapists but also explore more practical markers of the differences among therapists at the tails of the distribution of outcomes. Percentage of variance estimates will be used to understand the degree to which treatment effects have been overestimated.

Estimation of Therapist Effects

Luborsky et al.'s (1986) reanalysis of four studies was among the first to determine the size of therapists effects. They obtained the raw data from four major psychotherapy studies: the Hopkins Psychotherapy Project (Nash et al., 1965), the VA-Penn Psychotherapy Project (Woody et al., 1983), the Pittsburgh Psychotherapy Project (Pilkonis et al., 1984), and the McGill Psychotherapy Project (Piper et al., 1984). In the reanalysis, Luborsky et al. correctly considered the therapist as a random factor and performed the appropriate analysis. Although they did not estimate the proportion of variance accounted for by therapists, the results clearly showed that there were large therapist effects, much in excess of the treatment effects.

Blatt et al. (1996) reanalyzed the data from the NIMH Treatment of Depression Collaborative Research Program to determine the characteristics of effective therapists. This is an important analysis because the NIMH study was well controlled, used manuals, and employed a nested design in which therapists were committed to and skilled in the delivery of each treatment (see the proceeding). For the three active treatments (CBT; interpersonal psychotherapy, IPT; and imipramine-clinical management, IMI-CM) and the pill-placebo group (clinical management, CM), Blatt et al. divided therapists into three groups based on composite residualized gain scores: a) more effective therapists, b) moderately effective therapists, and c) less effective therapists. There was significant variation among therapists in this well-controlled study. Blatt et al. concluded:

> The present analyses of the data . . . indicate that significant differences exist in therapeutic efficacy among therapists, even within the experienced and well-trained therapists in the [NIMH study]. Differences in therapeutic efficacy were independent of the type of treatment provided or the research site and not related to the therapists' level of general clinical experience or in treating depressed patients. Differences in therapeutic efficacy, however, were associated with basic clinical orientation, especially about treatment. More effective therapists had a more psychological rather than biological orientation to the clinical process. . . . Additionally, more effective therapists, compared with less and moderately effective therapists, expect therapy to require more treatment sessions before patients begin to manifest therapeutic change. . . . Relatively few significant findings were obtained when comparing attitudes about the etiology of depression or about techniques considered essential to successful treatment.
>
> (pp. 1282–1283)

Interestingly, two therapists who achieved therapeutic efficacy with medication in the IMI-CM group also achieved success in the clinical management condition, suggesting that the relationship between client and therapist is vitally important even for treatment with medication. McKay, Imel, and Wampold (2006) found that there indeed was significant variability in treatment outcomes across the psychiatrists. Psychiatrists accounted for between approximately 6.7 and 9.1 percent of variability in outcomes on the Hamilton and Beck Measures of Depression, respectively, compared to 5.9 and 3.4 percent accounted for by treatment (i.e., medication vs. placebo). Essentially, psychiatrists accounted for at least as much (if not more) variability in outcomes than whether a patient received the medication or not. Indeed, the best psychiatrists had better outcomes giving a placebo than the poorer psychiatrists giving the medication (see Figure 6.5). While this finding is in need of further replication in larger samples, the finding that psychiatrist outcomes vary even in a manualized medication management protocol has important substantive and methodological implications for how the results of drug trials are interpreted. First, the psychiatrist is crucial even when the active ingredients of a treatment are supposedly pharmaceutical. Second, if provider effects are not

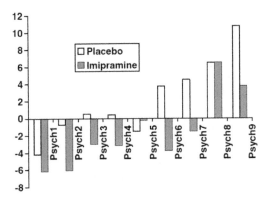

Figure 6.5 Bar chart illustrating provider variability in outcomes in the NIMH-TDCRP placebo-medication treatment arms. The y-axis indicates residualized gain scores for the BDI (lower = better treatment outcomes). Each set of bars represents a provider. Reprinted from "Psychiatrist effects in the psychopharmacological treatment of depression," by K.M. McKay, Z.E. Imel, and B.E. Wampold, 2006, *Journal of Affective Disorders, 92,* p. 289. Copyright 2006 by Elsevier B.V. Reprinted with permission from Elsevier.

being appropriately modeled in drug trials, the size of treatment effects will be overestimated. More importantly, this analysis demonstrates that qualities of the therapeutic interaction with a skilled clinician even in clinical management have effects on benefits of treatment, even if the treatment is pharmacological.

Luborsky, McLellan, Diguer, Woody, and Seligman (1997) conducted a reanalysis of seven samples of drug-addicted and depressed clients that is particularly informative, as the same therapists were used in several of the samples. Although Luborsky et al. did not provide estimates of the therapist effects, their conclusions were clear cut:

> *Therapists in all seven samples differed widely in the mean level of improvement shown by the patients in their caseloads.* . . . [The results] were somewhat surprising because (a) patients within each sample were similar in terms of diagnosis; (b) they were randomly assigned; (c) the therapists had been selected for their competence in their particular form of psychotherapy; and (d) the therapists were regularly supervised and were further guided by treatment manuals. Despite these steps that should have maximized skill and minimized differences, the range of percentages of improvement for the 22 therapists in the seven samples was from slightly negative change, to slightly more than 80% improvement.
>
> (emphasis added, p. 60)

An important finding of this study is that therapists who were successful in one sample were also successful in other samples. Luborsky et al. attributed this finding, based on this and previous research, to the fact that "the most effective therapists are rated by their patients, even after a few sessions, as being helpful and part of an alliance with them" (p. 62).

The final reanalysis involves the treatment of alcohol problems in the multisite study conducted by Project MATCH (see Chapter 5 for a description of this study; Project MATCH Research Group, 1997, 1998). This is a study in which therapists were selected for their competence and allegiance to the treatment and were well trained and supervised. Recall that in this study there were few differences among the treatments. However, in the reanalysis (Project MATCH Research Group, 1998), more than 6 percent of the variability in outcomes was due to therapists (range: 1 percent to 12 percent).

Meta-Analyses

In 1991, Crits-Christoph et al., based on the data from 15 previously published studies, provided the first meta-analytic estimate of therapist effects. In the 15 studies, they calculated the proportion of variability in outcomes attributable to therapists within 27 different treatments. For all outcome measures and all treatments, the mean proportion was 0.086; that is, overall, nearly 9 percent of the variability in outcomes was due to therapists.[2] In a recent meta-analysis of 46 studies with 1,281 therapists and 14,519 patients, 5 percent of the variability in treatment outcome was attributable to the therapist (Baldwin & Imel, 2013). However, the effects were larger in naturalistic settings (7 percent based on 17 studies) versus clinical trials (3 percent based on 29 studies).

A particularly interesting aspect of both the Crits-Christoph and Mintz (1991) and Baldwin and Imel (2013) meta-analyses is that the estimates of therapist variability ranged greatly from one study to another. In Baldwin and Imel, the percentage of variability accounted for by therapists was quite different across studies, ranging from 0 to .55, ($I^2 = 61.9$, suggesting that over half of the total variability in therapist ICC was attributable to between-study differences). This large amount of variability in ICC values means therapist differences depend on the study.

There are some general trends among this variability to report. The controlled studies that used treatment manuals and that were published more recently had smaller therapist effects than did the other studies, according to Crits-Christoph and Mintz (1991) who concluded that "this implies that the quality control procedures commonly implemented in contemporary outcome trials (e.g., careful selection, training, and supervision of therapists and the use of treatment manuals) to control for differences among therapists may have been quite successful" (p. 24). This finding is consistent with Baldwin and Imel (2013), who found that therapists accounted for less variability in outcomes in clinical trials than in naturalistic settings where controls such as manuals were less likely to be used.

While the trend towards homogenization of therapists does not imply that there is no evidence of therapist effects in clinical trials, it does raise the question of how meaningful therapist differences are to patients when the overall percentage of variance in outcomes accounted for is relatively small (e.g., 5 percent).[3] As can be seen in Figure 6.6, when comparing therapists in the middle of the distribution, the impact on patients is likely to be small—there is a relatively small improvement in outcome when a client moves from a therapist

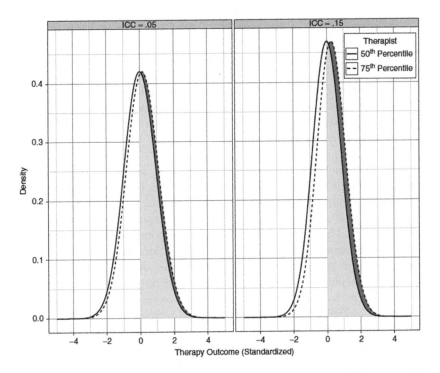

Figure 6.6 Distribution of outcomes for therapists at the 50th and 75th percentile assuming intra-class correlations of .05 or .15. In the figure, outcomes are standardized such that observations below zero are below average and above zero are above average. The light gray shading indicates the probability of an above average outcome for a patient seeing a therapist at the 50th percentile (i.e., the client has a 50 percent chance at a better than average outcome). The dark grey indicates the increase in the probability of an above average outcome for a patient seeing a therapist at the 75th percentile. Reprinted from S. A. Baldwin & Z.E. Imel. "Therapist effects: Findings and methods," 2013, in M.J. Lambert (Ed.), *Bergin and Garfield's handbook of psychotherapy and behavior change*, 6th ed., p. 279. Copyright 2013, Wiley. Reprinted with permission of Wiley.

at the 50th percentile to the 75th (Baldwin & Imel, 2013). However, as noted by Imel et al. (in press):

> Although the absolute amount of patient outcome variance attributable to therapists is small, small effects can some times have large impacts. For example, in a classic paper, Abelson and Rubin (1985) demonstrated that counter to the belief of most baseball fans, the individual hitter only explains about one third of 1% of the variance in getting a hit in a given at bat. However, when viewed cumulatively (over say 1,000 at bats), the difference in number of hits between a below average and above average hitter can become sizeable (hits are almost 50% more frequent in the above average hitter). Abelson's paradox of small explained variance and large cumulative impact has parallels in the evaluation of therapist outcomes. For example, a large study of therapist influences on patient outcomes in a managed care system found that therapists accounted for 5% of the variance in outcomes. However, the average effect size of patients who saw therapists in the top quartile of outcomes was over twice as large as the therapists in the bottom quartile (Wampold & Brown, 2005; see also Okiishi, Lambert, Nielsen, & Ogles, 2003).

Imel et al. (in press) conducted a Monte Carlo simulation study to more fully explore the expected differences in outcomes between therapists given different estimates of therapist variability. The authors assumed an average response rate of 50 percent across all patients, 30 patients per therapist, and 50 therapists. They examined differences in response rates across therapists for three different ICC values (.05, .10, .20). Outcomes (response vs. non-response) were generated for each of the 50 therapists' 30 clients, and this process was replicated 10,000 times. The average response rate and 95% confidence intervals for each of the 50 therapists for each of the ICC values are presented in Figure 6.7. Even when the ICC estimate is relatively low (.05), the difference in the response of patients to the treatment between the therapist with the best and worst outcomes is dramatic. The best therapist had a response rate of 80 percent (24 patients responded to treatment out of 30 patients) as compared to 20 percent (6 responses out of 30 patients) for the lowest performing therapist.

Imel et al.'s simulation is corroborated by a naturalistic study with a large database. Saxon and Barkham (2012) examined the outcomes of 119 therapists and 10,786 patients in the UK's National Health Service primary care counseling and psychological therapy and found that about 7 percent of the variability in outcomes was due to the therapists (equal to Baldwin & Imel's (2013) aggregate estimate for naturalistic studies), although this increased quite dramatically when the severity of the patients increased (i.e., therapists, variability in outcomes was greater when treating more severe clients). Importantly, Saxon and Barkham found that of 119 therapists in practice, 19 had outcomes that

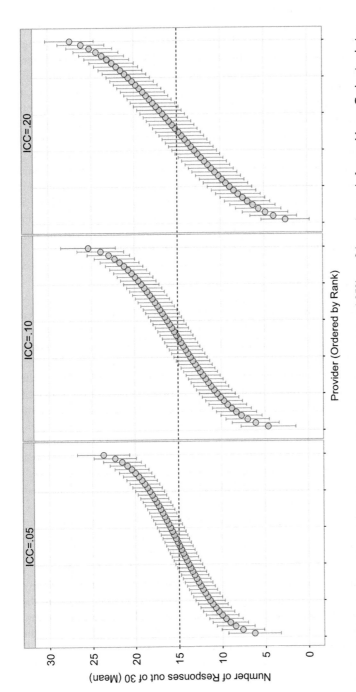

Figure 6.7 Dot plot showing variability in average therapist response rates and 95% confidence intervals from a Monte Carlo simulation (10,000 replicates) for the different ICC values. Figure generated from simulation data reported in "Removing very low-performing therapists: A simulation of performance-based retention in psychotherapy," by Z.E. Imel, E. Sheng, S.A. Baldwin, and D.C. Atkins, in press, *Psychotherapy*.

were considered "below average," and if these therapists' 1,947 patients had been seen by other therapists, an additional 265 patients would have recovered.

A case could be made that the variability of therapists in naturalistic settings is due to the fact that some therapists in such settings are providing evidence-based treatments and others are using untested or ineffective treatments. Consequently, it could be argued further that if therapists in practice were adequately trained to give an evidence-based treatment and properly supervised, then the variability among therapists would be small (Shafran et al., 2009). To investigate this issue, Laska, Smith, Wislocki, Minami, and Wampold (2013) examined therapist effects in a PTSD clinic in a Department of Veterans Affairs hospital, where all the therapists were trained by two national trainers to provide cognitive-processing therapy, an evidence-based treatment for PTSD, and were then supervised by one of the trainers. Despite this ideal situation that purportedly would minimize therapist effects, 12 percent of the variability in outcomes was due to the therapist, which is larger than the estimate for therapist effects in naturalistic settings (cf., Baldwin & Imel, 2013).

Conclusions

The essence of therapy is embodied in the therapist. Previously, we have seen that the particular treatment that the therapist delivers does not affect outcomes to a significant degree but that allegiance to the therapy was important. The results of the literature reviewed here are clear. Although some studies can be found that demonstrate therapist homogeneity, the preponderance of the evidence indicates that there are important therapist effects (in the range of 3 percent to 7 percent of the variability in outcomes accounted for by therapists, with substantial variability around these estimates). Therapist effects generally exceed treatment effects, which at most account for one percent of the variability in outcomes (see Chapter 5), as predicted by the Contextual Model. In addition, ignoring therapist effects inflates estimates of treatment effects, which suggests that importance of differences between treatments is inflated, making the importance of therapists relatively greater.

Now that we have reviewed evidence that supports the notion that some therapists consistently achieve better outcomes than others, despite the treatment provided, an important question results: What are the characteristics and actions of effective therapists? This question will be addressed in Chapters 7 and 8. There are two general classes of actions that might characterize effective therapists, those that are related to what is purported to be therapeutic in the Contextual Model, such as empathy and forming an alliance, and those that are purported to be important in the Medical Model, such as adherence to the protocol (i.e., delivering the specific ingredients) and competence at delivering the particular treatment. We will examine evidence for each of these two classes of actions in Chapters 7 and 8.

Notes

1. Here the proportion of variability due to treatment is reported using $\hat{\omega}^2$, to be consistent with Wampold & Serlin (2000). Essentially $\hat{\omega}^2$ is an unbiased estimator of R^2 discussed in Chapter 3.
2. Crits-Christoph and Mintz (1991) investigated the size of the treatment by therapist interaction effects in crossed designs in addition to the size of the therapist effect. This is important because, as discussed above, the interaction effect inflates the mean squares for treatment. They found that zero to ten percent of the variance in outcomes, as determined by aggregating the dependent measures in a study, was due to the interaction. However, when individual variables were considered, the interaction accounted for up to 38 percent of the variance. These values indicate that failing to correctly analyze crossed designs will result in liberal F tests and overestimation of treatment effects as the interaction term contained in the mean squares treatment is ignored.
3. Receiving treatment (vs. a waitlist) accounts for 14 percent of the variance in outcomes. Viewed in this context, 3 to 7 percent of variance in total outcomes appears quite important (see also Baldwin & Imel, 2013, p. 277).

Chapter 7

General Effects

Surviving Challenges and Anticipating Additional Evidence

As discussed earlier, general effects are the effects produced by the common factors. The Contextual Model posits that the common factors are therapeutic in that they are responsible for therapeutic change. Accordingly, indicators of the common factors should be associated with outcomes of psychotherapy. However, a global prediction of this sort is a weak conjecture for a number of reasons that will become apparent as we present the evidence for general effects in this chapter. Of course, one of the major challenges to the simple prediction of an association of this type is that "correlation does not mean causation," and an association may indeed be an artifact due to the fact that the outcome may well be causing the detection of the common factor, or it may be a third variable is causing both the common factor and outcome (DeRubeis, Brotman, & Gibbons, 2005). One of the characteristics of a progressive research programme, as discussed in Chapter 3, is that it responds to challenges with new conjectures that are then investigated. In this way, we will see that the Contextual Model is able to anticipate the results from studies designed to examine the challenges.

In this chapter, we focus most directly on the working alliance for several reasons. First, the alliance is a central construct in the Contextual Model—if it is not associated with outcome in a robust fashion, then the Contextual Model is, or should be, at risk for abandonment. Second, the alliance has long been theorized to be a pan-theoretical construct that is critical to the success of all treatments (Bordin, 1979). Third, there is more research on the alliance than on any other factor (Grencavage & Norcross, 1990; Norcross, 2011). Fourth, the alliance as a therapeutic factor has come under much scrutiny from adherents of the Medical Model, on a number of quite legitimate grounds (DeRubeis et al., 2005; Siev, Huppert, & Chambless, 2009). The criticisms have generated new conjectures that have been empirically examined, and a review of this research is very instructive about the progressivity of the two competing models.

A number of other general effects will be examined. Central to the Contextual Model are expectations, although unfortunately this is a difficult factor to examine within psychotherapy; here the research on placebo effects is particularly instructive, as well as what research there is on expectations and attributions in psychotherapy. Concepts related to the first pathway, real relationship, will also be reviewed, including empathy, positive regard/affirmation, congruence/ genuineness, and attempts to assess the real relationship directly.

Working Alliance

The concept of the alliance between therapist and client originated in the psychoanalytic tradition and was conceptualized as the healthy, affectionate, and trusting feelings toward the therapist, as differentiated from the neurotic component (i.e., transference) of the relationship. In the late 1970s, Ed Bordin (1979) proposed that the alliance between therapist and client was a pan-theoretical construct consisting of three components: a) agreement about the goals of therapy, b) agreement about the tasks of therapy, and c) the bond between the therapist and the client. The alliance refers to a working relationship, rather than simply an affective relationship between the two participants. Hatcher and Barends (2006) described the alliance as "the degree to which the therapy dyad is engaged in collaborative, purposive work" (p. 293) and provides the rationale for why the alliance is sometimes referred to as the "working alliance."

Over the years, there has been much confusion about the theoretical bases of the alliance (Hatcher & Barends, 2006; Horvath, 2006) and criticisms of the importance of the alliance in psychotherapy outcomes (e.g. remember Baker et al.'s 2008 observation that the alliance has a "marginal scientific status"). We first present the research evidence for the association of the alliance and outcome, including a discussion of each theoretical or methodological issue. As has been the case throughout, we give primacy to meta-analyses, although in several instances it is necessary to resort to narrative reviews of the evidence.

Association of the Alliance and Outcome

The typical design for assessing the association of alliance and outcome is quite simple. The alliance is measured some time during therapy and then correlated with an outcome assessed at the end of therapy. A variety of measures have been used to assess the strength of the alliance. This conceivably could be problematic, although a factor analysis of primary measures showed a general factor related to the collaborative relationship (Hatcher & Barends, 1996). Measures of the alliance can be completed by the client, the therapist, or observers, which could easily create some artifacts, which we address later. These studies usually measure the alliance at one or a few times, which also might influence the association between the alliance and outcome.

The evidence for the alliance-outcome association appears to be robust. The first meta-analysis of the correlation between alliance and outcome was conducted in 1991 and found an aggregate correlation of .26 for the 26 studies reviewed (Horvath & Symonds, 1991), which is a moderate-sized effect. Since then, three additional meta-analyses have been conducted (Horvath & Bedi, 2002; Horvath, Del Re, Flückiger, & Symonds, 2011b; Martin, Garske, & Davis, 2000)—the four

Table 7.1 Summary of Meta-analyses of the Correlation of Alliance and Outcome

Author (Year)	Number of Studies k	Aggregate correlation r	Equivalent d	R^2
Horvath & Symonds (1991)	26	.26	0.54	.07
Martin et al. (2000)	79	.22	0.45	.05
Horvath & Bedi (2002)	100	.21	0.43	.04
Horvath et al. (2011b)	190	.28	0.58	.08

meta-analyses are summarized in Table 7.1. For the purpose of understanding the magnitude of the alliance-outcome correlation, we will direct attention toward the latest and most comprehensive meta-analysis (viz., Horvath, Del Re, Flückiger & Symonds, 2011a, b). The 2011 meta-analysis was methodologically the most sophisticated, using a random effects model, aggregating outcome measures within studies, and using state-of-the-art methods. It is also the most comprehensive, in that 190 studies were included (involving more than 14,000 cases, see Del Re, Flückiger, Horvath, Symonds, & Wampold, 2012). Given the number of studies reviewed in the latest meta-analysis, the estimate of r = .28 is quite precise, with a 95 percent confidence interval ranging from .249 to .301. Clearly there is an association of moderate size between the alliance measured sometime during therapy and the final outcome. However, the alliance-outcome correlation appears to be attenuated by measurement issues and may be larger than meta-analytic results suggest (Crits-Christoph, Gibbons, & Hearon, 2006). It is noteworthy that the alliance is correlated with outcome in child and adolescent psychotherapy (Shirk, Karver, & Brown, 2011) and couple and family therapy (Friedlander, Escudero, Heatherington, & Diamond, 2011).

Although it is clear that the alliance is correlated with outcome, there are many threats to the conclusion that the alliance creates change, which we will discuss in some detail, beginning with more minor concerns and then addressing issues that cut to the core of the Contextual Model. Table 7.2 summarizes the evidence regarding threats to the validity of the alliance as an important factor in psychotherapy.

Methodological Issues

There are many methodological issues that are potentially problematic when considering the association of the alliance and outcome. First, it is not uncommon in these studies for the same person to rate both the alliance and the outcome, creating a "halo effect," which more technically is called method variance (correlation of two variables due to the fact that they are measured with the same method; see Cook & Campbell, 1979). This issue was addressed by Horvath et al. (2011a, b) by comparing correlations derived from the ratings

Table 7.2 Challenges to the Importance of the Alliance as a Therapeutic Factor

Threat or Clarification	Description	Evidence	Meta-analytic References
Method Variance ("Halo Effect")	Alliance and outcome rated by same person	Magnitude of correlation unaffected by whether alliance and outcome are rated by the same person	Horvath et al., 2011a, b
Alliance Rater	Perspective of rater (client, therapist, or observer) influences the magnitude of correlation	Magnitude of correlation based on client and observer rated alliance higher than therapist rated alliance, but difference not significant	Horvath et al., 2011a, b
Alliance-outcome Proximity	Measurements proximate in time (i.e., at the end of therapy) are more highly correlated	Correlation of studies that measured alliance later in therapy produced larger correlations; however, even when measured early, the alliance was moderately correlated with outcome	Horvath et al., 2011a, b Flückiger et al., 2012
Measure Used	Measurement artifact	No differences in magnitude of correlation for the various measures of the alliance	Horvath et al., 2011a, b
Publication Bias	Studies with significant results more likely to be published	No evidence of publication bias	Horvath et al., 2011a, b
Researcher Allegiance to Alliance	Researchers with an allegiance to the alliance concept will find larger alliance-outcome correlations	An interaction of allegiance and when alliance was measured was found; At earlier time points, allegiance to the alliance resulted in larger correlations	Flückiger et al., 2012

(Continued)

Table 7.2 (Continued)

Threat or Clarification	Description	Evidence	Meta-analytic References
Treatment and Disorder Specificity	Alliance more important for relational therapies (e.g., humanistic, relational dynamic therapies) than for other therapies (e.g., CBT)	No effect for treatment, CBT or not, disorder specific treatment or not, outcome was targeted symptom or not. Correlations for substance use disorders smaller than other disorders. However, there is some evidence that the alliance might work differently in different therapies	Flückiger et al., 2012 Flückiger et al., 2013
Bond not Distinct from Real Relationship	Alliance, primarily the bond, reflects simply relationship	Real relationship predicts outcome over and above alliance	None
Patient's Contribution to the Alliance	Alliance-outcome correlation due to patient's contribution to the alliance	Therapist's contribution, not the patient's contribution, predicts outcome	Del Re et al. (2012)
Prior Symptom Improvement	Early symptom improvement creates better alliances and better final outcomes	Most studies find alliance predicts outcome over and above early change, but some studies have not found this.	None
Growth of the Alliance and Tear and Repair	Strength of the alliance varies over the course of therapy; repairs of ruptures therapeutic	Repairing ruptures related to outcome	Safran et al. (2011)

by the same person (usually the client) to correlations derived from rating of different persons (e.g., the therapist rated the alliance and the client rated the outcome). Although the correlation from the same raters (viz., $r = .29$) was larger than the correlation from different raters (viz., $r = .25$), the difference was not statistically significant. Relatedly, the magnitude of the correlation was higher when the alliance was rated by the client or an observer ($r = .28$ and $.29$ respectively) than compared to when the alliance was rated by the therapist ($r = .20$). However, these differences were not statistically significant either.

A second problem is the proximity of the ratings. If the alliance is measured toward the end of therapy, then there will be a tendency for the two measures to reflect a general outcome of the case—if the case were successful then there would be a tendency to rate all aspects of the therapy positively (a variant of the "halo effect"; Crits-Christoph, Gibbons, Hamilton, Ring-Kurtz, & Gallop, 2011). The alliance effect would be much more persuasive if the alliance was measured early in therapy before much of the work of therapy has began. Horvath and colleagues examined this issue and found that indeed for the studies in which alliance was measured late in therapy (about 20 percent of the studies) correlation of the alliance with outcome was extraordinarily large ($r = .39$). However, the majority of the studies in which the alliance was measured early and the studies in which the alliance was measured mid-therapy produced significantly smaller correlations ($r = .25$ in both cases). Although proximate measurements typically yield larger correlations, making the result not surprising, the magnitude of the correlation of alliance and outcome was moderate and approximately equal to the value established for this effect. Moreover, using a longitudinal meta-analysis specifically designed to examine the effect of when alliance was measured, Flückiger, Del Re, Wampold, Symonds, and Horvath (2012) found an interaction of the time alliance was measured and researcher allegiance to the alliance concept (see discussion later in this chapter).

Another issue is that many different measures are used to assess the alliance, as mentioned previously, and that they might well measure various theoretical aspects of the alliance. However, Horvath et al. (2011a, b) found that the particular alliance measure had no effect on the magnitude of the correlation. Another methodological issue is publication bias, which is the effect on meta-analyses as a result of under-publication of research with null results (Sutton, 2009). Horvath et al. addressed this issue in several ways, including a) searching literature in English, German, Italian, and French; b) searching theses and book chapters as well as journal articles; c) calculating the fail-safe N (the number of studies with null finding that would be needed to change the conclusion, which in this case was more than 1,000); and d) examining the funnel plot to detect publication bias. There was no evidence that publication bias affected the results.

The final methodological threat is the allegiance of the researcher. Recall that in terms of efficacy of treatment, researcher allegiance to the treatment being delivered influenced the efficacy of the favored treatment (see Chapter 5); the same phenomenon may be true in terms of the alliance as well because some researchers are affiliated with the alliance as an important therapeutic factor. As mentioned above, Flückiger et al. (2012) did indeed find an interaction between allegiance and the time when the alliance was measured. At the earliest time point, researchers with an allegiance to the alliance reported larger correlations than those without an allegiance; however, the magnitude of the correlation was in excess of .20 for those *without* an allegiance when the alliance was measured early in therapy.

It appears that methodological issues do not threaten the conclusion that the alliance is an important factor in psychotherapy outcome. However, there are more severe and substantive threats to identifying alliance as an important therapeutic factor, which are addressed in the following sections.

Treatment Specificity and the Alliance: Alliance as an Active Ingredient, Clarification of the Bond in the Alliance, and Direct/Indirect Effects

An important question is whether the alliance is an important factor in some treatments but not in others. According to Siev et al. (2009), some therapies emphasize the alliance as a therapeutic tool, raising it to the level of a specific ingredient for that therapy:

> Overall, alliance may have the greatest relationship to outcome if the therapist makes it a central focus of treatment. However, in such treatments, the distinction between alliance and technique is blurred. As others have noted (Beutler, 2002; Crits-Christoph et al., 2006), if one addresses alliance directly in treatment sessions, the very focus on alliance becomes a treatment technique.
>
> (p. 74)

This is an observation that reasonably applies to most humanistic therapies, relational psychodynamic therapies, and hybrid treatments such as motivational interviewing (e.g., a cognitive behavioral therapy with humanistic roots), although clearly the Contextual Model suggests that the alliance is important for treatments that do not focus on the relationship through the mechanisms discussed previously. However, in contrast to Siev et al.'s prediction, in their meta-analysis, Horvath et al. (2011a, b) found no differences in the magnitude of the alliance-outcome correlation among CBT, interpersonal therapy, dynamic therapy, and substance abuse treatments, although there is some question about how the alliance functions in the treatment for patients with substance-use problems (see the following). Flückiger et al. (2012), using the same data set, examined this and some related issues in greater depth by examining whether the research was conducted in the context of an RCT, whether the treatment was guided by a manual for a specific disorder, whether the treatment was CBT or not, and whether the outcome variable was a symptom measure or not. If indeed the alliance was less important in treatments that used specific ingredients (other than the alliance) to address particular deficits, then it would be expected that one or more of these factors would have an effect on the magnitude of the alliance-outcome correlation. However, none of these factors moderated the size of the alliance-outcome correlation.

There is some evidence that the treatment of substance-use disorders has a smaller alliance-outcome correlation than treatments for other disorders ($r = .18$ for substance-use disorders compared to, e.g., depression $r = .34$ and anxiety $r = .31$; Flückiger et al., 2013). However, in this sample of studies, the substance-use disorder variable was associated with higher proportions of racial and ethnic minority patients, confusing the interpretations of the role of the alliance in substance-use disorders. In addition, factors such as therapist empathy are central (and may be considered specific ingredients) to primary treatments for substance abuse disorders (i.e., motivational interviewing), and thus it is unlikely that the working alliance is unimportant in substance treatment (see e.g., Moyers, Miller, & Hendrickson, 2005).

The meta-analyses of the alliance for different treatments may not fully capture the complexity of how the alliance works for different treatments. Bordin (1979), when he proposed the alliance as a pan-theoretical construct, recognized that while crucial to all therapies, the bond might work in different ways in different kinds of treatment: "Different approaches to psychotherapy are marked by the difference in the demands they make on patient and therapist. . . . One bond may not be necessarily stronger than the other, but they do differ in kind" (p. 253, 254). Hatcher and Barends (2006) were more explicit:

> Successful collaboration is based on a level of trust and attachment (bond) that is commensurate with the task. This assumption implies that the level of bond required to engage successfully in treatment will vary across therapy approaches depending on the degree of personal involvement expected of the client.
>
> (p. 293)

It seems that these theorists are focusing on differences in how the bond works in therapy, and there is at least one study that addressed this directly. It appears that avoidance of affect in psychodynamic treatments suppressed the bond and negatively influenced the outcome of therapy whereas in cognitive therapy avoidance of affect was positively related to the bond and to outcome (Ulvenes et al., 2012). In psychodynamic therapy, where engaging with difficult material is endemic to the treatment, often with affective arousal, requiring a strong bond with the therapist, exemplified by trust in the therapist personally and trust that engaging in this difficult work will be therapeutic, is necessary. Bordin referred to this early on:

> For example, the kind of bond developed when a therapist gives a patient a form and asks him to make a daily record of his submissive and assertive acts and of the circumstances surrounding them, appears quite different

from the bond developed when a therapist shares his or her feelings with a patient, in order to provide a model, or to provide feedback on the patient's impact on others.

(1979, p. 254)

This point was reiterated by Hatcher and Barends (2006): "This . . . implies that the level of bond required to engage successfully in treatment will vary across therapy approaches depending on the degree of personal involvement expected of the client" (p. 254).

The discussion of the bond in different therapies brings up a thorny theoretical issue and one about which there is scant, but emerging, evidence. Bordin (1979) referred to two kinds of bonds, the first kind involving affective attachment involving liking, trust, and respect, and a second kind referring to the bond required to do the difficult work of therapy, whether it be dealing with difficult affective material or participating in prolonged exposure. Hatcher and Barends (2006) make the distinction clear:

It is possible to like and admire someone who is nevertheless not working with you effectively (Hatcher & Barends, 1996). Bordin's second concept views the bond as supporting the therapy's goals and tasks, and so is perhaps better named the "work-supporting bond." The question is not "Do you like and respect your therapist?" but rather "Do you like and respect your therapist enough to do the work you expect to do in your therapy?" and "Does your therapist respect and appreciate you enough to permit you to work effectively in therapy?"

(p. 296)

The distinction is important for the Contextual Model, as the former appears to be what Gelso (2014) call the real relationship, which is defined as "the personal relationship between therapist and patient marked by the extent to which each is genuine with the other and perceives/experiences the other in ways that befit the other" (p. 3) and the latter a "work-supporting bond" (Hatcher & Barends, 2006, p. 296), which is part of the alliance and operates to create change through the second two pathways of the Contextual Model. Interestingly, measures of the real relationship predict outcome over and above measures of the alliance (Gelso, 2014), indicating that there is some evidence that the real relationship and the alliance are distinct constructs, although more work is needed in this regard.

As well, in cognitive therapy for depression, there is some evidence that the strength of the collaborative bond is not related to outcome, but rather it is agreement about the tasks and goals of therapy that seem to be important (Webb et al., 2011); for exposure treatments for PTSD it also appears that the task component of the alliance is important (Hoffart, Øktedalen, Langkaas, & Wampold, 2013). These findings are understandable by examining the pathways in the Contextual Model, where CBT is focused on therapeutic activities and is very explicit about the rationale for the treatment, which emphasize two pathways, expectations and specific ingredients, with particular emphasis on the participation in the specific ingredients. For these two pathways, agreement about the goals of therapy and the tasks of therapy are particularly salient. Indeed, as emphasized by Hatcher and Barends (2006), "Alliance cannot happen without techniques. . . . If technique fails to engage the client in purposive work, technique is not working properly, and changes must be made as to engage the client effectively" (p. 294).

The manner in which the alliance and specific ingredients work together is unclear at this point in time. Moreover, research examining this question is difficult to conduct. A notable exception is a study by Barber et al. (2006), who examined the interactions of adherence, competence, and alliance in 95 patients receiving an evidence-based cocaine treatment and found complex results. When the alliance was particularly strong, adherence to the treatment model was not predictive of outcome. However, when the alliance was weaker, a moderate level of adherence, as opposed to either a low level or a high level of adherence, was predictive of outcome. One interpretation is that the alliance may be sufficient for improvement despite the absence of specific ingredients if it is exceptionally strong, but the flexible use of the treatment is needed otherwise (see also Owen & Hilsenroth, 2014), an interpretation not incompatible with the Contextual Model. However, because the alliance in substance-use treatments is not as highly related to outcome as it is in treatments for other disorders, and because this result has not been replicated, conclusions from this study should be considered tentative. These issues are reminiscent of Horvath's (2006) distinction between the alliance as "active ingredient" and as "facilitative ingredient" (see p. 259). In some ways, the use of the term "active ingredient" is reminiscent of Siev et al. (2009) in that it conveys that the alliance acts directly to produce benefits, although the mechanism involved is somewhat mysterious (although, as Siev suggests, it is explicit in some therapies, e.g., Safran & Muran, 2000). In the Contextual Model, the alliance exerts its direct influence through the mechanism related to expectations, discussed later in this chapter (pathway two of the Contextual Model). Horvath's "facilitative ingredient" refers to idea that the alliance is need as a foundation to allow the use of specific ingredients, which then are beneficial (pathway three of the Contextual Model). Nevertheless, the two pathways interact, as it is not possible to have agreement about tasks and goals without specific ingredients. Clearly, investigating the relationship of alliance and specific ingredients is difficult due to the complexity of the phenomenon.

Patient and Therapist Contributions to the Alliance

Descriptions of the alliance emphasize the collaboration between the therapist and the patient and consequently alliance is a dyadic phenomenon, even when it is rated by one of the participants. Nevertheless, both patient and therapist contribute to the development of the alliance. It may well be that it is the patient's contribution to the alliance that is important for therapeutic change.

Some patients come to therapy motivated (ready for change in Prochaska and Norcross's model, see Prochaska & Norcross, 2002) and have relatively developed interpersonal skills, functional attachment styles, adequate social support, and sufficient economic resources. Such patients will likely be able to form a working alliance with any reasonably competent therapist and will benefit from therapy. On the other hand, patients who have dysfunctional attachment styles (say, with borderline personality disorder features), have little social support, live with economic deprivation, and are not ready to make changes will have difficulty forming an alliance with their therapist and will also have a poor prognosis. Consequently, if this is true there would be an alliance-outcome correlation, but both the alliance and outcome would be a consequence of patient characteristics, rather than something the therapist provides to the patient. Such a case would be contrary to the Contextual Model, as the focus there is on therapeutic conditions provided by the therapist, as pointed out by DeRubeis et al. (2005).

An alternative view is that it is the therapist who facilitates formation of the alliance. It is the therapist's contribution to the collaborative working relationship that is important for outcome. According to this view, more effective therapists would be those who were able to form strong alliances across the range of patients relative to less effective therapists, a result that would be consistent with the Contextual Model.

The meta-analyses of the alliance-outcome correlations reviewed so far have aggregated the correlations of alliance and outcome disregarding the fact that patients in psychotherapy are nested within therapists (see Chapter 6). That is, the alliance-outcome is a "total" correlation that contains, in a sense, correlations due to the patient and contributions due to the therapists. This total correlation may be due entirely, largely, or to some extent to the patient's contribution to the alliance. On the other hand, the total correlation may be mostly due to the influence of the therapist. The conjecture that the alliance-outcome correlation largely will be due to the patient's contribution to the alliance is a threat to "nonspecific" factors, forming a protective belt, in Lakatosian terms, for the Medical Model; on the other hand, the Contextual Model, when confronted with this criticism, would predict that the total alliance-outcome correlation would be due to a large extent to the therapist's contribution to the alliance.

Investigating patients' and therapists' contribution to the alliance involved using multilevel modeling techniques to account for the nesting of patients within therapists. Such methods allow for examining the correlation of the alliance and outcome within therapists (i.e., the patient's contribution, expressed as a within therapist regression coefficient pooled over all therapists) as well as the correlation of the therapist's average alliance over all of his or her patients and outcomes (i.e., the therapist's contribution, expressed as a between therapist regression coefficient). Recently, Baldwin, Wampold, and Imel (2007) examined the alliance and outcome of 80 therapists and 331 patients to examine the within-therapist and between-therapist coefficients. The outcome measure was the Outcome Questionnaire 45 (OQ; Lambert, Gregersen, & Burlingame,

2004, lower scores indicate better psychological functioning) and alliance was measured early in therapy (viz., fourth session with the Working Alliance Inventory, WAI; Horvath & Greenberg, 1989).

Baldwin et al. (2007), using multilevel models with the pretreatment OQ score as a covariate in all models, found that about 3 percent of the variability in outcomes was due to the therapist, which is slightly smaller than the average therapist effect in naturalistic settings (see Chapter 6). The total alliance-outcome correlation with post-treatment OQ was −.24, which is approximately equal to the value found in the meta-analyses discussed earlier in this chapter for early assessments of the alliance (the effect was negative becuause of lower scores on the OQ indicate better psychological functioning). The results of the multilevel regression analysis are illustrated in Figure 7.1. As is clear

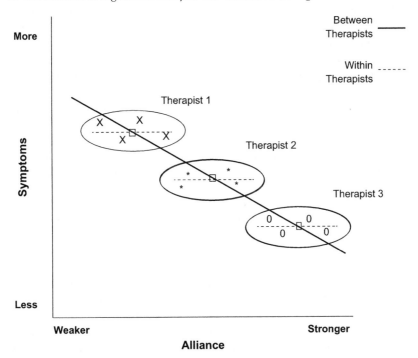

Figure 7.1   An illustration of the within- and between-therapist alliance-outcome correlations. Within- and between-therapist correlations are illustrated with only three therapists using simulated data to aid in the presentation of the correlations. The Xs refer to the alliance scores for Therapist 1's patients; the asterisks refer to the alliance scores of Therapist 2's patients; open circles refer to the alliance scores of Therapist 3's patients; open squares refer to each therapist's mean alliance score. Reprinted from "Untangling the alliance-outcome correlation: Exploring the relative importance of therapist and patient variability in the alliance," by S.A. Baldwin, B.E. Wampold, and Z.E. Imel, 2007, Journal of Consulting and Clinical Psychology, 75, p. 847. Copyright 2007 by the American Psychological Association. Reprinted with permission.

from the figure, the better therapist (viz., Therapist 3) generally had stronger alliances with his or her patients and had better outcomes, in comparison to the other therapists (say, Therapist 1). The regression coefficient for the between-therapist effect was −0.33, which was statistically significant, indicating that therapists contributed to the alliance-outcome correlation, as anticipated by the Contextual Model. After entering the therapist's contribution to the alliance, variability in outcomes due to therapist was essentially zero, indicating that the differences among therapists in terms of outcome was due to their ability to form alliances with their patients—therapists who form better alliances with a range of patients get better outcomes. This is evidence that relates to the question: What are the characteristics and actions of effective therapists? And it turns out that one of the answers to this question centers on the alliance, a key construct in the Contextual Model.

The results for the patient's contribution to the alliance are more difficult to explain. As illustrated in Figure 7.1, the regression line within therapists is horizontal, indicating that there is no relationship between the patient's contribution to the alliance and outcome (actually, the coefficient was −0.08, very small and non-significant). Some patients come to therapy better able to form relationships in general and report better alliances with a particular therapist than other patients of the same therapist, but these patients do not have better outcomes than the other patients of the same therapist. As an example, consider a difficult patient with chaotic interpersonal relationships, who has difficulty trusting others, including the therapist. This patient will have a relatively poor alliance with Therapist X relative to other patients of Therapist X. Yet, if Therapist X (e.g., Therapist 3 in Figure 7.1) is able to form strong alliances with a range of patients, then this patient's alliance is stronger *than it would have been with another less skilled therapist* and consequently would have a better outcome with Therapist X than with another therapist. For this patient, even though the alliance was fairly low for that therapist, it may have been one of the few persons with whom the patient has ever been able to form a strong alliance. As well, the magnitude of the therapist's contribution to the alliance-outcome (−0.33) was significantly greater than the patient's contribution (−0.08).

The results of Baldwin et al. (2007) were anticipated by the Contextual Model and were contrary to attempts to nullify the importance of the alliance. Nevertheless, as we know from the various reconstructions of science, and particularly Lakatos, a single study should not lead to abandonment of a theoretical perspective. Nevertheless, the importance of the therapist contribution to the alliance has been replicated several times (Crits-Christoph et al., 2009; Dinger, Strack, Leichsenring, Wilmers, & Schauenburg, 2008; Zuroff, Kelly, Leybman, Blatt, & Wampold, 2010), although not always (Falkenström, Granström, & Holmqvist, 2014). Importantly there is a meta-analytic result that supports Baldwin et al.'s conclusions. The correlations reported in the primary studies of the meta-analyses of alliance and outcome report only the total correlation. However, Del Re et al. (2012) observed that the ratio of patients to therapists (PTR) varied greatly. When the PTR is large (many patients per therapist), then most of the alliance is due to the patient, whereas when PTR equals one, the variability in the alliance is due to the therapist. As expected if Baldwin et al.'s results hold, then PTR should be associated with the size of the total correlation reported in each primary study: the larger the PTR, the smaller the total correlation. The expected association was found, was not due to various other moderators that posed confounds, and quantitatively the estimates produced by the meta-analysis were approximately equal to Baldwin et al.'s results (Del Re et al., 2012).

Early Symptom Change Creates Better Alliance and Better Final Outcome

DeRubeis et al. (2005) raised the possibility that early symptom change may cause both the rating of the alliance and the later outcome of psychotherapy. It is possible that the patient makes particularly commendable progress early in therapy, which creates a positive view of therapy and the therapist by both the patient and the therapist, resulting in a strong working alliance, but the factors that induced the early change, and not the alliance, create additional benefits. This is a complex phenomenon to investigate, but nearly 20 studies have used a variety of statistical methods to control for symptom reduction before the alliance is measured to assess whether the alliance predicts the progress of therapy accounting for the effects of the early change. Most of these studies, conducted by researchers of disparate perspectives, have concluded that indeed the alliance is predictive of outcome over and above what is due to the early symptom change (Arnow et al., 2013; Baldwin et al., 2007; Barber, Connolly, Crits-Christoph, Gladis, & Siqueland, 2009; Crits-Christoph et al., 2011; De Bolle, Johnson, & De Fruyt, 2010; Falkenström, Granström, & Holmqvist, 2013; Falkenström et al., 2014; Flückiger, Holtforth, Znoj, Caspar, & Wampold, 2013; Gaston, Marmar, Gallagher, & Thompson, 1991; Hoffart et al., 2013; Klein et al., 2003; Tasca & Lampard, 2012; Zuroff & Blatt, 2006), although a few have found this not to be so (DeRubeis & Feeley, 1990; Feeley, DeRubeis, & Gelfand, 1999; Puschner, Wolf, & Kraft, 2008; Strunk, Brotman, & DeRubeis, 2010; Strunk, Cooper, Ryan, DeRubeis, & Hollon, 2012). Unfortunately, there have been no meta-analytic studies to address this issue, and conducting such a meta-analysis would be difficult given the variety of statistical methods used to investigate how early progress and alliance function to produce final change. It is beyond the scope of this chapter to review all these studies, but one study (viz., Falkenström et al., 2014), which used particularly sophisticated methods with an adequate sample, is discussed).

Falkenström et al. (2014) used a naturalistic setting involving 719 patients treated by 69 therapists in the context of primary care in Sweden for problems related to, for the most part, anxiety, relationships, depression, grief, work-related issues, and somatic complaints. The alliance scores at the third session were used as well as weekly measures of psychological functioning using the Clinical Outcomes in Route Evaluation Outcome Measure (CORE-OM). The authors used a piecewise longitudinal model that included the intercept and the slope of the CORE-OM prior to the alliance measurement as well as the slope of the CORE-OM after the alliance was measured. As suggested by DeRubeis et al.

(2005), initial distress and early change predicted the alliance scores at session three: less initial distress and greater change were associated with better alliances. The goal of the analyses however was to predict patient progress after the alliance was measured, controlling for various factors, including a) association of initial distress and session 3 alliance, b) association of prior progress and session 3 alliance, c) the association of early progress (before session 3) and progress after session 3, d) association of initial distress and progress after session 3, and e) therapist variability in rates of change before and after the alliance was measured and in the alliance scores. After controlling all of these possible influences on the rate of change, alliance at session 3 predicted improvement after the session 3, suggestion that the alliance is not simply an artifact of early change.

Although the evidence related to the issue of prior symptom change leading to higher ratings of the alliance and improved outcomes is not definitive, there is insufficient evidence to discount the importance of the alliance as a therapeutic factor on this basis.

Growth of the Alliance Over the Course of Therapy

The final aspect of the alliance to be considered is related to the growth of the alliance over the course of therapy. For much of the research reviewed, the alliance measured was conceptualized as reflective of the collaboration of the therapist and the client in therapy without considering that the alliance may well fluctuate during the course of therapy, depending on various aspects of therapy or because of external events (e.g., infidelity of the client's spouse may result in a general decrease in trust). Horvath (2006) cautioned against considering the alliance to be static (see Gelso & Carter, 1994, for how the alliance and other aspects of the relationship may unfold during therapy). Nevertheless, there has been little research examining the growth of the alliance over the course of therapy.

One notable exception to the tendency to ignore changes in the alliance involves research on ruptures in the alliance and their repair (often referred to as "tear and repair," see Safran & Muran, 2000). According to this psychodynamic model, participating in the difficult work of therapy puts strains on the alliance, particularly the bond, and one of the tasks of therapy is to address and repair some the ruptures that will naturally occur. According to this view, such strains occur not only in therapy, so the repair is also a corrective experience for the patient. Safran, Muran, and Eubanks-Carter (2011) meta-analyzed studies that examined the extent to which ruptures were repaired in relationship to outcome and found an aggregate correlation of .24, which was significantly greater than zero. However, this evidence should be considered in light of the difficulty in measuring ruptures and repairs and given that this concept has not yet survived the scrutiny that has been paid to the alliance in general. Nevertheless, this result buttresses the idea that the alliance is an important factor in psychotherapy.

Researchers are beginning to attend to the growth of the alliance and how it is related to the outcome of therapy. Advances in longitudinal methods now allow for disaggregating between-client variability and within-client variability over time (Curran & Bauer, 2011). With regard to the alliance, between-client variability is the relative standing of the alliance for a client relative to other clients (either all other clients or within a given therapist—see Baldwin et al., 2007). In the studies reviewed to this point, the correlations of alliance and outcome have been based on between-client variability in the alliance—clients who have a stronger alliance with their therapist relative to other clients have better outcomes in the basic design. As many clinicians understand, it is changes that the client makes during therapy that are important. For example, a client who has had a tenuous working relationship with his or her therapist might begin to trust the therapist at some point in therapy, which is then followed by treatment gains. Thus, within-client variability in the alliance may well be critical to understanding how the alliance works in therapy. Of course, this variability also may be related to rupture and repair, although the methods discussed in this section have not yet been applied to the "tear and repair" area yet.

There is evidence that different alliance patterns are associated with outcome. An early study used cluster analysis to identify three patterns: stable alliance, linear alliance growth, and quadratic alliance growth (high, followed by low, returning to high alliance; Kivlighan & Shaughnessy, 2000). As hypothesized by Gelso and Carter (1994) and consistent with the "tear and repair" conjecture, quadratic alliance growth was related to client improvement. However, the nature of the relationship between alliance and symptoms over time can only be examined when both alliance and symptoms are measured regularly. Tasca and Lampard (2012), in a day-treatment program for eating disorders, measured weekly the alliance to the group as well as the urge to restrict. They detected a reciprocal effect where growth in the alliance predicted a subsequent reduction in the urge to restrict. In addition, reduction in the urge to restrict predicted a subsequent improvement in the alliance. Falkenström et al. (2013), using the same data set for the between-client analysis discussed above (viz., Falkenström et al., 2014), found that alliance predicted subsequent symptom change and that prior symptom change predicted alliance. Hoffart et al. (2013) examined the alliance and symptoms measured weekly in two treatments for PTSD. They found that when the task component of the alliance was greater than expected for a given client, subsequent symptoms were reduced. However, they did not find the reciprocal pattern—when a given client's symptoms improved, subsequent alliance for that client did not strengthen.

The evidence from these recent studies that have examined within-client fluctuations in the alliance indicate that when the alliance is stronger than usual for a given client, a reduction in symptoms will follow; there is some evidence for reciprocal influence of symptoms on the alliance. It appears that the within-client perspective provides evidence that the influence of alliance on outcome is not an artifact.

Conclusions—The Importance of the Alliance Established

Meta-analyses since the 1990s have indicated a robust moderate correlation between the alliance and outcome. However, a number of challenges to the importance of the alliance have been raised, which has given rise to additional research. A hallmark of a progressive research programme is that challenges create new conjectures. As the evidence has accumulated, the predictions of the Contextual Model have been consistent with observations. More sophisticated methods have allowed for unpacking how the alliance works in psychotherapy, and in each instance there is insufficient evidence to support the challenges.

As discussed in this chapter (and Chapter 2), the alliance is a collaborative working relationship and as such creates benefits through the collaborative work. That is, the alliance, with a possible exception of the bond, is not directly therapeutic. Agreement on the goals and tasks of therapy are needed to ensure that collaborative work proceeds in therapy. In the later stages of therapy, the alliance is likely a reflection that therapeutic work has been proceeding. One of the primary consequences of the alliance is the creation of expectations, which is now discussed.

Expectations, Placebos, and Attributions

The second pathway of the Contextual Model, as discussed in Chapter 2, proposes that acceptance of an explanation for one's disorder and agreement about the actions needed to overcome one's difficulties creates expectations that have a powerful and direct influence on subjective experiences (e.g., emotions and cognitions; see Kirsch, 1985) In this section, evidence is presented to support this notion, with an emphasis on research on placebos but also the available research on expectations in psychotherapy.

Placebos

As discussed in Chapter 1, the placebo has had a long and controversial history in medicine and psychotherapy, with regard to its definition, the effects that it produces, and the research designs that are employed to understand it (Shapiro & Shapiro, 1997a, b). In 1955, Beecher reviewed 15 studies and estimated that in clinical practice placebos lead to significant improvement in approximately one-third of cases for outcomes that were subjective. Despite the nefarious reputation of placebos, the title of Beecher's article "The Powerful Placebo" was generally accepted as truth until it was challenged by the results of a meta-analysis entitled "Is the Placebo Powerless?" (Hróbjartsson & Gøtzsche, 2001). Despite this controversy, which will be reviewed in the following, the effect of placebos constitutes a research field in itself, spanning the areas of medicine, psychology, anthropology, and neuroscience. In this chapter, we present an abbreviated review, but the literature on placebos has been reviewed extensively elsewhere (e.g., Benedetti, 2009, 2011; Guess, Kleinman, Kusek, & Engel, 2002; Harrington, 1997; Price, Finniss, & Benedetti, 2008; Shapiro & Shapiro, 1997a, b).

Placebo Effects in Medicine

As mentioned above, Beecher's (1955) conclusions about the clinical effectiveness of placebos were challenged by Hróbjartsson and Gøtzsche (2001). Hróbjartsson and Gøtzsche reviewed clinical trials in which patients were randomly

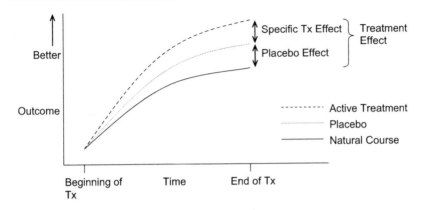

Figure 7.2 Additive model for placebo effects. Reprinted from "The placebo is powerful: Estimating placebo effects in medicine and psychotherapy from clinical
trials," by B.E. Wampold, T. Minami, S.C. Tierney, T.W. Baskin, and K.S. Bhati,
2005, *Journal of Clinical Psychology, 61*, p. 838. Copyright 2005 by John Wiley
and Sons. Reprinted with permission.

assigned to a placebo condition or to a no treatment condition. Placebos were
varied, including pharmacologies (e.g., pill), physical (e.g., manipulation), or
psychological (e.g., psychotherapy). Effects of the placebo were assessed by
comparing the placebo condition to the no treatment condition.

To understand the results of this meta-analysis it is important to understand
the various effects due to treatments, placebos, and natural course of the disorder, as shown in Figure 7.2. In this illustration, the natural course of the
disorder is toward improvement, although that need not be the case, as some
disorders are naturally deteriorating (e.g., cancer) or stable (e.g., some forms of
arthritis). A critically important effect in medicine is the specific effect—the difference between the active treatment and the placebo at the end of treatment.
This is the effect that is necessary for the approval of a drug by the Food and
Drug Administration (FDA). The validity of this effect depends on the treatment and placebo being indistinguishable and the double blinding of the treatments, two conditions that are not present in psychotherapy trials (Wampold,
Minami, Tierney, Baskin, & Bhati, 2005). The placebo effect is the difference
between the placebo and the natural course of the disorder. Hróbjartsson and
Gøtzsche (2001) estimated the placebo effect by estimating the effect from comparisons of placebo to no treatment.[1]

Based on 114 studies, Hróbjartsson and Gøtzsche (2001) concluded basically
that the placebo was "powerless." They analyzed the primary "objective" or
"subjective" outcome for each study, preferring binary outcomes (e.g., smoking or not) over continuous outcomes. They found that for studies with binary
outcomes (e.g., mortality or recovered), there were no statistically significant
placebo effects. Nevertheless, there was a small but significant placebo effect for

studies with continuous outcomes (d = 0.28), larger for "subjective" outcomes (d = 0.36) than for "objective" outcomes (a difference of d = 0.12, which was not statistically significant). The effect was largest for pain (d = 0.27). Based on these results, they stated, "In conclusion, we found little evidence that placebos in general have powerful clinical effects" (p. 1599).

Because Hróbjartsson and Gøtzsche's (2001) results were contrary to what was commonly accepted as truth, their evidence was challenged. Vase, Riley, and Price (2002) noted that the objective of the trials reviewed by Hróbjartsson and Gøtzsche was to show the efficacy of the active treatment and, therefore, not optimally designed to detect a placebo effect. Of particular importance, according to Vase et al., is the instruction given to the patients in these trials, as they are told that they may or may not, depending on randomization, receive a placebo—that is, there is a 50 percent chance they were not getting the active medication. However, in studies designed to test the mechanisms of placebos, subjects are often led to believe they are receiving a substance that has potent ingredients, and then their response can be compared to subjects who do not receive the substance. In a meta-analysis of 23 clinical trials that used placebo as a control for analgesic medications and 14 studies that investigated placebo analgesic mechanisms, using pain intensity ratings only, Vase et al. (2002) found that the effect size for the clinical studies was quite small (d = 0.15) compared to the effects for the mechanism studies (d = 0.95).

Hróbjartsson and Gøtzsche (2006) found several errors in Vase et al.'s coding and analysis and severely criticized their conclusions. However, Hróbjartsson and Gøtzsche (2006) did report that even after correcting for these errors, the mechanism studies produced considerably larger effects (d = 0.51 than did the clinical trials not investigating mechanisms (d = .19).

Wampold and colleagues (2005) also criticized Hróbjartsson and Gøtzsche (2001) on a number of grounds. Consistent with Vase et al. (2002), Wampold et al. contented that many of the trials included in Hróbjartsson and Gøtzsche (2001; also see update, Hróbjartsson & Gøtzsche, 2004) were not well designed to detect a placebo effect. For example, one trial in the 2004 update compared the analgesic effects of various treatments (viz., injection of glucose or sucrose, pacifier, and combination of injection and pacifier), a placebo (viz., injection of sterile water), and no treatment for pain in neonates (Carbajal, Chauvet, Couderc, & Oliver-Martin, 1999)—no extant theory of placebo action would predict that an injection of sterile water would have an effect in neonates. Wampold et al. reanalyzed the trials included in Hróbjartsson and Gøtzsche but considered critical variables that would moderate the placebo conditions. First, disorders being treated were classified based on their amenability to the placebo effect, relying on Papakostas and Daras's (2001) criteria: "Generally, the presence of anxiety and pain, the involvement of the autonomic nervous system, and the immunobiochemical processes are believed to respond favorably to placebo, whereas hyperacute illnesses (i.e., heart attack), chronic degenerative diseases, or hereditary diseases are expected to resist" (pp. 1620–1621).

Second, building on Vase et al. (2002), Wampold et al. examined research designs to determine whether the design disadvantaged the placebo treatment or not. Third, the size of the placebo effect was compared to the size of the treatment effect to determine the degree to which the treatment is due to the placebo, assuming the effects are additive (see Figure 7.2). Finally, measures were defined as subjective if they relied on the report of the patient (nb., Hróbjartsson and Gøtzsche did not define "subjective" and "objective") and the difference in effects between subjective and objective measures was compared *within* studies only, to be able to rule out various between-study confounds.

The results of Wampold et al.'s (2005) reanalysis generally demonstrated the placebo effects were detected when they were expected. When the disorder was amenable to placebo and the design was adequate, the placebo effect was significantly greater than zero (d = 0.29). As predicted, as the amenability to placebo decreased, the size of the placebo effect decreased. Finally, there were no differences in the magnitude of the placebo effect for subjective and objective measures. Most interestingly, the placebo effect (d = 0.29), when the disorder was amenable to placebo and the design was adequate, was comparable to (actually slightly larger than) the treatment effect (d = 0.24), implying that the effect of treatment was completely due to the placebo (again, assuming additivity). Not surprisingly, Hróbjartsson and Gøtzsche found fault with the reanalysis and a lively debate ensued (Hróbjartsson & Gøtzsche, 2007a, b; Hunsley & Westmacott, 2007; Wampold, Imel, & Minami, 2007a, b). A careful reading of this debate will require the historical perspective that the placebo is an anathema to modern medicine and indeed to the Medical Model of psychotherapy.[2]

We now turn to evidence about one of the most widely used medical practices, antidepressants. Approximately 270 million prescriptions are written each year for antidepressant medications, generating $12 billion in sales in 2008, although gross sales receipts are declining as antidepressants patents expire and generics become available. To be approved by the FDA, each antidepressant must have demonstrated separation from a placebo (i.e., a statistically significant specific effect, as illustrated in Figure 7.2) in two clinical trials.[3] A number of antidepressants have been approved over the years based on this separation, but a major issue is that there may well be many trials that do not show a superiority of the antidepressant, but these results are irrelevant as far as the FDA is concerned. Moreover, the FDA is concerned with the primary measure of depression, typically the clinician-rated Hamilton Rating Scale for Depression (HRSD), and ignores measures rated by the patient, including, for example, quality-of-life measures (Spielmans & Kirsch, in press). Over the years, Irving Kirsch and colleagues, through Freedom of Information Act requests, have obtained data from published and unpublished trials to examine the treatment and placebo effects (Kirsch, 2002, 2009; Kirsch et al., 2008; Kirsch, Moore, Scoboria, & Nicholls, 2002; Kirsch & Sapirstein, 1998; Kirsch, Scoboria, & Moore, 2002), the results of which are discussed in an indictment of antidepressants entitled *The Emperor's New Drugs: Exploding the Antidepressant*

Myth (Kirsch, 2010). The interest here is not on the controversy about the use of the antidepressants but rather on the effects of a pill placebo for depression. The results of the most recent meta-analysis of antidepressants will be briefly discussed here.

Kirsch and colleagues (Kirsch et al., 2008) obtained data from clinical trials investigating the effectiveness of four new-generation antidepressants submitted to the FDA. Because the FDA, as part of the licensing process, requires that drug companies report all controlled trials, whether or not the results are published (Spielmans & Kirsch, in press), these data were not influenced by publication bias. Because these trials did not contain no-treatment controls, comparisons involved the effects from before treatment to end of treatment for the placebo condition and for the treatment conditions. The weighted mean improvement on the HRSD in the antidepressant and the placebo conditions were 9.60 and 7.80, respectively; that is, the effect of the placebo was greater than 80 percent of the change in the drug condition. In terms of effect sizes, the pre- to post-effect size for the drug conditions was 1.24 and for the placebo was 0.92, a difference of 0.32. These trials when aggregated show a superiority of antidepressants to placebo—a debate can be made about whether the separation is clinically meaningful, particularly given the side effects of antidepressants (Kirsch, 2002, 2009, 2010; Kirsch et al., 2002; Spielmans & Kirsch, in press). However, it is also clear that pill placebos have a powerful influence on depression. For the purposes of the Contextual Model, this suggests that generating an expectation of improvement, providing a (biological) explanation and related actions (take a pill—albeit a chemically inert pill), and having a relationship with a provider who listens empathically results in an improvement in mental health that approaches the efficacy of the standard medical treatment for depression.

The final illustration of the placebo effect is from a meta-analysis of the association of patient adherence to a drug treatment and mortality (Simpson et al., 2006). Because about one in four patients do not adhere to the treatment protocol, it is important to examine outcomes for patients who are adherent and who are not adherent. The results for the eight trials that contained placebo conditions are presented here; in six of the trials, the treatment was effective (i.e., drug was more effective than the placebo) and in two of the trials the treatment was harmful (drug was less effective than placebo). The conditions examined in these trials were either cardiac conditions or diabetes, conditions not generally considered amenable to placebos; moreover, the outcome (mortality) is generally thought to be an objective measure and not influenced by patient self-report.

The results of this meta-analysis are shown in Figure 7.3. Not surprisingly for beneficial drugs, the mortality rate for patients who adhered to the treatment protocol was lower than for patients who did not adhere to the protocol. However, a similar reduction in mortality was observed for patients who adhered to the placebo, although the drug, as reflective of the classification

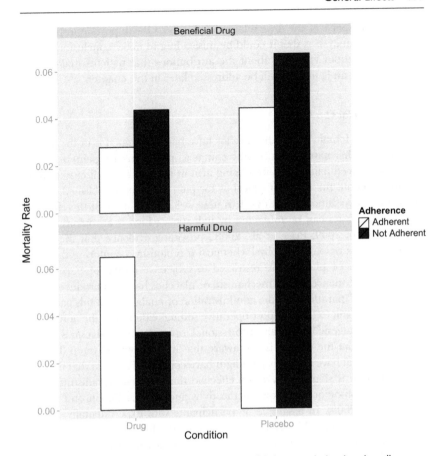

Figure 7.3 Mortality rates for beneficial and harmful drugs and placebos by adherence status. Adapted from "A meta-analysis of the association between adherence to drug therapy and mortality," by S.H. Simpson, D.T. Eurich, S.R. Majumdar, R.S. Padwal, S.T. Tsuyuki, J. Varney, and J.A. Johnson, 2006, *BMJ: British Medical Journal*, pp. 3–4.

as beneficial, was more effective than the placebo. This result could be due to the "powerful" placebo, but it could also be due to the fact that patients who adhere to the treatment protocol are generally "better" patients in that they have better health habits—a "healthy adherer" effect, according to the authors.

The results for the harmful drugs are what are particularly interesting. Again, not surprisingly, the mortality rate for patients who adhered to a harmful drug protocol was higher than for those who did not adhere. However, those in the placebo condition who adhered had lower mortality rates than any of the other conditions, suggesting believing that the drug was beneficial (i.e., took the drug as prescribed), when in fact it was a placebo, had a powerful impact on mortality. Here the "healthy adherer" is less likely as it did not counter the effect of the harmful aspects of the drug relative to placebo. One important implication of this meta-analysis is that it could be misleading to make conclusions about treatments without knowing about the attributions that patients make about the treatment, an issue that will be addressed later in this chapter.

Theories of Placebo Action

The primary domain in which placebos have been examined is in the area of pain, using either naturally occurring pain (e.g., post-operative pain) or experimentally induced pain (e.g., submerging arm in ice water). As discussed in the previous section, the effect of placebos for pain has been established in both clinical and experimental settings. It is now well established that the effects of placebo analgesics can be mitigated by naloxone, which is an opioid antagonist (Benedetti, 2009; Price et al., 2008), providing evidence that the release of endogenous opioids is a physiochemical mechanism, countering the claim that the effects of placebo are restricted to subjective ratings of participants. Interestingly, evidence for the mechanism of placebos has been produced in the "open-hidden" paradigm for the administration of analgesics. In this paradigm, patients with pain (often in a post-operative setting) either view the administration of the analgesic by a health professional (open) or the analgesic is administered such that the patient is not aware that it has been delivered (hidden). The studies that have used this paradigm have consistently shown that the open administration is significantly more effective than hidden administration, for opioid and non-opioid analgesic medications and also for Parkinson's patients (Price et al., 2008). In a sample of participants with experimentally induced pain, Amanzio, Pollo, Maggi, and Benedetti (2001) found a similar advantage for the open administration of a non-opioid analgesic ketorolac. The interesting part of this experiment was that naloxone eliminated the advantage of the open administration of ketorolac, even though ketorolac is not an opioid analgesic, indicating that the advantage of the open administration of the analgesic was due to release of endogenous opioids created by the awareness that analgesic was administered, suggesting that expectations are involved. As we will see, expectations appear to be the primary mechanism involved with placebo effects.

There is possibly a conditioning component to placebo action. Suppose a pill contains an active ingredient that reliably produces a biological effect. The pill itself (i.e., its appearance, taste, and smell) is an unconditioned stimulus, but because it is paired with the biological effect, it becomes a conditioned stimulus (CS). There is evidence that after several trials with an active medication, a placebo can produce effects through this conditioning mechanism (Ader, 1997; Benedetti, 2009; Price et al., 2008). Such conditioned placebo effects can occur in infrahuman animals as well. However, there are some issues with conditioning models of placebo effects. First, whether classical conditioning in humans is mediated by expectations has been a perennial and vexing issue in behavioral psychology. Second, there is experimental evidence for the primacy of expectations. In a classic experiment, Montgomery and Kirsch (1997) examined the effects of conditioning and expectation. They induced cutaneous pain (pain of the skin as opposed to deep pain) in participants and a placebo cream was then applied. The application of the cream was associated with reduced pain by a simultaneous reduction in the pain stimulus, a manipulation about which the participants were unaware. In this way, the placebo cream became a CS. The participants were then assigned to one of two conditions—in the first, the participants were informed about the experimental manipulation that reduced the intensity of the pain and learned that the cream was inert and in the second no explanation was given. A placebo effect for the cream occurred only in the second group, demonstrating that knowledge of the effect overrode the conditioned response. Benedetti (2011), based on this and other evidence, made the following conclusion:

> This is very important point because it suggests that expectation play a major role, even in the presence of a conditioning procedure [*sic*]. In other words, expectation and conditioning are not mutually exclusive—they may represent two sides of the same coin.
>
> (p. 190)

A third consideration is that various medical practices become culturally imbedded. A pill or an inoculation, or for that matter a physician in a white coat, are cultural symbols that have power through cultural pathways. What is powerful in one culture may be meaningless in another, and indeed placebos work differently in different cultures (Morris, 1997, 1998).

An issue that is raised by the results of various placebo mechanism studies relates to the additivity assumption that was discussed earlier. The model described in Figure 7.2, with regard to clinical trials of treatments, assumes that the specific treatment effect is a quantity that is added to the placebo effect. This assumption actually involves independence as well—the effect due to the placebo is independent of the effect due to the treatment. Irving Kirsch (2000) questioned this assumption, and there is evidence to support the notion that the two effects are neither independent nor additive. One problem is that there is not *one* placebo effect. Analgesic placebo effects created by expectations and by conditioning may be comparable in size yet have very different mechanisms. As summarized by Price et al. (2008), "In fact, if the placebo response is induced by means of strong expectation cues, it can be blocked by the naloxone, [but] conversely . . . if the placebo response is induced by means of prior conditioning with a non-opioid drug, it is naloxone-insensitive" (p. 578). In fact, the same placebo may affect different sensations in different ways, as summarized by Price et al.:

> In a pharmacological study in healthy volunteers, it was found that placebo analgesia in experimental ischemic arm pain was accompanied by a reduction of heart rate. Both the placebo analgesic effect and the

concomitant heart rate decrease were reversed by the opioid antagonist naloxone, whereas the β-blocker propranolol antagonized the placebo heart rate reduction but not placebo analgesia.

(p. 581)

In an intriguing study, Kong et al. (2009) investigated how expectations and a treatment can interact. Participants were administered either sham acupuncture or genuine acupuncture. For both groups, participants' expectations were increased by surreptitiously decreasing the painful stimuli on the "meridian" side of the hand, where participants had been informed that the acupuncture should be effective (high expectancy side), and leaving the pain stimuli constant on the "non-meridian" side, where participants were informed that the acupuncture would be not be effective (the control side). (The explanations of differences between these two conditions presented to the participants were bogus.) In this way, the participants were led to believe the acupuncture (either sham or genuine) was effective. Finally, pain was induced and acupuncture (sham and genuine to the respective groups) was administered, pain ratings were obtained, and fMRI data was obtained. Consistent with many studies of acupuncture, participants reported analgesic effects with sham as well as genuine acupuncture but no differences in reported pain between the two conditions. Moreover, greater analgesic effects were found on the "meridian" side than the "non-meridian" side, a difference clearly created by expectations. Although these results were not unexpected given the importance of expectations and the results of previous acupuncture studies, what was curious was that the fMRI data indicated that different neural networks were involved:

> For the verum [genuine] acupuncture group, there were only a few small differences between the high expectancy side and control side. For the sham acupuncture group, however, a more complicated network, particularly involving a number of areas in the frontal gyrus, was significantly involved. *These results suggest that expectancy may involve distinct mechanisms under different circumstances.*

(emphasis added, p. 945)

That is, analgesic expectancy effects, induced experimentally through the same experimental manipulations and producing equal subjective reports of pain relief, may involve different mechanisms depending on the treatment with which it is associated. Consequently, there is an interaction between treatment and expectancy, which creates suspicion about the viability of interpreting specific treatment effects to be independent from placebo effects due to expectancy.

An important issue about the mechanism of placebos is related to the importance of the verbal interaction between the patient and the healers. Clearly, a placebo effect can be induced through conditioning without the presence of a healer and certain symbols, such as a pill or syringe, can induce a placebo effect.

However, this does not indicate the interaction of the healer and the patient is unimportant in producing the placebo effect. This is an important issue because the Contextual Model emphasizes that the expectations for improvement in psychotherapy occur in the interaction between the therapist and client. Here the evidence also seems to indicate the verbal suggestion as well as characteristics of the healer are important factors in the creation of placebo effects.

The classic study on the importance of what is said to the patient involved treatment of pain in patients who underwent thoracic surgery for lung cancer (Pollo et al., 2001). All patients were treated with an opioid analgesic (viz., buprenorphine) given with an intravenous infusion of saline solution. At the point of the intervention, the patients were only given the saline solution and then were assigned to one of three verbal statement conditions: a) patients received no verbal statements (natural history); b) patients were told that they were receiving either a painkiller or a placebo (classic double-blind instruction); and c) patients were told that they were indeed receiving a painkiller (deceptive instruction). The patients were then able to request the painkiller if needed; the dependent variable was the number of requests made during a 3-day period. In this experiment only the verbal instructions were different. The patients in the double-blind condition made significantly fewer requests for the painkiller than did the patients in the natural history condition, but the patients in the deceptive condition made even fewer requests than those in the double-blind condition. This result harkens back to the claim that the clinical effects of placebos are underestimated because of the double-blind instructions. However, importantly, it also indicates that what is told to patients can have a dramatic effect.

The power of the relationship in healing was beautifully revealed in a study of placebo acupuncture for patients with irritable bowel syndrome (IBS) (Kaptchuk et al., 2008). IBS is a prevalent disorder in primary medical care and it is thus a suitable domain in which to situate this study because IBS is responsive to placebos. In this study, the relationship with the acupuncturist was manipulated by assigning IBS patients to one of three conditions: a) a wait-list condition, which served as a natural history control; b) a limited interaction condition, in which sham acupuncture was administered with limited interaction with the acupuncturist; and c) an augmented condition, in which the acupuncturist provided a "warm, empathic, and confident patient-practitioner relationship" (p. 2). In the limited interaction condition, the acupuncturist met with the patient for a brief period (less than 5 minutes), explained that he or she "knew what to do" but because of the nature of the study was not allowed to converse with the patients, placed the placebo needles, and left the patient in the room for 20 minutes, as is customary. In the augmented relationship condition, the initial visit was 45 minutes and the practitioner followed a structure that involved four content areas and contained five elements related to style. Content included questions concerning symptoms, the relationship of IBS to lifestyle and relationships, as well as the patient's understanding of the cause and meaning of her disorder. This conversation was delivered in a warm and friendly manner, using active listening, appropriate silences for reflection, and a communication of confidence and positive expectation. However, specific cognitive or behavioral interventions, education, or counseling were proscribed. The acupuncture was delivered in the same 20-minute procedure as the limited relationship group. Both acupuncture groups received additional sessions of the sham acupuncture over a 3-week period. The results of this study are shown in Figure 7.4 for the four dependent variables: a) global improvement, b) adequate relief, c) symptom severity, and d) quality of life. Clearly, the augmented relationship was superior to limited relationship, but even the limited relationship was superior to the no-treatment condition; the effects were most

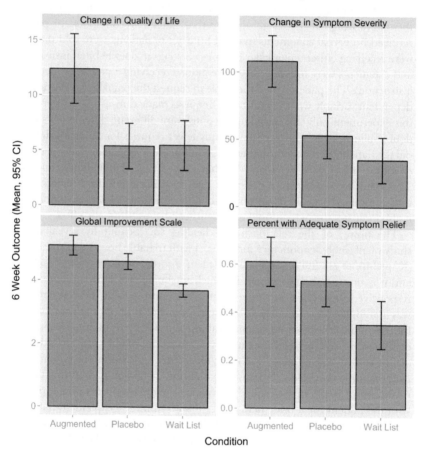

Figure 7.4 Outcomes for waitlist, acupuncture placebo with limited interaction, and acupuncture placebo with augmented interaction at 6-month time point. Adapted from "Components of placebo effect: Randomised controlled trial in patients with irritable bowel syndrome," by T.J. Kaptchuk, J.M. Kelley, L.A. Conboy, R.B. Davis, C.E. Kerr, E.E. Jacobson, ...A.J. Lembo, 2008, *BMJ: British Medical Journal, 336(7651)*, p. 1001.

pronounced for quality of life. A follow-up analysis examined the characteristics of the patients that predicted a placebo response as well as differences among the practitioners (Kelley et al., 2009). Patient extraversion was reliably related to placebo response. Despite the structured nature of the interaction, there were significant practitioner effects—in fact, practitioner effects were twice as large as the effect due to differences in conditions. An analysis of videotapes found that more effective practitioners facilitated relationships that were similar to what has been determined to be the ideal interaction in healthcare, based on psychotherapy models. The results of this study, both in terms of the effects of the augmented relationship condition, particularly on quality of life, and the practitioner effects, are consistent with predictions of the Contextual Model.

Based on the evidence produced by many placebo and related studies, most theorists place expectations at the center of these models. After reviewing the evidence and having been involved in much research on placebos, Price et al. (2008) developed a model to explain the conditions necessary to produce a placebo effect. Key to the placebo effect, according to this model, is a) the desire to feel relief or the desire to achieve some pleasure; b) an induction of an expectation that the goal (relief or pleasure) can be achieved by the placebo; and c) the presence of emotional arousal. In the definition of psychotherapy provided in Chapter 2 we emphasized that the client is seeking therapy, which fulfills the desire component of Price et al.'s model. In addition, expectations are central to the Contextual Model, created by an explanation provided by the therapist, which interacts with the patient's pre-therapy belief that therapy may be helpful.

According to Kirsch (Kirsch, 2005; Kirsch & Low, 2013), placebos are effective because of a change in response expectancies:

> Response expectancies are anticipations of automatic subjective reactions, such as changes in depression, anxiety, pain, etc. Kirsch has argued that response expectancies are self-confirming. The world in which we live is ambiguous, and one of the functions of the brain is to disambiguate it rapidly enough to respond quickly. We do this, in part, by forming expectations. So what we experience at any given time is a joint function of the stimuli to which we are exposed and our beliefs and expectations about those stimuli (Kirsch, 1999; Michael, Garry, & Kirsch, 2012).
>
> (Kirsch & Low, 2013, p. 221)

According to Kirsch, placebos as well as psychotherapy change patients' response expectancies. In this way, a patient no longer expects what he or she believed would be the inevitable outcome of certain experiences or situations. In the Contextual Model, this change in response expectancies is predicted to be a core psychological process across treatments—a primary mechanism on which the effectiveness of psychotherapy partially depends.

We now turn our attention to what can be learned from studies that have utilized placebos with psychotherapy. This will facilitate an understanding of how expectations and attributions are involved in producing the benefits of psychotherapy. These studies are different from studies that compare the effects of psychotherapy vis-à-vis a placebo-like control, as will be clear.

Establishing the Importance of Attributions in Psychotherapy Using Placebos

We focus our review on two studies, one from 1978 (Liberman, 1978) and a recent one (Powers, Smits, Whitley, Bystritsky, & Telch, 2008), which will show the consistency of results but also offers a historical perspective. In the older study, Bernard Liberman and Jerome Frank were interested in mastery, which was defined as "control over one's internal reactions and relevant external events" (p. 35), a concept not too different from Kirsch's response expectancies. According to Liberman and Frank, psychotherapy is a means to attain a healthy sense of control, particularly over aspects of life that are problematic to the patient. The relevance of the therapeutic activity and the patient's attributions about their performance are critical therapeutic components and particularly important in the design and interpretation of the experiment to be described here. Liberman hypothesized the performance of a therapeutic task that was attributed to one's own efforts would be more beneficial than the same performance attributed to an external source. To test this hypothesis, neurotic outpatients in the Johns Hopkins outpatient clinic were randomly assigned to two conditions: a mastery condition, in which the benefits of treatment would be attributed to one's own efforts, and a placebo condition, in which the benefits were attributed to an external source (in this case, a placebo). The Hopkins Symptom Checklist (HSCL) was administered before the treatment, at termination, and importantly for this study, at 3-months follow-up.

The treatment given to the patients at the clinic might seem quite odd. The patients' treatment involved performing three tasks: a) discriminating as quickly as possible between different colored stimuli, b) a perception task based on thematic apperception test cards for which patients answered content and mood questions about what they saw; and c) modification of physiological responses to stressful and non-stressful visual and auditory stimuli based on purported biofeedback. They were given feedback, independent of how they actually performed, that their performance on the tasks was improving.

In the mastery condition, patients were told that "work on the tasks would enable the patient to gain greater control over important physical and mental abilities and that this increased control would enable him [sic] to better handle his [sic] problems" (p. 51) and that benefits were due to one's own efforts. In the placebo condition, an inert pill was given and the patients were told that the medication would improve their physical and mental abilities, the medication would help them feel better generally, and the tasks were measures of their abilities and an indicator of the medication's effectiveness. Because the researchers wanted the patients to make attributions relative to the tasks and not the therapist actions, there was no relationship with a therapist, although the patients made audiotapes after the session and staff wrote supportive notes to the patients (blind to the condition).

The results of this study supported the power of the attribution to one's own efforts. At the end of treatment, patients in both groups improved equally, even though the treatment contained no ingredients thought to be therapeutic. However, when the treatment was discontinued and the placebos withdrawn from patients in the placebo condition, patients in the placebo condition relapsed at a greater rate than the mastery condition. Consistent with the research on placebos, but here demonstrated in a treatment of psychological problems, one's beliefs about the treatment affect the benefits derived from therapy. Also interesting of course is that the treatment contained no known scientific ingredients, yet when the patients were led to believe that the tasks would be effective, they benefited. As noted by Liberman, "The presentation by senior staff therapists at the Johns Hopkins Medical Institution provided an element of status and prestige which facilitated acceptance of these explanations" (p. 52).

The second study (Powers, Smits, Whitley, Bystritsky, & Telch, 2008) involved a one-session treatment for claustrophobia, a treatment previously found to be effective. Participants who displayed claustrophobic fear were randomly assigned to waitlist condition, a psychological placebo, or exposure plus an inert pill condition. The interesting part of the experiment involves the explanations given to the exposure or the exposure + pill placebo groups. Participants in this pill placebo condition were randomized to one of three explanations: a) the pill was a sedating herb that made the exposure treatment easier, b) the pill as a stimulating herb that made exposure more difficult, or c) the pill was a placebo that had no effect on the participant. Participants in the three pill placebo conditions were able to complete the exposure protocol but fear returned for the sedating description condition (39 percent relapsed), whereas there was no return of fear for the other two instructional conditions (zero percent for each). The return of fear for the sedating herb condition was mediated by the participants' ratings of self-efficacy to tolerate small enclosures. These results replicated Liberman's (1978) finding that attributing successful completion of therapeutic tasks, whether bogus in Liberman's case or based on current scientific knowledge, as in Powers et al.'s case, to an external source (here, the sedating herb), are not maintained. Clearly, the acquisition of the belief that one's efforts are responsible for improvement is critical; that is to say, it is the attribution made about the treatment, in addition to or perhaps rather than the treatment itself, that is important.

Expectation Research in Psychotherapy

Examining the role of expectations in psychotherapy is problematic. In medicine, expectations can be induced verbally and then physicochemical agents or procedures (e.g., acupuncture, as discussed earlier), can be administered making the two components (creation of expectations and the treatment) independent, as was the case of many of the placebo studies reviewed earlier. In psychotherapy, creating the expectations, through explanation of the patient's disorder, presenting the rationale for the treatment, and participating in the therapeutic actions are part of therapy. Because it is difficult to manipulate the expectations for therapy, there is little experimental research in this area that is informative. This has left researchers assessing expectations through self-report of the patient and correlating with outcome, which raises well-known issues that were discussed earlier in this chapter, including the inducement of positive expectations by patient improvement prior to when it was measured. In addition, expectations are often measured *prior* to when the rationale for the treatment is provided to the patient.

Despite these issues, there have been comprehensive reviews, both narrative (Greenberg, Constantino, & Bruce, 2006) and meta-analysis (Constantino, Glass, Arnkoff, Ametrano, & Smith, 2011), both of which concluded that the expectations of patients were predictive of psychotherapy outcome. The meta-analysis, involving 46 studies and 8,016 patients, found a correlation of the expectation variables and outcome to be quite small ($r = .12$, equivalent to $d = .24$) but statistically significant. The authors of the expectation meta-analysis note the poor quality expectation measures in psychotherapy:

> In fact, of the 46 studies in our meta-analysis, we coded 31 (67.4%) as involving 'poor' expectancy measurement. Problems included, but were not limited to, the use of one-item scales, measures that confounded expectancy and another construct, scales that confounded outcome and treatment expectations, measures that used the same questions for both expected outcome and actual outcome, and the use of projective measures to assess outcome expectations . . . [and expectations are] often assessed at baseline or early treatment only.
>
> (Constantino, Arnkoff, Glass, Ametrano, & Smith, 2011, p. 189)

As explained in Chapter 2 and the discussion of placebos in this chapter, expectations of psychotherapy are created through the explanation for the disorder and the presentation of the treatment. However, expectations are only created if the patient accepts the explanation (Wampold & Budge, 2012; Wampold, Imel, Bhati, & Johnson Jennings, 2006). As mentioned previously, the Contextual Model predicts that the explanations must be, to use Vygotskyian terms, in the zone of proximal development for a given patient—that is, the explanation and treatment must be compatible with the patient's cultural beliefs. According to this view, an evidence-based treatment will be more effective if it is adapted to the patient's cultural group, which is contrary to the Medical Model, which stipulates that as long as the psychological deficit underlying a disorder is addressed, which is assumed to be culturally invariant, the treatment will be effective. There have been a number of meta-analyses examining the effectiveness of culturally adapted treatments (see Huey, Tilley, Jones, & Smith, in press, for a review of these meta-analyses). Recently, Benish, Quintana, and Wampold

(2011) meta-analyzed only direct comparisons of a culturally adapted treatment to a bona fide evidence-based treatment and found that the culturally adapted treatment was superior (d = 0.32 for all measures), a result consistent with previous meta-analyses (Huey et al., in press). Benish et al. coded whether the adaptation involved adapting the explanation to be congruent with the patient's cultural belief with regard to mental illness, which they call the *illness* myth, rather than other adaptations, such as language. It turned out that illness myth moderator was statistically significant—culturally adapted treatments that specifically used the illness myth had better outcomes compared to the evidence-based treatment than did other cultural adaptions (d = 0.21). This evidence appears to be in line with conjectures of the Contextual Model.

Other Common Factors

Over the years, as reviewed in Chapter 2, there have been a number of common factors identified. Although these factors are not distinct, many have been investigated, including empathy (Elliott, Bohart, Watson, & Greenberg, 2011), goal consensus/collaboration (Tryon & Winograd, 2011), positive regard/affirmation (Farber & Doolin, 2011), and congruence/genuineness (Kolden, Klein, Wang, & Austin, 2011). The results of meta-analyses that have aggregated the correlation of these factors with outcomes are found in Table 7.3. In none of these cases have confounds been investigated in the manner in which they have for the alliance, but nevertheless the size of the effects for these factors are impressive.

One of the issues prominent in Chapter 6 on therapist effects is related to what are the characteristics and actions of effective therapists. As discussed earlier in this chapter, more effective therapists are better able to form alliances

Table 7.3 Effect Sizes for Common Factors

Factor	# Studies	# Patients	Effect Size d	% of variability in outcomes
Common Factors				
Alliance[a]	190	>14,000	0.57	7.5
Empathy[b]	59	3599	0.63	9.0
Goal Consensus/Collaboration[c]	15	1302	0.72	11.5
Positive Regard/Affirmation[d]	18	1067	0.56	7.3
Congruence/Genuineness[e]	16	863	0.49	5.7
Expectation in Therapy[f]	46	8016	0.24	1.4
Cultural Adaptation of EBT[g]	21	950	0.32	2.5

a Horvath et al. (2011a, b)
b Elliott et al. (2011)
c Tryon & Winograd (2011)
d Farber & Doolin (2011)
e Kolden et al. (2011)
f Constantino et al. (2011)
g Benish, Quintana, & Wampold (2011)

with a variety of patients than are less effective therapists. Unfortunately, as reviewers have noted, there has been limited research on this question (Baldwin & Imel, 2013; Beutler et al., 2004), particularly using proper methods to disaggregate therapist and patient variables, as was the case with the alliance. However, such studies are beginning to emerge, and they have revealed some informative results with regard to the mechanisms of change inherent in the Contextual Model.

In a landmark study, Anderson, Ogles, Patterson, Lambert, and Vermeersch (2009) identified a set of interpersonal skills that predicted therapist outcomes. In the usual psychotherapy design, aspects of the psychotherapy are examined either by observing therapists in action—that is, with clients in therapy—or by using self-report measures. Unfortunately, this strategy is problematic because the client has an influence on the apparent skill of the therapist, as will be discussed in Chapter 8. Consequently, when identifying therapist actions, variability in clients must be considered (similar to Baldwin et al., 2007). Instead of observing therapists in action, Anderson et al. provided each therapist a standard stimulus, which consisted of a video of a client, and then coded therapist responses to this stimulus. Therapists who scored higher on a set of facilitative interpersonal skills in response to the vignette were found to have better outcomes with their actual clients. Anderson et al.'s facilitative skills included verbal fluency, interpersonal perception, affective modulation and expressiveness, warmth and acceptance, empathy, and focus on other. That is to say, therapists who scored higher on these skills in the responses to an experimental stimulus also had better outcomes with patients. What is interesting is that all of these skills are related to aspects described in the Contextual Model and supported by correlations of process variables and outcome (see Table 7.3).

There have been a few other studies that have examined characteristics of therapists outside of therapy as a predictor of therapist effectiveness. The countertransference literature suggests that therapists should reflect on his or her own reaction to the client to determine if these reactions are reasonable given the patient presentation or are based on therapist issues (Gelso & Hayes, 2007). Nissen-Lie and colleagues (2010) found that therapist self-doubt, a type of reflection about practice, was a good predictor of a strong alliance as well as outcomes. Moreover, they found that using relational skills in the presence of a negative personal reaction to clients was deleterious.

Summary of Evidence for General Effects

The Contextual Model makes several conjectures about what evidence should be observed under certain conditions. Variables that would be classified as *common factors* have been shown, in several meta-analyses, to be correlated with outcome, and the size of the effects could be characterized as moderate or larger (in Chapter 8 evidence for specific effects will be presented and then the relative size of the common factor effects can be discussed). Nevertheless, making sense of these correlations is difficult for several reasons. First, as discussed, conceptually and empirically, the common factors are not distinct. For example, agreement about goals and tasks overlaps with goal consensus and collaboration and empathy overlaps with congruence and genuineness. Second, only the alliance has been examined extensively to address threats to validity of the conclusion that common factors are important in psychotherapy. Third, the Contextual Model makes more complex predictions than simply that the common factors are important.

The Contextual Model, as presented in Chapter 2, is consistent with the research evidence in psychotherapy and other social science areas. More rigorously said, there is little if any research that is sufficiently discrepant from what the Contextual Model predicts that one should consider abandoning it. It is helpful to look at the evidence related to the three pathways of the Contextual Model. The first pathway involves the benefits purportedly gained by the human interaction with an empathic and caring therapist. Recall that in Chapter 2, it was noted that social connection is necessary for psychological and mental well-being (Baumeister, 2005; Cacioppo & Cacioppo, 2012; Cohen & Syme, 1985; Lieberman, 2013)—indeed perceived loneliness is a greater risk factor for death than smoking, obesity, lack of exercise, environmental pollution, or excessive drinking (Holt-Lunstad, Smith, & Layton, 2010). To show that the real relationship in psychotherapy is critical to the benefits of psychotherapy is more difficult. Nevertheless, in this chapter we presented evidence that the real relationship predicts the outcome of psychotherapy over and above the alliance. Furthermore, empathy, a critical variable in the social connection between humans (de Waal, 2008; Niedenthal & Brauer, 2012; Preston & de Waal, 2002), is more highly correlated with outcome than any other variable studied in psychotherapy. In psychotherapy, control treatments that involve *only* a relationship with the therapist produce benefits, often approaching the benefits produced by the very best evidence-based treatments (as will be seen in Chapter 8). As well, as discussed in this chapter, when placebo treatments are augmented by an empathic interaction with the practitioner, benefits are increased. Finally, the actions that characterize effective therapists, including warmth and acceptance, empathy, and focus on other, as discussed here, are critical features of closer interpersonal relationships. There is no doubt that people can make changes in their life without a real relationship with a therapist (e.g., with bibliotherapy, see e.g., Cuijpers, 1997; or as was the case in the Liberman, 1978 study reviewed in this chapter); the Contextual Model only says that *in psychotherapy*, the human connection between the patient and the therapist creates some of the benefits of psychotherapy.

The second pathway in the Contextual Model involves the expectations created by the acceptance of the explanation that is provided to the patient and the treatment. The importance of the collaborative working relationship in psychotherapy, which is indicative of the acceptance of the explanation and the treatment, is clearly established by the research on the alliance that was reviewed in this chapter. Importantly, more effective therapists are those that are able to create a working relationship across a range of patients. Although research on benefits of expectations in psychotherapy is difficult to conduct, meta-analyses have established an association between expectation and outcome. Perhaps the best evidence for the power of expectations comes from the research on placebos, which was reviewed extensively in this chapter. Importantly, the expectations that are created in the context of a social interaction are particularly powerful. Moreover, two studies (viz., Liberman, 1978; Powers et al., 2008), separated by 30 years, demonstrated that the attributions one makes about the treatment are crucial to the maintenance of the benefits of psychotherapy.

The final pathway of the Contextual Model, which involves participating in therapeutic actions that lead to healthy and desirable changes, also involves the alliance. Agreement about the tasks of therapy is critical to the engagement in and completion of these therapeutic tasks. That the alliance is predictive of outcomes across various treatments suggests that regardless of the treatment, engagement in the therapeutic activities is critical. As will be reviewed in the next chapter, therapies without *any* therapeutic actions are not as effective as therapies with therapeutic actions. However, the most important issue for the final pathway is whether some therapeutic actions—the ones that address specific deficits related to the patient's difficulties—are more effective than others and that those specific ingredients are responsible for the benefits of psychotherapy. Such evidence would be difficult to assimilate into the Contextual Model. However, as reviewed in Chapter 5, all treatments intended to be therapeutic appear to be equally effective. In the next chapter, the issue of specificity of ingredients is addressed.

Notes

1. The model presented in Figure 7.2 is an additive model in which the treatment effect and the placebo effect are independent and additive. That is, the specific effect is added to the placebo effect from the treatment effect, which is the difference between the treatment and natural course of the disorder. The assumption of additivity may not be true, however (Benedetti, 2011; Kirsch, 2000; Kirsch, Scoboria, & Moore, 2002. This issue will be discussed later in this chapter.

2. Another interesting meta-analysis reviewed 13 clinical trials of acupuncture, placebo acupuncture, and no acupuncture for pain (Madsen, Gøtzsche, & Hróbjartsson, 2009), producing results similar to Wampold et al. (2005). A small but significant difference between acupuncture and placebo was found ($d = 0.17$) and a moderate and statistically significant effect for placebo versus no treatment ($d = .42$). Again, much, although not all, of the analgesic effect of acupuncture was due to a placebo effect. Although acupuncture is not a conventional treatment for pain, there are some informative meta-analyses of treatments that are approved and widely used.

3. For a detailed and informative discussion of the how psychiatric drugs are approved by the Food and Drug Administration see Spielmans and Kirsch (in press).

Chapter 8

Specific Effects

Where Are They?

In this chapter we examine the evidence for specific ingredients—are the purported ingredients of an effective treatment responsible for the benefits of the treatment? The most direct way to examine the importance of a specific ingredient is in a *component* study, in which a critical ingredient is removed from an existing treatment or a component is added to an existing treatment to determine the effects of the deleted or added component. Next, designs that attempt to use some type of "placebo" control to examine the specific effects are reviewed, but it will become apparent that these placebo-type designs are inadequate for this purpose. Then, designs that attempt to match treatments to patients with a particular psychological deficit are reviewed. We also examine adherence and competence, as these are important auxiliaries in the Medical Model related to specific ingredients. Finally, we will look at attempts to identify mediating processes for specific treatments, including adherence to the treatment protocol, although there have been few attempts to synthesize this literature, which makes it difficult to present.

Component Studies

Design Issues

There are two types of component studies. In the first, the researcher removes the specific ingredient from the treatment and determines whether the efficacy of the treatment is attenuated, as would be expected. This design is called a *dismantling design*, as it "dismantles" an effective treatment to identify the effective ingredients. In a dismantling study, attenuation of the benefits when a critical specific ingredient is removed provides evidence that the specific ingredient is indeed therapeutic. Such a result would provide evidence for specific effects and would thus be supportive of the Medical Model of psychotherapy. Borkovec (1990) described the advantages of the dismantling study:

> One crucial feature of the [dismantling] design is that more factors are ordinarily common among the various comparison conditions. In addition to representing equally the potential impact of history, maturation, and so

on and the impact of nonspecific factors, a procedural component is held constant between the total package and the control condition containing only that particular element. Such a design approximates more closely the experimental ideal of holding everything but one element constant. . . . Therapists will usually have greater confidence in, and less hesitancy to administer, a component condition than a pure nonspecific condition. They will also be equivalently trained and have equal experience in the elements relative to the combination of elements in the total package. . . . At the theoretical level, such outcomes tell what elements of procedure are most actively involved in the change process. . . . At the applied level, determination of elements that do not contribute to outcome allows therapists to dispense with their use in therapy.

(pp. 56–57)

Dismantling studies are discussed thoroughly in clinically oriented research design texts (e.g., Heppner, Kivlighan, & Wampold, 2008; Kazdin, 2002).

The second component strategy to demonstrate specificity is to add an ingredient to an existing treatment package. In this design, which is called an *additive design* (Borkovec, 1990), there typically is a theoretical reason to believe that a specific ingredient will augment the benefits derived from the treatment:

The goal is ordinarily to develop an even more potent therapy based on empirical or theoretical information that suggests that each therapy [or component] has reason to be partially effective, so that their combination may be superior to either procedure by itself. In terms of design, the [dismantling] and additive approaches are similar. It is partly the direction of reasoning of the investigator and the history of literature associated with the techniques and the diagnostic problem that determine which design strategy seems to be taking place.

(Borkovec, 1990, p. 57)

We now review the evidence produced by component studies.

Evidence From Component Studies

A classic dismantling study will be presented first, followed by two meta-analyses. In a study discussed earlier in this volume, Jacobson et al. (1996) dismantled cognitive therapy for depression. The purpose of this study was to "provide an experimental test of the theory of change put forth by A. T. Beck, A. J. Rush, B. F. Shaw, and G. Emery (1979) to explain the efficacy of cognitive-behavioral therapy (CT) for depression" (p. 295). To accomplish this goal, patients with major depression were randomly assigned to one of three treatment conditions: a) CT in its entirety, including behavioral activation (BA), automatic thought modification (AT), and modification of core schemas; b) BA and

AT; and c) only BA. The authors made a specific prediction: "According to the cognitive theory of depression, CT should work significantly better than AT, which in turn, should work significantly better than BA" (p. 296). Contrary to expectations, no significant differences among the three conditions were found and various auxiliaries that might have accounted for this unexpected result could not be invoked: "Despite excellent adherence to treatment protocols by the therapists, a clear bias favoring CT, and the competent performance of CT, there was no evidence that the complete treatment produced better outcomes, at either the termination of acute treatment or the 6-month follow-up, than either component treatment" (p. 295). The lack of differences in outcomes led the authors to make the following conclusions:

> These findings run contrary to hypotheses generated by the cognitive model of depression put forth by Beck and his associates (1979), who proposed that direct efforts aimed at modifying negative schema are necessary to maximize treatment outcome and prevent relapse. These results are all the more surprising, given that they run counter to the allegiance effect (Robinson, Berman, & Neimeyer, 1990), which is quite commonly related to outcome in psychotherapy research.
>
> (p. 302)

The unexpected result suggested a reconsideration of both the mechanisms of change in CT:

> If BA and AT treatments are as effective as CT and also are as likely to modify the factors that are thought to be necessary for change to occur, then not only the theory but also the therapy may be in need of revision.
>
> (pp. 302–303)

In this classic study, the results cast doubts on the specificity of the specific ingredients of CT for depression. If this result were to be replicated across component studies, then doubt would be created about the specificity of psychotherapy more generally. Ahn and Wampold (2001) conducted a meta-analysis of component studies of psychotherapeutic treatments that appeared in the literature between 1970 and 1998. They located 27 comparisons that attempted to isolate a specific component to test whether that component produced effects above those produced by the same treatment without the component. For each study, an effect size was calculated by comparing the outcomes for the two groups (treatment vs. treatment without component) aggregated over all dependent variables within the study (i.e., targeted and non-targeted variables), using the within-study aggregation method used previously (Hedges & Olkin, 1985; Wampold et al., 1997b). Then the aggregate effect size across the 27 studies was calculated. The aggregate effect size was found to be equal to −0.20. Although the effect size was in the opposite direction of what was predicted (i.e., the treatment without the component outperformed the complete treatment), it was not statistically different from zero. However, the effect sizes were homogeneous, suggesting that there were no moderating variables affecting the results. Thus, adding or removing a purportedly effective component did not seem to increase the benefit of psychotherapeutic treatments, as would be expected if the specific ingredients were remedial, as predicted by the Medical Model.

There were a few issues with the Ahn and Wampold (2001) meta-analysis. First, they did not segregate targeted and non-targeted variables. Typically, specific ingredients of treatments should have a direct effect on targeted measures, and thus component studies, unless the component involves some "enrichment" activity focused on general well-being, should demonstrate effects on targeted variables. Second, Ahn and Wampold analyzed dismantling studies and additive studies together. Finally, the corpus of studies is now quite dated, as they included studies only to 1998.

Bell, Marcus, and Goodlad (2013) replicated and extended the previous meta-analysis, including studies published between 1980 and 2010, which included three times as many studies as Ahn and Wampold had available at the end of 1998. Additionally, they examined dismantling designs and additive designs separately, as well as segregating targeted variables and non-targeted variables. The results of their analysis are summarized in Table 8.1. All effects

Table 8.1 Summary of Effects from Component Studies

Variables	K	D	95% CI
	Dismantling		
Termination			
Targeted	30	0.01	(−0.11, 0.12)
Non-Targeted	17	0.12	(−0.04, 0.28)
Follow-up			
Targeted	19	0.08	(−0.07, 0.22)
Non-Targeted	11	0.15	(−0.05, 0.36)
	Additive		
Termination			
Targeted	34	0.14	(0.03, 0.24)
Non-Targeted	24	0.12	(−0.02, 0.25)
Follow-up			
Targeted	32	0.28	(0.13, 0.38)
Non-Targeted	24	0.14	(−0.00, 0.28)

Note. Reprinted from "Are the parts as good as the whole? A meta-analysis of component treatment studies," by E.C. Bell, D. K Marcus, and J.K. Goodlad, 2013, *Journal of Consulting and Clinical Psychology, 81*(4), p. 728. Copyright 2013 by the American Psychological Association. Reprinted with permission.

detected by Bell et al. were negligible to small (viz., ranged from 0.01 to 0.28), and only the effects for targeted variables in the additive studies (at termination and at follow-up) were significantly different from zero, replicating Ahn and Wampold (2001), with the exception of targeted variables for additive studies. The most important result from the perspective of specificity is seen in the dismantling studies for targeted variables. Taking out the ingredient hypothesized to target the purported deficit of the patient should attenuate the targeted symptoms at the end of treatment, which this meta-analysis did not find (viz., d = 0.01). Even the largest effect (targeted variables for additive studies at follow-up) accounted for less than 2 percent of variability in outcomes. In terms of theory about why an added component may add to the effect at follow-up for targeted variables, Bell et al. referred to this as a "sleeper effect," but it is also possible that it is an artifact (see Flückiger, Del Re, & Wampold, in press). On the other hand, later in this chapter, a study will be discussed that might explain this result. Bell et al. made the following recommendation for practice: "If this [added] component does not lead to increased attrition or significantly increased costs, it may be worth the effort" (p. 731). The results of Bell et al. as well as Ahn and Wampold displayed relatively little heterogeneity, making the results quite robust, without concern for moderating variables, such as the nature of the treatment being investigated.

In terms of component design, neither Ahn and Wampold (2001) nor Bell et al. (2013) provided compelling evidence for specific effects. The latter found small effects for targeted variables for additive studies only, results that in the context of other findings from these two meta-analyses are difficult to interpret in terms of evidence for specificity.

Controlling for Common Factors in Psychotherapy Research: Logic of Placebos in Medicine and in Psychotherapy

In medicine, the double-blind randomized placebo control group design is used to test for specificity. In psychotherapy research, researchers have attempted to use placebo-type control groups to establish the specificity of various psychotherapeutic treatments, but unfortunately, as we will see, they cannot adequately function to establish specificity.

In the Medical Model in medicine, there are two types of effects. The first type consists of physicochemical effects due to specific medical procedures and thus are called specific effects. The second type of effects are placebo effects, which are effects due to aspects of the medical treatment that are incidental to the treatment and are non-physicochemical—that is, psychological. The field of medicine recognizes the presence of placebo effects but, for the most part, finds them of little interest (see Chapter 7). In medicine, the existence of specific effects can be established by comparing a medical treatment to a placebo. To be valid, the placebo needs to be identical to the treatment in all respects, except that the placebo does not contain the specific ingredient of the medical treatment. For example, the efficacy and specificity of an ingested pharmacological pill is established by comparing its effects to a placebo pill that resembles the active pill in size, shape, color, taste, smell, and texture. The pill and the placebo are indistinguishable, except the active pill contains a chemical compound that is purported, by theory, to be remedial for the disorder being treated; the placebo, however, contains no ingredients thought to be physicochemically remedial for the disorder. The placebo is the proverbial "sugar pill." The equivalence of the drug and the placebo can be maintained only if the patient and the experimenter, as well as the evaluators, are unaware of the status of the pill administered to the patient. Consequently, medical placebo trials are double-blinded in that the patient, the experimenters (or administrators), and the evaluators do not know whether a given patient is receiving the drug or the placebo (more of a triple blind, actually). The field of medicine recognizes that expectations of the patient, administrator of treatment, and evaluators have an effect on the measured effect of the treatment, and, therefore, maintaining the blind in medical research is critical to the integrity and validity of the research. To accomplish the blind, the active medication and the pill placebo must be indistinguishable (Wampold, Minami, Tierney, Baskin, & Bhati, 2005).

The logic of the placebo study in medicine is straightforward. If the drug condition is found to be superior to the placebo, then the efficacy of the specific ingredient is established because the only difference between the drug and the placebo is the specific ingredient. All other effects are controlled because they should logically be equivalent in the two conditions. Expectancy, for example, is controlled, because neither the patient nor the experimenter knows whether or not the patient received the drug.[1]

Adherents of the Medical Model of psychotherapy use "placebo-type" control psychotherapies to claim that the ingredients characteristic of a particular treatment are responsible for the benefits derived from the particular treatment. Unfortunately, using medical placebos as an analogue in psychotherapy research is flawed, and, consequently, the claim that placebo-type controls can be used to establish specificity is unjustified. Before discussing the problems with psychotherapy placebos, it should be noted that the popularity of the term placebo has waned and in lieu of it are the more in vogue (and vague) terms *alternate treatment, nonspecific treatment, attention control, minimal treatment, supportive counseling, nondirective counseling,* or *supportive therapy.* The logic of all these treatments is the same in that the researcher attempts to control for the incidental aspects of treatments. To denote these types of controls, we use the term *pseudo-placebo* generically to be inclusive of the various types of controls used by psychotherapy researchers.

It is difficult to define a psychotherapy placebo because the specific effects and the general effects are both derived through psychological processes (Wampold et al., 2005; Wilkins, 1983, 1984). In medicine, specific effects are physicochemically based and placebo effects are psychologically based. The ingredients of the placebo are uncontroversial because there is general agreement about which ingredients have the potential to be remedial physicochemically and which are inert physicochemically. For example, the lactose in a placebo pill used as a control for a drug indicated for HIV would not, by any reasonable physicochemical theory, be remedial for HIV; moreover lactose is not necessary for the treatment of HIV. Consequently, lactose is an appropriate compound for the placebo and an inequivalence in the dosage of lactose in the drug and placebo would not be a threat to the validity of the study. On the other hand, psychotherapy placebos must contain ingredients that are necessary for the delivery of the treatment and which are, according to many psychological theories, as least partially remedial for the disorder. The most perspicuous example of such an ingredient is the relationship between the therapist and the client. This relationship technically is necessary because psychotherapy by definition involves a relationship between therapist and client (see Chapter 2). Moreover, most theories of change recognize the importance of the relationship; even strict behaviorists classify the relationship as necessary but not sufficient.

Having to include ingredients in pseudo-placebos that are necessary and remedial dictates that the ingredient must be comparable across the two conditions (treatment and placebo). To be valid logically, for example, the treatment and the placebo must involve comparable relationships between therapists and clients. But the therapeutic relationship is only one such ingredient that must be equalized; others include the credibility of the treatment to the client, client expectation that the therapy will be beneficial, the skill of the therapist, the preference of the client for the therapy, and the therapist's belief that the treatment is beneficial. Recall from Chapter 5 that Jacobson claimed that behavioral marital therapy (BMT) was at a disadvantage relative to insight-oriented marital therapy (IOMT) because BT contained fewer "nonspecific" elements than did IOMT (Jacobson, 1991). The same could be said for all placebos unless the equivalence of the treatment and the pseudo-placebo vis-à-vis all non-specific ingredients is established. But it is logically and pragmatically impossible to create pseudo-placebos that contain, in terms of the quality and quantity, the same non-specific ingredients contained in the psychotherapeutic treatment.

Many psychotherapy researchers have defined pseudo-placebos in terms of a subset of the incidental aspects of psychotherapy treatments. For example, Bowers and Clum (1988) defined "nonspecific treatments . . . as having two primary components: a discussion of the client's problems and the manipulation of the belief that one is getting an effective treatment" (p. 315). Borkovec (1990) argued that "perhaps the best description of the placebo condition, then, is that it involves contact with a therapist who engages in methods that the client believes will be helpful, even though the therapist (or investigator) believes that the method will be of only limited effectiveness relative to the therapy condition to which it is compared [and] whatever active ingredients it contains are common across many forms of psychosocial therapy" (p. 53).

Others have defined pseudo-placebos solely in terms of expectancy, the relationship, support, or other related factors. Clearly, defining and developing placebo control groups in psychotherapy that are equivalent to treatment groups on *all* of the factors that are incidental to the theoretical approaches would be difficult, if not impossible, so researchers resort to making the treatment and placebo groups equivalent on one or a few common factors.

Not only is designing a pseudo-placebo to control for all incidental aspects of treatment practically impossible, it is logically impossible. The logical problems in the development of placebo groups in psychotherapy research can be explicated by examining the double blind in medical research. Recall that the double blind in medical research requires that neither the patient nor the administrator be aware of whether a given patient is receiving the treatment or the placebo. In psychotherapy research, one of the blinds will necessarily be absent. In psychotherapy research, it is obvious that therapists logically must be aware of the treatment being delivered; they have to be trained to deliver the active treatments as well as the pseudo-placebo treatment in a manner consistent with the protocols for those treatments. As noted by Seligman (1995), "Whenever you hear someone demanding the double-blind study of psychotherapy, hold on to your wallet" (p. 965).

The fact that therapists are cognizant of whether they are delivering a treatment that was intended to be therapeutic or a placebo is critical to tests of the Contextual Model of psychotherapy. Recall that a required element of the Contextual Model is that the therapist believes that the therapy is beneficial. Pseudo-placebos are designed by therapist-experimenters so that they are *not* intended to be therapeutic; trained therapists who deliver the placebos will also know that they are not intended to be therapeutic: "Therapist expectation, comfort, and enthusiasm [in placebo groups] are quite likely to vary considerably from those associated with active forms of treatment" (Borkovec, 1990, p. 54). The allegiance of the therapist was discussed in Chapter 5.

The failure to maintain blinds has been shown empirically to have considerable effects on assessed outcomes. Carroll, Rounsaville, and Nich (1994) conducted a study to assess how often psychotherapy and pharmacotherapy blinds are broken relative to evaluators of clinical functioning and how such breaks affect the assessment of clients. Cocaine-dependent subjects were randomly assigned to four conditions: relapse prevention plus desipramine; clinical management (the psychotherapy placebo) plus desipramine; relapse prevention plus pill placebo; or clinical management and pill placebo. The clinical evaluators were unaware of assignments and subjects who informed the evaluators of their assignment were dropped from the study. The subject's true assignment was guessed correctly by the evaluator over half the time and greater than would be expected by chance; for those in the psychotherapy condition, the evaluators correctly guessed 77 percent of the time. For the subjective measures in the study, the pattern of ratings "worked in favor of the active psychotherapy condition" (p. 279), whereas no bias was detected for more objective measures. So, not only were evaluators able to guess the psychotherapy conditions with some regularity, subsequent subjective evaluations were biased in favor of active treatments.

Finally, there is inevitably a fatal flaw in the design of pseudo-placebos from a Contextual Model perspective. According to the Contextual Model, expectations are created through providing an explanation to the patient for their problems (and not simply a rationale for treatment) as well as a treatment. Moreover, the treatment facilitates the client's involvement in performing some actions that help him or her reach the goals of therapy. An explanation and therapeutic actions are common factors. *Consequently, for this reason and the previous discussion, comparison of a treatment intended to be therapeutic and a pseudo-placebo, no matter how well designed, does not yield an effect that reflects the importance of a particular specific effect—it simply indexes the difference between a treatment that has structure, rationale, explanation, treatment actions, and a "treatment" without any of these qualities that are purported to be intrinsic to psychotherapy effectiveness according to the Contextual Model.*

A persuasive case that placebos have not controlled for the incidental factors of psychotherapy can be made by reviewing several studies that have used pseudo-placebos. First, consider the placebo control group used by Borkovec and Costello (1993) to establish the efficacy of applied relaxation and cognitive-behavioral therapy in the treatment of generalized anxiety disorder. The two treatments intended to be therapeutic, applied relaxation (AR) and CBT, contained many specific ingredients, whereas the placebo, labeled nondirective (ND) therapy, did not contain these ingredients. In all three conditions, the rationale for the treatment was given to the clients. The initial rationale given to the ND clients was created to sound plausible and reasonable:

> Clients were told that therapy would involve exploration of life experiences in a quiet, relaxed atmosphere; the goal was to facilitate and deepen knowledge about self and anxiety. Therapy involved an inward journey that would change anxious experience and increase self-confidence. The therapist's role would be one of providing a safe environment for self-reflection and of helping to clarify and focus on feelings as the therapeutic vehicle to facilitate change. The clients' role was described to emphasize their unique efforts to discover new strengths through introspection and affective experiencing.
>
> (p. 613)

Therapists were instructed to create an "accepting, nonjudgmental, empathic environment, to continuously direct client attention to primary feelings, and to facilitate allowing and accepting of affective experience using supportive statements, reflective listening, and empathic communications" (p. 613). However, any direct suggestions, advice, or coping methods were not allowed.

At the end of the first session, the researchers assessed clients' perceptions of the credibility of the treatment and their expectancy of their improvement. No significant differences between the treatments were found on these variables.

They also assessed relationship constructs at several points during therapy; again there were no significant differences. In addition, they measured experiencing, for which the ND subjects experienced deeper emotional processing.

ND in this study was superior to most other pseudo-placebos in the literature but nonetheless was deficient on a number of dimensions. To begin with, the therapists were trained in the laboratory of the researcher, an advocate of the two treatments in the study. Furthermore these therapists delivered all of the treatments, were certainly aware that ND was not intended to be therapeutic, and knew that the laboratory in which the study was conducted had an allegiance to the active treatments (see Chapter 4). Moreover, the authors recognized that the treatment was not intended to be therapeutic: "We chose a simple, reflective listening ND only to provide a nonspecific condition for control purposes: our intention was not to do a comparative outcome study contrasting the best available experiential therapy with cognitive-behavioral therapy" (p. 612). So, the therapists were forbidden to use methods that most nondirective therapists would use and could not give any suggestions, advice, or discuss how the clients might cope with their anxiety. While credibility and expectancy may have been comparable at the end of the first session, it is not clear that such ratings would be maintained throughout the therapy, given the proscriptions on the ND therapists. The placebo ND condition did not resemble either of the other two treatments with their active ingredients removed; rather it was a degraded form of a different therapy, experiential therapy, conducted by therapists who knew it was not intended to be therapeutic, and who had allegiance to the treatments to which it was compared.

In spite of these problems, Borkovec and Costello concluded that "from these results, we have drawn the conclusion that the behavioral therapy [viz., AR] and the CBT contain active ingredients in the treatment of GAD, independent of nonspecific factors" (p. 617). But there are issues in addition to the pseudo-placebo group that make this conclusion tenuous. First, expectancy ratings at the end of the first session correlated, on average, .43 with outcome.[2] That is, almost 20 percent of the variability in outcomes was accounted for by one simple common factor (viz., expectancy) measured at the first session. The average effect size for AR versus ND was .50, which indicates that treatment accounted for about 6 percent of the variability in outcome (see Table 3.1). This indicates, assuming that the ND did control for all incidental aspects of AR and CBT, that a single common factor, measured very early on, accounted for more than three times the sum total of the variability accounted for by all specific ingredients! There is another anomaly in these findings that casts doubt on the necessity of the specific ingredients. CBT contained all of the ingredients of AR as well as cognitive ingredients, but the results showed that AR and CBT were equivalent, which is a clear indication that the ingredients in CBT are not necessary to produce benefits (similar to the components studies reviewed above). However, the frequency of practicing relaxation and relaxation-induced anxiety during training showed no relationship with outcome, discounting the specific ingredients in AR. Finally, at the end of 12 months, the three therapies were equivalent in their outcomes, even when clients who sought additional treatment were eliminated from the analysis. So, this study, which has an exemplary placebo group, provided only very weak evidence for specific effects.

If the Borkovec and Costello study was a commendable attempt at constructing a pseudo-placebo that, although equal to the active treatments minus the specific ingredients, contained factors incidental to the active treatments, then consider the following ill-advised attempt. In this case, the placebo was labeled "supportive psychotherapy" and was compared to interpersonal psychotherapy for the treatment of depressed HIV clients (Markowitz et al., 1995):

> Supportive psychotherapy, defined as noninterpersonal psychotherapy and noncognitive behavioral therapy, resembles the client-centered therapy of Rogers, with added psychoeducation about depression and HIV. Unlike interpersonal psychotherapists, supportive psychotherapists offered patients *no explicit explanatory mechanism for treatment effect and did not focus treatment on specific themes.* Although supportive psychotherapy may have been hampered by the proscription of interpersonal and cognitive techniques, it was by no means a nontreatment, particularly as delivered by empathic, skillful, experienced, and dedicated therapists. Sixteen 50 minute sessions of interpersonal therapy were scheduled within a 17-week period. The supportive psychotherapy condition had between eight and 16 sessions, determined by patient need, of 30–50 minute duration.
>
> (Emphasis added, p.1505)

Here the treatments explicitly differ along the dimensions of a) whether or not a rationale for treatment was provided, b) the structure of treatment, c) the length of treatment, and d) the duration of treatment. Not surprisingly, it was found that the supportive psychotherapy was less beneficial than the interpersonal psychotherapy. These differences were attributed to the specific ingredients: "Our findings follow clinical intuition in showing an advantage for a treatment that targets depression over a nonspecific alternative" (p. 1508).

A placebo control group used by Foa, Rothbaum, Riggs, and Murdock (1991) falls between the commendable placebo designed by Borkovec and Costello (1993) and ill-designed placebo designed by Markowitz et al. (1995). Foa et al. compared stress inoculation training (SIT), prolonged exposure (PE), and supportive counseling (SC), the placebo, for the treatment of PTSD resulting from a recent rape. SC consisted of the following:

> Supportive counseling followed the nine-session format [as the other treatments], gathering information through the initial interview in the first session and presenting the rationale for treatment in the second session. During the remaining sessions, patients were taught a general problem-solving technique. Therapists played an indirect and unconditionally supportive role.

Homework consisted of the patients keeping a diary of daily problems and her attempts at problem solving. Patients were immediately redirected to focus on current daily problems if discussions of the assault occurred. No instructions for exposure or anxiety management were included.

(Foa et al., 1991, pp. 171–718)

Clearly, SC was not intended to be therapeutic, as "in the absence of other components, few would accept deflecting women from discussing their recent rape in counseling as therapeutic" (Wampold, Mondin, Moody, & Ahn, 1997a, p. 227). Moreover, the therapists were supervised by Foa, whose allegiance was to the SIT and PE. Finally, no attempt was made to determine whether the subjects found SC credible or if they expected SC to be beneficial. Nevertheless Foa et al. (1991) included supportive counseling "to control for nonspecific therapy effects" (p. 716).

The basic problems with pseudo-placebos have been discussed in this section. Logically and pragmatically, psychotherapy placebos cannot control for the incidental aspects of psychological treatments. More complete discussions of the problems with pseudo-placebos are found in the literature (Baskin, Tierney, Minami, & Wampold, 2003; Brody, 1980; Budge, Baardseth, Wampold, & Flückiger, 2010; Critelli & Neumann, 1984; Grünbaum, 1981; Horvath, 1988; Laska, Gurman, & Wampold, 2014; Shapiro & Morris, 1978; Shepherd, 1993; Wampold et al., 2010; Wampold et al., 2005; Wilkins, 1983, 1984). What is interesting, however, is how controls for psychotherapy trials have evolved, given some trends in the field. First, typically funding requires manualization of and adherence to treatments protocols, even if the treatment is a pseudo-placebo, and, consequently, researchers have more deliberately designed pseudo-placebo treatments.[3] Second, since Wampold et al. (1997b) made a distinction between treatments that were intended to be therapeutic and those that were not (see Chapter 5), researchers have made an attempt to include the necessary features so that a control treatment meets the classification for a treatment intended to be therapeutic. In many cases, the treatment consists of some form of "Rogerian Client-Center Counseling" or "Supportive Therapy," citing primarily Rogers (1951a). The line between a treatment that might meet the requirements of the Contextual Model and what constitutes a treatment intended to be therapeutic is not clear, as noted by Markowitz, Manber, and Rosen (2008):

To control for therapist contact and nonspecific elements of attending treatment, psychotherapy trials increasingly compare an experimental treatment to another form of psychotherapy, rather than to a waiting list. Among the more robust examples of a psychotherapy control condition is brief supportive psychotherapy (BSP), which has been used as a comparator in several randomized controlled outcome trials. Brief supportive psychotherapy involves the "common factors" of psychotherapy (Frank,

1971), which constitute the core of all therapies and have been credited with most of the outcome variance of efficacious specific therapies such as CBT and IPT (Wampold, 2001; Zuroff & Blatt, 2006). These common factors include emotional arousal, an understanding and empathic therapist, a structure and ritual to the treatment, success experiences, and provision of therapeutic hope and optimism. These factors are sufficiently active that BSP has at times worked "too well" as a control condition, keeping pace with more elaborate treatments (e.g., Markowitz, Kocsis, Bleiberg, Christos, & Sacks, 2005; Hellerstein, Rosenthal, Pinsker, Samstag, Muran, & Winston, 1998; McIntosh et al, 2005). Hence, it has been proposed not only as a control condition, but also as a treatment of choice (Hellerstein, Rosenthal, & Pinsker, 1994).

(p. 68)

Despite the description of BSP as having a "a structure and ritual to the treatment," BSP lacked many aspects of what the Contextual Model requires:

The BSP therapists used an unpublished treatment manual based on supportive psychotherapy principles (Pinsker, 1997; Navalis et al., 1993), which emphasize reflective listening and elicitation of affect. Therapists allowed patients to determine the focus of each session, pulling for emotion, validating emotions when possible, and offering empathic comments. They underscored thematic continuities as they arose from session to session, but did not provide other structure. They refrained from delineating any theoretical framework other than implicitly recognizing the importance of the patient's emotions. Moreover, they avoided cognitive and behavioral techniques and interpersonal problem solving that might overlap with [the active treatment].

(p. 70)

For all their problems, it should be recognized that pseudo-placebo treatments do contain one or more of the aspects of the Contextual Model. Pseudo-placebos are sufficiently credible to clients that the clients continue in treatment. Although the therapists know that they are delivering a treatment not intended to be therapeutic, they create and maintain some degree of therapeutic relationship with the clients. Being naturally desirous to help those in distress, the therapists likely take an empathic stance toward their clients in the pseudo-placebo treatments. According to the Contextual Model, pseudo-placebos create change primarily through the first pathway involving the real relationship, as well as perhaps a modicum of expectancy that can be created with explanation or treatment actions. Thus it is expected that pseudo-placebo treatments will be more beneficial than no treatment but less beneficial than treatments fully intended to be therapeutic. Consequently, both the Medical Model and the Contextual Model posit that placebo treatments will be more beneficial than no treatment but less beneficial than treatments intended to be therapeutic, and thus the expected results are not particularly informative in differentiating the progressivity of the two research programs. Nevertheless, it is not uncommon for researchers to conclude that the superiority of Treatment A to a pseudo-placebo is evidence that the ingredients of Treatment A are specific in treating a particular disorder, a conclusion that is frankly incorrect. As we shall see, some of this evidence is difficult to interpret due to the ambiguity about whether a treatment has the components of the Contextual Model (i.e., is intended to be therapeutic) or is a pseudo-placebo dressed up to look like a legitimate treatment.

Meta-Analyses of Pseudo-Placebos

Because both the Contextual Model and the Medical Model make essentially the same prediction about pseudo-placebos, the review of the meta-analyses will be relatively brief, although there are some interesting interpretations to be made.

Bowers and Clum (1988) reviewed 69 studies published from 1977 to 1986 that contained at least one behavioral psychotherapy intended to be therapeutic as well as groups designated as placebo, attention, or nonspecific controls. Each placebo was rated as to its credibility compared to the active treatment. The overall efficacy of the treatments versus no-treatments was 0.76, consistent with absolute efficacy meta-analyses reviewed in Chapter 4. The comparison of treatment to placebo yielded an effect size of 0.55, indicating that the placebo was 0.21 effect size units superior to no treatment. In another meta-analysis of placebo effects, Barker, Funk, and Houston (1988) reviewed only studies in which the placebo treatments generated a reasonable expectation for change. Their review of 17 studies containing 31 treatments found that the comparison of a treatment to the pseudo-placebo produced an effect size of 0.55 and the comparison of placebo to no treatment produced an effect of 0.47, indicating that treatments were clearly superior to pseudo-placebos with adequate expectation for change and that such placebos were also superior to no treatment.

In 1994, Lambert and Bergin reviewed 15 meta-analyses and arrived at the following effect sizes:

Psychotherapy versus no-treatment:	0.82
Psychotherapy versus pseudo-placebo	0.48
Pseudo-placebo versus no-treatment	0.42

These effects are in line with the prediction of both the Contextual Model and the Medical, so not much is learned. However, a few additional meta-analyses are interesting.

Stevens, Hynan, and Allen (2000) examined 80 studies that contained a complete treatment, a "common factor control," (CF) and a no-treatment condition. "Common factor controls" included "false feedback, progressive muscle relaxation, pill placebos, nondirective counseling, meetings with untrained 'therapists,' and discussion groups" (p. 276). Their findings were quite different from those of Lambert:

Psychotherapy versus no-treatment:	0.28
Psychotherapy versus "common factor controls"	0.19
"Common factor controls" versus no-treatment	0.11

Given the heterogeneity of the CF controls, some concern is raised about the conclusions. However, Stevens et al. examined the credibility of the CF interventions and surprisingly found that credibility was not related to the effects of the CF interventions. They also examined the effects across various outcome domains, including subjective well-being, symptoms, and life-functioning. Here we might expect that the CF controls would have greater effect on subjective well-being and active psychotherapies would have greater effect on symptoms, as suggested by the Contextual Model (see Chapter 2), but no such effects were found; however, the degree of focus on symptoms for treatments was not examined (e.g., CBT versus dynamic therapies). Nevertheless, Stevens et al. found a very small effect for CF controls, even when they were credible, contrary to what might be expected by the Contextual Model.

It is clear from the Stevens et al. (2000) meta-analysis that placebo type controls for psychotherapy vary widely. Baskin et al. (2003) examined the adequacy of these control groups by looking at the structural equivalence of the control condition to the active psychotherapy. A control condition was defined to be *structurally equivalent* to the active treatment provided they did not differ on the following dimensions: "(a) the number of sessions, (b) the length of sessions, (c) the format (i.e., group or individual), (d) the training of the therapists, (e) whether interventions were individualized to the clients, and (f) whether clients could discuss topics logical to the treatment (e.g., were trauma victims allowed to talk about their trauma?) or whether they were restricted to neutral topics" (p. 975). Based on 21 studies, Baskin et al. calculated the effect size between the active psychotherapy and the pseudo-placebo. For the eight studies where the pseudo-placebo was not equivalent to the active treatment, the active treatment was superior (d = 0.47, 95% CI 0.31 to 0.62), an effect in the neighborhood of Lambert and Bergin's (1994) estimate (see the proceeding) and one which was homogeneous. However, for the 13 studies of structurally equivalent pseudo-placebos, the active treatment was not significantly superior to the pseudo-placebo (d = 0.15, 95% CI 0.01 to 0.29). In the latter case, the effects were heterogeneous, suggesting that there is something interesting (and unknown) moderating the effects within the set of structural equivalent controls. Nevertheless, these results suggest that when the pseudo-placebos are well designed, their efficacy approaches that of the active treatment.

Despite the foregoing discussion about the inadequacies of using pseudo-placebos to establish the specificity of ingredients, there is a continued practice of citing differences between active treatments and pseudo-placebos to bolster the case for specific ingredients. A particularly egregious example is a recent meta-analysis of CBT for depression (Honyashiki et al., in press). In this meta-analysis, CBT treatments for depression were compared to no treatment and pseudo-placebos (called *psychological placebos* by the authors). In all, the meta-analysis contained 13 trials that compared CBT to no treatment, 6 trials than compared CBT to pseudo-placebos, and 1 trial that compared pseudo-placebo to no treatment. None of the pseudo-placebo treatments had any structure, goal setting, cogent therapeutic actions, and offered little more than minimal empathic responding and sometimes not even that. All of the controls contained proscriptions of what the therapist could do. In one control condition, which we classify as failing to faithfully allow the therapist to be empathic, to avoid behavioral strategies, if the patient stated, "'My daughter does not like me as she never comes to visit me,' the therapist would ask, 'How many children do you have?'" (Honyashiki et al., (2014), see Table 2). With regard to the effect of CBT versus pseudo-placebos, the researchers conducted both a pairwise meta-analysis (i.e., with the six trials that directly compared these two conditions) as well as a network meta-analysis (see Chapter 5). In neither meta-analysis was CBT shown to be significantly more effective than the pseudo-placebo, but the authors found evidence that the separation between CBT and pseudo-placebo controls grew over the course of therapy, which is not surprising given the inane composition of the pseudo-placebos. Despite the non-significant differences between CBT and pseudo-placebos, which should create concern on the part of advocates of CBT for depression, the authors, based on point-estimates that favored CBT and which increased over time, claimed that this meta-analysis established the specificity of CBT for depression. Indeed, the authors went further and suggested that the results cast serious doubt on the Dodo bird conclusion.

As noted in Chapter 5, there are some meta-analyses that have shown marginal superiority of one class of treatments to a class called "supportive therapy" (Braun, Gregor, & Tran, 2013; Cuijpers et al., 2012). As discussed in Chapter 5, the status of treatments in the class "supportive therapy" may actually be pseudo-placebos and certainly lack aspects that would qualify them as fully therapeutic according to the Contextual Model. Given the results of those meta-analyses and the ones discussed in this section, two conclusions are warranted. First, logically and empirically, the evidence from designs using pseudo-placebos provides little if any evidence to support specificity. The results that pseudo-placebos, when well designed—and even sometimes when they are not well designed—perform nearly as well as evidence-based treatments, ought to create skepticism about the necessity of specific ingredients that address particular psychological deficits. Second, it is also clear, on the other hand, that completely unstructured treatments, without therapeutic goals and therapeutic actions, despite the fact that the therapist is emphatically engaged with the patient, are insufficient. As Jerome Frank noted decades ago, an explanation and a treatment (myth and ritual) are needed in psychotherapy.

Interactions Between Patient Variables and Treatment

The Medical Model claims that specific ingredients are needed to remediate particular deficits and consequently some treatments will be more effective than others. Nevertheless, the results reviewed in Chapter 5 indicated that there is little evidence that any particular treatment that is intended to be therapeutic is superior to any other. If the Medical Model is indeed adequate to explain the benefits of psychotherapy, then the uniform efficacy of treatments for particular disorders must require some auxiliary claim. One auxiliary is related to issues with DSM diagnoses:

> Treatment outcome studies based on selecting subjects using DSM-like criteria consistently fail to show significantly large treatment differences that would help us understand etiology and inform treatment selection. Take, for example, the results of the NIMH Treatment of Depression Collaborative Research Program (Elkin, Parloff, Hadley, & Autry, 1985). The results of this multimillion dollar study suggest that it makes relatively little difference what treatment depressed clients receive (Elkin et al., 1989). This is hardly a surprise. A syndromal classification system assumes that a depressive is a depressive is a depressive. However, there are several well-developed accounts for how depression might come about (e.g., biological, behavioral, cognitive-behavioral, and interpersonal theories, etc.). If one assumed that depressive symptoms were one possible endpoint from a number of etiological pathways and that any group of persons with depression contained a number from each pathway, then comparative outcome studies are forever doomed to get equivalent results because those who have had a biological cause might respond to medication but not those who were interpersonally unskilled, and so on. So far there is little evidence that there are common etiological pathways that describe a uniform course or response to treatment for any reasonable proportion of the DSM-IV categories. Even the notion of uniqueness of symptoms clustering to reveal an underlying problem finds little support. In the National Comorbidity Study (Kessler et al., 1994), over half of the participants who received one diagnosis over the course of a lifetime had at least one other diagnosable disorder as well.
> (Follette & Houts, 1996, p. 1128)

The thesis here is clear: The commonly used diagnostic categories do not correspond to entities with uniform psychological/biological etiologies and consequently various treatments for disorders that have multiple determinants will produce similar outcomes. That is, clients within disorders are heterogeneous with regard to the causal factors creating the disorder and, therefore, different specific ingredients are needed to address specific deficits, regardless of diagnosis.

The heterogeneity of clients with regard to etiology premise purports that a specific treatment (say Treatment A) that targets a particular causal process (A′)

will have superior outcomes for those clients for whom it can be demonstrated that the disorder is caused by A' than will other treatments targeted toward other causal processes. This is a *causal moderation* hypothesis. If the Medical Model is correct, then a treatment by psychological deficit interaction should be found in studies that match treatment to clients based on theoretical grounds. It should be noted that this is a "weak" interaction effect and stronger ones have been predicted. For example, Hofmann and Lohr (2010) indicated the following condition for specificity: "A treatment T1 may be more efficacious than T2 for treating symptoms S1 but not for treating symptoms S2" (p. 14).

Evidence for Treatment by Psychological Deficit Interaction

As we shall see, the evidence for a treatment by psychological deficit interaction is weak, at best. Early narrative reviews remarked about how little evidence existed for the predicted interaction between treatment and client psychological deficit (Clarkin & Levy, 2004; Dance & Neufeld, 1988; Garfield, 1994; Smith & Sechrest, 1991), despite an emphasis on aptitude by treatment interactions (ATIs) during the period following Cronbach and Snow's (1977) seminal work on the topic. Despite the flurry of activity to find ATIs in psychotherapy in the 1980s and 1990s, the chapter on client variables (Bohart & Wade, 2013) in the most recent edition of *Bergin and Garfield's Handbook of Psychotherapy and Behavior Change* (Lambert, 2013) did not contain *any* discussion of the interaction of treatment and patient deficits. Perhaps the focus on interactions of this type has been avoided because two very large trials designed to detect treatment by deficit interactions failed to find any support for this conjecture.

For many years, there has been speculation that client characteristic/treatment interactions would exist in the area of substance abuse, as the treatments are conceptually diverse, encompassing such approaches as twelve-step programs, cognitive therapies, and motivation enhancement therapies. To test various hypotheses about such interactions, Project MATCH, a collaborative clinical trial, including 952 clients receiving outpatient therapy and 774 clients in aftercare treatment, was sponsored by the National Institute on Alcohol Abuse and Alcoholism (Project MATCH Research Group, 1997; see Chapter 5 for a discussion of this study as it pertains to relative efficacy). In this study, 16 matching (i.e., client/treatment interaction) hypotheses were developed, based on theory and research. Subjects, in the outpatient arm and in the aftercare arm, were assigned to cognitive behavioral coping skills therapy (CBT), motivational enhancement (MET), and twelve-step facilitation therapy (TSF). Client characteristics studied included alcohol involvement, cognitive impairment, conceptual level, gender, meaning seeking, motivation, psychiatric severity, sociopathy, support for drinking, and type of drinking. Some of these hypotheses were clear instances of causal moderation; for example, responsiveness to the cognitive therapy would be predicted by degree of cognitive impairment. Whether other hypotheses could be construed as evidence for causal moderation was ambiguous, however. Because the study was designed to test matching effects, special attention was given to design issues related to interactions, including importantly a sufficient number of patients to have adequate power to detect an interaction, should it be present.

The results of Project MATCH indicated that the three treatments were, for the most part, equally effective in both the aftercare and outpatient arms of the study, as discussed in Chapter 5. Of the 16 matching hypotheses in each arm, only one significant result was detected: for outpatients, clients whose psychiatric severity was relatively low had more abstinent days in the TSF condition than in the CBT condition. Clearly, the limited support for theoretically relevant interactions must be interpreted as lack of support for the premise that the specific ingredients of alcohol treatments are differentially active with various types of clients. Project MATCH involved an enormous effort to detect theoretically derived interactions—yet very limited evidence for the hypothesized interactions was found.

Project MATCH was followed up by the UK Alcohol Treatment Trial (UKATT; UKATT Research Team, 2007), a multicenter randomized controlled trial with more than 700 clients, whose primary purpose was to investigate two approaches for treating alcohol disorders, motivational enhancement therapy (MET) and a more intensive treatment based on social networks (social and behavior network therapy, SBNT). Consistent with Project MATCH and the Imel, Wampold, Miller, and Fleming (2008) meta-analysis, no differences between the two treatments were found. Five specific interaction hypotheses were specified, three of which fell into the class of treatment by client deficit interactions: clients with weak social networks would benefit more from SBNT; clients with low levels of readiness for change would benefit more from MET; and clients with higher levels of anger would benefit more from MET. Given that there were multiple tests involving different follow-up points, the few significant interaction effects were regarded to be a "consequence of multiple comparisons and as having occurred by chance [and] any adjustment for multiple testing would render all apparently significant results nonsignificant at the 5% level" (p. 231), and two of the significant results were in the opposite direction to the matching hypotheses. The UKATT Research Team made the following conclusion:

> No hypothesized matching effects were observed. . . . The conditions in question here are that two large, rigorous, multi-centre randomized controlled trials in two different health systems [viz., Project MATCH and UKATT] have failed to demonstrate any clinically meaningful increment to treatment effectiveness. It therefore seems warranted to consider the possibility that there were no substantial matching contingencies waiting to be discovered.
>
> (pp. 232–234)

Interactions between treatments and characteristics of the clients that support the specificity of treatments has been a cornerstone of the Medical Model of psychotherapy since 1969 when Paul asked the question, "What treatment, by whom, is most effective for this individual with that specific problem, under which set of circumstances, and how does it come about?" (p. 111). In the subsequent 30 years, there has been virtually no evidence to support theoretically derived inter-action of hypothesized client deficits and treatment. There has been absolutely no demonstration of the stronger interaction effect put forth by Hofmann and Lohr (2010), hypothesized a priori: "A treatment T1 may be more efficacious than T2 for treating symptoms S1 but not for treating symptoms S2" (p. 14).

Smith and Sechrest (1991) were, in our view, prescient in their observation of treatment by client characteristic psychotherapy research, an observation saturated with Lakatos' philosophy of science (see Chapter 3, Lakatos, 1970; Lakatos & Musgrave, 1970; Larvor, 1998):

> Despite the fairly consistently negative outcomes of the search for ATIs, the search is unabated. . . . If type of therapy does not appear to be related to outcome of therapy, then the effect of type of therapy must lie in an interaction with other variables. All that remains is to ferret out and display the interaction. . . . To a metascientist the movement toward ATI research might be viewed as a symptom of a degenerating program of research. Pro-grams can be said to be degenerating if they (a) fail to yield new predictions or empirical successes and/or (b) deal with empirical anomalies through ad hoc maneuvers that overcomplicate rather than clarify the problem of interest (Gholson & Barker, 1985). Perhaps psychotherapy researchers should be seriously and dispassionately reconsidering the core assumptions of their theories rather than building an elaborate ATI structure on a crum-bling theoretical foundation.
>
> (p. 237)

Evidence for Other Treatment by Client Interactions

The treatment by client deficit interaction was a Medical Model auxiliary prop-osition used to explain the apparent uniformity of outcomes across treatments. The lack of evidence to support this auxiliary does not imply that all treatment by client characteristic interactions might be non-existent.[4] The Contextual Model predicts that clients may prefer and have better outcomes in some types of therapy than others based on their characteristics, including personality, cul-tural attitudes, values, and identity, context, and demographics. In Chapter 7, evidence was presented that showed that culturally adapted treatments were more effective than non-adapted treatments for racial and ethnic minority cli-ents, which is a treatment (culturally adapted or not) by client characteristic (culture) interaction. Although this current chapter is focused on evidence for specificity, some treatment by client characteristic evidence is presented here that could be interpreted to be consistent with Contextual Model predictions.

In 2011, John Norcross edited the book *Psychotherapy Relationships that Work: Evidence-based Responsiveness* (Norcross, 2011), which contained a section entitled

"Tailoring The Therapy Relationship to the Individual Patient: What Works in Particular." This section contained chapters that presented meta-analyses on adapting psychotherapy to types of clients. Here we briefly discuss the evidence for two of these interactions (an additional chapter reviewed cultural adaptations, which were discussed in Chapter 7).

Beutler has hypothesized that clients who have resistance as a personality characteristic will benefit from relatively less structured treatments or less directive therapists whereas those clients who are not resistant will benefit relatively more from structured treatments and directive therapists (Beutler & Clarkin, 1990; Beutler & Harwood, 2000; Beutler, Harwood, Michelson, Song, & Holman, 2011). Beutler, Harwood, Michelson, et al. (2011) meta-analyzed 12 studies that investigated this hypothesis and reported a large effect size (d = 0.82). Beutler and colleagues also hypothesized that client coping style would interact with treatment (Beutler & Harwood, 2000; Beutler, Harwood, Alimohamed, & Malik, 2002; Beutler, Harwood, Kimpara, Verdirame, & Blau, 2011). Specifically, it was hypothesized that externalizing clients would benefit relatively more from symptom-focused treatments, whereas internalizing clients would benefit relatively more from insight-oriented treatments. Based on a review of 12 studies, Beutler, Harwood, Kimpara, et al. (2011) reported a medium-sized effect for this interaction (d = 0.55). Although the effects for these two interactions are quite large, there were some fundamental issues with how the primary studies assessed interactions and how these were coded in the meta-analyses. Consequently, these results are not central to the case for the Contextual Model, but clearly the idea that client personality or demographic characteristics interact with the features of the treatment are intriguing. Moreover, the evidence from the Beutler meta-analyses, however flawed, are not consistent with the Medical Model, which gives prominence to psychological deficits rather than to personality characteristics. Specifically, it is possible to conceive of a cognitive therapy that relies on the same underlying theory of cognitive dysfunction but is administered in a less directive manner in order to accommodate certain types of patients.

Adherence and Competence

In various chapters, it has been indicated that adherence and competence are Medical Model auxiliaries that are used to interpret the results of clinical trials. To properly make conclusions about the effectiveness of a treatment, the therapeutic ingredient purported to be remedial for the disorder needs to be delivered as specified in the protocol (i.e., adherence) and to be delivered skillfully (competence). Together, these two aspects are referred to as the *integrity* or *fidelity* of the treatment. As we have discussed, many clinical trials, including those finding differences among treatment and those that do not, have been impugned based on the integrity (primarily on basis of adherence) issue. It is now virtually required that clinical trials of psychotherapy assess and report adherence and competence.

Theoretical Considerations

As discussed in Chapter 2, adherence refers "to the extent to which a therapist used interventions and approaches prescribed by the treatment manual, and avoided the use of interventions procedures proscribed by the manual" (Waltz, Addis, Koerner, & Jacobson, 1993, p. 620). Even though the Medical Model requires adherence to the protocol and predicts that adherence is necessary for the benefits of the treatment, the Contextual Model also requires the delivery of ingredients consistent with the rationale for treatment provided to the client. However, the Contextual Model clearly is less dogmatic about the ingredients and certainly allows eclecticism, so long as there is a rationale that underlies the treatment and that the rationale is cogent, coherent, and psychologically based. Sol Garfield (1992), a prominent proponent of a common factors approach, in discussing the results of a survey of eclectic therapists, described the role of adherence in a Contextual Model context:

> These eclectic clinicians tended to emphasize that they used the theory or methods they thought were best for the client. In essence, procedures were selected for a given patient in terms of that client's problems instead of trying to make the client adhere to a particular form of therapy. An eclectic therapy thus allows the therapist potentially to use a wide range of techniques, a view similar to my own in most respects. . . . This approach is clearly opposite to the emphasis on using psychotherapy manuals to train psychotherapists to adhere strictly to a specific form of therapy in order to ensure the integrity of the type of psychotherapy being evaluated.
>
> (p. 172)

Thus, according to the Contextual Model, adherence to a manualized treatment is not required and is not thought to be related to outcome. Nevertheless, therapists working from a Contextual Model perspective necessarily will have a cogent rationale for the treatment and consequently the therapeutic actions will be consistent with that rationale. Consider the case of a therapist with a PTSD client who has little psychological mindedness, who approaches the world from a scientific perspective, and who conceives of the therapist as a doctor who will provide a cure. Although there are many approaches that the therapist could use, the therapist believes that prolonged exposure (PE; Foa, Hembree, & Rothbaum, 2007) would be well received by this client and consequently administers the treatment in a manner consistent with the rationale. However, this therapist, who ascribes to a Contextual Model of psychotherapy, presumes that the efficacy of the treatment is due to many factors unrelated to the exposure as specifically outlined in Foa et al.'s manual.[5] So, although this therapist would not be concerned about precisely following the manual, the treatment would be broadly consistent with such a protocol. Thus, the Contextual Model suggests that treatments should be coherent and consistent but it does not require technical adherence to a protocol.

According to Waltz et al. (1993) *competence* "refers to the level of skill shown by the therapist in *delivering the treatment*. By skill, we mean the extent to which the therapists conducting the interventions took the relevant aspects of the therapeutic context into account and responded to these contextual variables appropriately" (emphasis added, p. 620). In this definition an emphasis is on the skills delivering particular ingredients, rather than on a general competence as a therapist:

> According to this definition, competence presupposes adherence, but adherence does not necessarily imply competence. . . . With our definition of competence, we move away from a notion of general therapeutic competence and focus instead on competence in performing a certain type of treatment. . . . We suggest that the conception of competence be derived from the treatment manual and the theory of change specified in it.
>
> (pp. 620–622)

From the Medical Model perspective, competence involves delivering the specific ingredients specified skillfully. On the other hand, the Contextual Model would predict that the competent therapist is interpersonally skilled, able to work collaborative with a range of clients, express empathy, and effectively engage the client in the treatment actions. The two perspectives might overlap in that both would emphasize therapist skill in explaining the basis of a treatment.[6]

It should be noted that adherence and competence generally are thought of as characteristics of therapists. Therapists adequately adhere to the protocol and do it skillfully or they do not. Until recently, the client's influence on ratings of adherence and competence has been ignored, an issue discussed below.

Evidence for Adherence and Competence

As mentioned earlier, typically adherence and competence are assessed and reported in clinical trials. In some instances, correlations of adherence and competence with outcomes are reported. Recently Webb, DeRubeis, and Barber (2010) performed a meta-analysis on all studies that reported these correlations. Based on 28 effects, the aggregate correlation between adherence and outcome was small and non-significant (r = .02, 95% CI: −.07 to .10) and based on 16 studies, the aggregate correlation of competence and outcome also was small and non-significant (r = .07, 95% CI: −.07 to .20). Clearly, these results are inconsistent with what would be expected from a Medical Model perspective and call into question the adherence auxiliary so prominently invoked by Medical Model advocates (see e.g., Beck & Bhar, 2009; Bhar & Beck, 2009; Clark, Fairburn, & Wessely, 2008; Perepletchikova, 2009).

There are some limitations to the Webb et al. (2010) meta-analysis that have to be considered before accepting these small and non-significant effects as true reflections about the importance of adherence and competence in psychotherapy. Sample sizes across studies were quite small. In addition, the effects were heterogeneous, so there is unexplained variability in the effects that needs explaining, which Webb et al. did by examining several moderators. Of course, treatment might be an important moderator—adherence particularly might be more important in focused treatments, such as CBT, than in more unstructured treatments, such as dynamic therapies. However, treatment did not moderate the effects for either adherence or competence. Problems targeted did seem to make a small difference for the competence-outcome correlation, as competence seemed to be more important for the treatment of depression ($r = .28$ for depression). Controlling for the temporal relationship between the adherence and symptoms (i.e., controlling for prior symptom change—see Chapter 7 for a discussion of this issue with regard to the alliance) did not affect the size of the effects. However, examination of the studies in this meta-analysis revealed that although adherence and competence were measured at various times during therapy, sometimes early, middle, or late, or using an average of measures at various times, the effect of time of measurement was not investigated. Finally, studies that adequately controlled for alliance produced smaller competence-outcome correlations, but this was not confirmed by examining within-study comparisons.

One of the surprising results of Webb et al.'s (2010) meta-analysis was that competence was not correlated with outcome. This result should shake one's confidence about what it means to be competent, as for many "competent" means achieving excellence (see Tracey, Wampold, Lichtenberg, & Goodyear, 2014 for a discussion of this issue). However, examining how competence is conceptualized and measured will provide some clarification. Recall that Waltz et al. (1993) conceptualized competence as being treatment specific—how well a therapist is delivering the particular treatment—rather than how competent the therapist is generally. Most competence rating scales use this therapy-specific conceptualization and are rated by experts in the particular therapy. Most of the studies in Webb et al. used this therapy-specific definition of competence, and, consequently, their results could be interpreted as competence *in the particular treatment* is unrelated to outcome. On the other hand, in Chapter 7, we saw that competence in particular "common factors," such as forming an alliance across a range of patients or having a high level of facilitative impersonal skills, was indeed related to outcome. Still, it is disturbing that expert rating of therapist competence is not related to outcome.

Many of the concerns about the alliance-outcome correlation (see Chapter 7) apply to the adherence and competence correlations with outcome as well. One of the most prominent issues is that the assumption that adherence and competence are therapist characteristics (see Baldwin & Imel, 2013). When Waltz et al. (1993) rigorously defined adherence and competence, they realized that the context of therapy—characteristics of the client and what was happening in therapy—were important: "When clients like their therapist and improve substantially, it is easier for therapists to look competent" (p. 624). In Webb et al.'s (2010) meta-analysis, only the total correlation between adherence and competence with outcome was assessed, obscuring the effects due to the therapist or the client considered separately. As discussed in Chapter 7 with regard to the alliance, disaggregating the effects of patient and therapist requires sophisticated statistical analyses with at least two levels—therapists and patients. Several studies have shown that ratings of adherence and competence are influenced by who the patient is (Barber et al., 2006; Imel, Baer, Martino, Ball, & Carroll, 2011). Indeed, difficult patients— either because of initial severity, comorbidity, or personality—could well make therapists look relatively less competent and have poorer outcomes, creating a correlation that is due to patients rather than therapists.

There is one exemplary attempt to disaggregate therapist and patient contributions to adherence and competence in relation to outcomes. Boswell et al. (2013) examined the process and outcome of 276 patients receiving CBT from 21 therapists for panic disorder in a multisite RCT. Measures of adherence, competence, and symptoms were assessed during the course of therapy, creating a three-level model: observations over the course of therapy nested within patients and patients nested within therapists (i.e., level 1: observations within patients; level 2: patients nested within therapists; level 3: therapists). Rather than predicting the outcome at the end of therapy, Boswell et al. examined the relationship of adherence and competence at a particular session with symptoms reported at the next session. Consistent with Webb et al., the overall correlation between adherence and subsequent level of symptoms was non-significant (r = .08, 95% CI: −.02, .07). There was a small but significant correlation between competence and subsequent symptoms (r = .15, 95% CI: .05, .25).

From here the results become more complex; these total correlations were unraveled. Consistent with past studies, there was significant variability in adherence and competence ratings both between and within therapists. That is, some therapists adhered more and were rated as more competent than other therapists, but therapists appeared to adhere more and appeared more competent with some of their patients than with others, as well. Unexpectedly, adherence and competence ratings decreased over the course of therapy. With regard to patient characteristics, the patient's level of trait interpersonal aggression at the beginning of therapy was associated with adherence and competence ratings— therapists' adherence and competence ratings were lower for patients with more trait aggression. Trait aggression explained much of the within-therapist adherence variability and some of the within-therapist competence variability. In terms of disaggregating the total correlations for adherence and competence with outcomes, for both adherence and competence, neither the between- or within-therapist adherence or competence ratings were associated with panic severity: "This indicates that even when a more proximal indicator is used and variability is accounted for at multiple levels, the associations between adherence and competence and outcome can be rather meager" (Boswell et al., 2013, pp. 449–450). Recall that there was a significant total correlation between competence and outcome. When this correlation was disaggregated into between- and within-therapist, it turns out that the between-therapist coefficient was negative (regression coefficient = −0.17), indicating that therapists rated as more competent obtained poorer outcomes, although the coefficient was not significant. On the other hand, the within-therapist coefficient, which was due to variability in competence among the patients of the same therapist, was positive (regression coefficient = 0.76). Although not quite statistically significant, it does show that it is the patient's contribution to competence ratings that is related to outcome rather than the therapists' competence relative to other therapists.[7]

Taken together, findings like those presented in the Boswell et al. study and the null effects for adherence and competence found in Webb et al. (2010) highlight the complexity of determining the true effect of therapist actions on client outcomes during an ongoing dyadic interaction. As an illustration of how adherence may be related to treatment outcome, Baldwin and Imel (2013) constructed a visualization of possible patient- and therapist-level associations (see Figure 8.1). We refer the reader to Baldwin and Imel (2013) for a full discussion of these

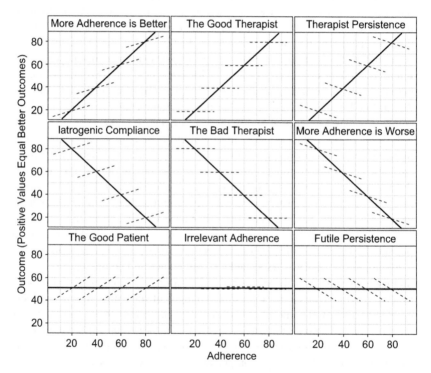

Figure 8.1 Different ways in which adherence and outcome might be associated between and within therapist caseloads. Solid lines represent between-therapist relationships (i.e., how therapist differences in levels of adherence are associated with outcome) and dashed lines represent patient-level associations (i.e. within-therapist associations). Reprinted from S. A. Baldwin & Z. E. Imel, "Therapist effects: Findings and methods," 2013, in M. J. Lambert (Ed.), *Bergin and Garfield's handbook of psychotherapy and behavior change*, 6th ed., p. 288. Copyright 2013, Wiley. Reprinted with permission of Wiley.

issues, but we do highlight several important issues here. The Contextual Model would be broadly consistent with adherence-outcome associations that are due to patients (i.e., the first and third columns). However, the Medical Model would posit associations that are in the first row—the more a therapist adheres to the treatment model the better and would generally be agnostic with respect to within therapist correlations. The Boswell et al. finding broadly maps onto the "good patient" panel, wherein observed associations between adherence and outcome are attributable to patients and not the potency of the adherence itself (i.e., therapists who were more adherent did not have better outcomes). However, as noted by Webb et al., negative total associations between adherence and outcome also could be due to patients (see "therapist persistence" panel). Specifically, a Medical Model would predict that therapists may use more specific interventions (i.e., be more adherent) because a patient is struggling and needs to improve. Essentially, the therapist is attempting to provide a stronger dose of treatment. Here, therapists with better adherence scores have patients with better outcomes, but patients with higher adherence scores within therapists may have worse outcomes. While we are not aware of any existing evidence for this pattern of results, it is clear that detecting the true association of adherence and outcome will require sophisticated modeling and larger sample sizes that are currently not generally available due to the labor intensiveness of human behavioral coding (Atkins, Steyvers, Imel, & Smyth, under review; Imel, Steyvers, & Atkins, in press).

Conclusions—Adherence and Competence

The Medical Model predicts that adherence and competence will be associated with better outcomes in psychotherapy. Indeed, these two variables, and particularly adherence, comprise a central auxiliary in the Medical Model, necessary to properly interpret the results of clinical trials. Presumably, one cannot make conclusions about the efficacy of a treatment if the treatment is not provided competently in the way the protocol stipulates. Nevertheless, the evidence seems to indicate that adherence and competence, as measured in clinical trials, are not related to outcome, creating uncertainty about the validity of the adherence and competence conjectures.

It is useful to compare the evidence for the alliance, a central construct in the Contextual Model, to the evidence for adherence and competence (see Chapter 7). The alliance is robustly correlated with outcome, across numerous studies. When the alliance was disaggregated into patient and therapist contributions, it was the therapist's contribution that predicted outcomes. That is, therapists who are better able to form alliances with patients have better outcomes with their patients than other therapists. Most other threats to the validity of the alliance have been investigated—the alliance has been put to the severest tests and to this point has survived as an important factor in psychotherapy effectiveness. Adherence and competence, on the other hand, do not appear to be robustly correlated without outcome—a comprehensive meta-analysis failed to find an association of adherence and alliance with outcome. In the Boswell et al. (2013) study, which found a relatively weak but significant correlation between competence and outcome, it appeared that the competence-outcome association was due to the patient's contributions to the competence ratings—that is, therapists who generally had higher competence ratings did not have better outcomes. Chapter 7 presented evidence that suggested that what makes a therapist competent (i.e., a therapist who achieves better outcomes) are factors central to the Contextual Model, such as forming a strong alliance and using a facilitative set of interpersonal skills.

There is a bit more material for speculation regarding adherence and competence. Boswell et al. (2013) observed, "Over half of the variance in adherence and competence was explained at the session level, suggesting that fidelity is contextually driven" (p. 451). To Medical Model adherents, this is a problem that must be addressed and highlights the need "for continued supervision or consultation for sustainability" (Boswell et al., p. 451). This conclusion is understandable if dependable adherence and competence scores are the goal but incomprehensible if indeed it is true that adherence and competence are not critical features in achieving better outcomes—why utilize interventions (viz., supervision and consultation) to achieve "satisfactory" levels of a variable that is not related to outcome? Interestingly, the variability of adherence scores from session to session, which was concerning to Boswell et al. and to dissemination researchers who seek to maintain fidelity to a specific approach, actually has been found to predict better outcomes—that is, patients of therapists who were flexible in their degree of adherence from one session to another achieved better outcomes (Owen & Hilsenroth, 2014). Boswell recognized that their results supported this idea: "Using sophisticated methods, this demonstration of mutual influence provides, albeit indirect, statistical support for the responsiveness hypothesis (Stiles et al., 1998)" (p. 452).

There is an older literature, which was reviewed in the first edition of this volume, that suggested that achieving high levels of adherence to a protocol can have deleterious consequences (Castonguay, Goldfried, Wiser, Raue, & Hayes, 1996; Henry, Schacht, Strupp, Butler, & Binder, 1993; Henry, Strupp, Butler, Schacht, & Binder, 1993). Here we review one of these studies that shows the problem with placing adherence as a goal to be achieved. Castonguay et al. (1996) compared the relative predictive ability of two common factors, working alliance and emotional experiencing, to an adherence variable, therapist's focus on the impact of distorted cognitions on depression (labeled "intrapersonal consequences"). In this study, four therapists, who received from 6 to 14 months of training and who were supervised throughout the study, delivered cognitive therapy (CT) for depression to 30 clients. The three predictor variables (viz., working alliance, experiencing, and intrapersonal consequences) were measured in the first half of treatment and then correlated with mid-treatment and post-treatment outcome scores, partialling out pre-treatment scores for each of the variables. Generally, the two common factors were correlated with outcome, as expected. However, the focus on intrapersonal consequences (i.e., the specific ingredient) was positively correlated with depressive symptoms; that is, there were higher rates of therapist focus on distorted cognitions in cases in which depressive symptoms were highest. Moreover, this latter relationship seemed to be accounted for by the working alliance, as the association between distorted cognitions and depressive symptoms was absent when working alliance scores were entered into the model. Descriptive analyses of representative cases with low alliance and high in intrapersonal consequences revealed the following:

> Although therapists dealt with these alliance problems directly, they did not do so by investigating their potential source. Instead, they attempted to resolve the alliance problems by increasing their adherence to the cognitive therapy model. (p. 501) . . . Some therapists dealt with strains in the alliance by increasing their attempts to persuade the client of the validity of the cognitive therapy rationale, as the client showed more and more disagreement with this rationale and its related tasks.
>
> (p. 502)

Thus, it appears that when the client was resistant to treatment (i.e., low agreement about goals and tasks), the therapist attempted to increase their adherence to the protocol by attempting to persuade the client to comply—and this was detrimental. This suggests that perhaps there is a curvilinear relationship between adherence and outcome—too much or too little is detrimental. Indeed, as discussed in Chapter 7, Barber et al. (2006) found that when alliance was high, adherence was irrelevant, but when it was low, moderate levels of adherence were most effective, which supports conjectures of the Contextual Model.

Mediators and Mechanisms of Change

Design Issues

Alan Kazdin, a luminary in the field of psychotherapy research, recently clarified the core logic of how we understand how psychotherapy works:

> A randomized controlled trial may show that treatment compared with no treatment leads to therapeutic change. From the demonstration we can say that the treatment caused the change, as that term is used in science. Demonstrating a cause does not say why the intervention led to change or how the change came about.
>
> (Kazdin, 2009, p. 419; see also Kazdin, 2007)

Kazdin defined the terms *cause*, *mediator*, and *mechanism* to differentiate various ways we can understand psychotherapy, as presented in Table 8.2. He then went on to describe the evidence that would be needed to establish mediators and mechanisms of change, as presented in Table 8.3. Clearly the requirements

Table 8.2 Mediators and Mechanisms of Change

Concept	Definition
Cause	A variable or intervention that leads to and is responsible for the outcome or change.
Mediator	An intervening variable that may account (statistically) for the relationship between the independent and dependent variables. Something that mediates change may not necessarily explain the processes of how change came about. Also, the mediator could be a proxy for one or more other variables or be a general construct that is not necessarily intended to explain the mechanisms of change. A mediator may be a guide that points to possible mechanisms but is not necessarily a mechanism.
Mechanism	The basis for the effect (i.e., the processes or events that are responsible for the change; the reasons why change occurred or how change came about).

Note. Reprinted from "Understanding how and why psychotherapy leads to change," by A. E. Kazdin, 2009, *Psychotherapy Research*, 19(4–5), p. 419. Copyright The Australian and New Zealand Association of Psychology and Law, reprinted by permission of Taylor & Francis Ltd, www.tandfonline.com on behalf of The Australian and New Zealand Association of Psychology and Law.

Table 8.3 Requirements for Demonstrating Mediators and Mechanisms of Change

Evidence	Definition
Strong Association	Demonstration of a strong association between the psychotherapeutic (A) intervention and the hypothesized mediator of change (B) and an association between the proposed mediator (B) and therapeutic change (C). Strong might be measured in effect size or percentage of variance but usually is addressed statistically through mediation analyses that show how the relation between A and C depend on B.
Specificity	Demonstration of the specificity of the association among the intervention, proposed mediator, and outcome. Ideally, many plausible constructs do not account for therapeutic change, with the exception of one, which strengthens the argument that the proposed construct mediates change.
Consistency	Replication of an observed result across studies, samples, and conditions (i.e., consistency in the relation) contributes to inferences about mediators. Inconsistency might result from operation of a moderator and not controvert interpretation of the critical construct. Yet consistency across studies greatly facilitates drawing inferences about whether a particular mediator may be involved.
Experimental manipulation	Direct experimental manipulation of the proposed mediator to show the impact on outcome (C).

Evidence	Definition
Time line	Demonstrating a time line or ordering of the proposed mediator and outcome (i.e., the mediator changes before the outcome).
Gradient	Showing a gradient in which stronger doses or greater activation of the proposed mediator is associated with greater change in the outcome can help make the case for a particular mediator. No dose-response relation (e.g., a qualitative or on-off gradient) or a relation that is not linear does not refute the role of the construct but may make inferences more difficult to draw.
Plausibility or coherence	A plausible, coherent, and reasonable process that explains precisely what the construct does and how it works to lead to the outcome. The steps along the way (from construct to change) can be tested directly.

Note. Reprinted from "Understanding how and why psychotherapy leads to change," by A. E. Kazdin, 2009, *Psychotherapy Research*, *19*(4–5), p. 420. Copyright The Australian and New Zealand Association of Psychology and Law, reprinted by permission of Taylor & Francis Ltd, www. tandfonline.com on behalf of The Australian and New Zealand Association of Psychology and Law.

to establish mediation and mechanisms of change are rigorous and demanding. Consequently, as Kazdin suggested, and others have documented (e.g., Johansson & Høglend, 2007), there is a paucity of evidence to establish mediation or mechanisms of change, despite decades of process research.

To illustrate the complexities of establishing mechanisms of change, cognitive therapy (CT) for depression is used as an example. In Figure 8.2, the hypothesized mechanisms of change of CT as well as five alternatives are presented. The hypothesized process of change involves CT changing cognitions, which subsequently reduces the symptoms of depression. The first alternative is that CT does not affect cognitions but does have an effect on depression through other means. The second alternative is that CT indeed does have an effect on cognitions, but the change in cognitions does not cause a decrease in depression symptoms, but rather CT acts through another mechanism. The third alternative is that other treatments that do not target cognitions also change cognitions, which in turn causes a decrease in depression symptoms. The fourth alternative is that CT is a beneficial intervention for depression, and a change in depressive symptoms then causes a change in cognitions.

The final alternative is one that is derived from the Contextual Model. Two of Kazdin's (2007, 2009) criteria of establishing mediating mechanisms were specificity and timeline. All of the models, except for the reciprocal model, consider only one mediator or class of mediators (here, cognitions) and consider variables as static in that they are measured at one or a few points in time and causality is unidirectional. As we have seen, characteristics of the patient as well as the patient's engagement and progress in therapy affect the manner in

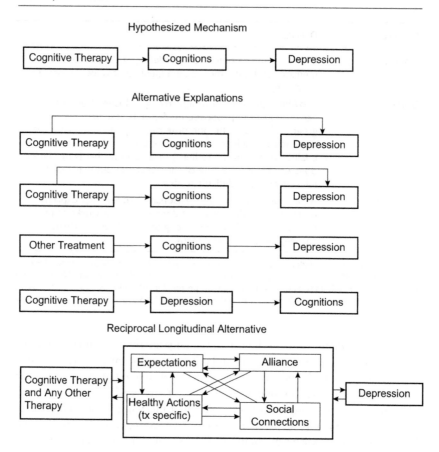

Figure 8.2 Possible mechanisms of change in cognitive therapy for depression.

which the treatment is given, various specific and common factors interact during the course of treatment, and symptom progression affects various processes as well. Every (effective) treatment has a set of therapeutic elements. Successful cases will involve patients who engage in the therapeutic activities and benefit from the treatment, so in most cases the purported mediating constructs for that treatment will appear to act as hypothesized—so all treatments might well appear to work through hypothesized mechanisms. The real test is when two treatments in the same study work through the respective hypothesized mediators and not through the mediators of the other treatment, as suggested by Kazdin. Of course, testing the reciprocal longitudinal model requires sophisticated methods (e.g., longitudinal multilevel models)—such methods are available and are beginning to be used. However, as we will see, the evidence for mediators and mechanisms has not coalesced.

Evidence for Mediators and Mechanisms

Cognitive Therapy

The discussion of evidence for mediators and mechanisms of change is focused primarily on CT for depression, and for CBT in general, for the primary reason that this search has had a long journey—and is a continuing one. Clearly, CT is an effective therapy for depression (see Chapters 4 and 5)—it is the most validated psychotherapy ever developed. However, to conclude that these benefits are mediated by a change in cognitions requires that evidence for the mediated model be produced as well as evidence that the benefits are not due to one of the alternative models in Figure 8.2.

One alternative to be ruled out is that cognitive therapy does not change cognitions. That is, cognitive therapy does not modify cognitions but decreases depression through some other mechanism. This alternative was convincingly ruled out early by a meta-analysis of the role of cognitions in cognitive therapy conducted by Oei and Free (1995), who reviewed 43 studies of various treatments of depression that included measures of cognitive style. The most common cognitive measures employed in the studies were the Dysfunctional Attitude Scale and the Automatic Thoughts Questionnaire, two measures developed to assess the cognitions hypothesized to be targeted by cognitive therapy. In this meta-analysis, it was found that there was a relationship between change in cognitions and cognitive therapy, strengthening the case for the specificity of cognitive therapy. There is no question that cognitive therapy, cognitions, and depression are interrelated; the issue is to understand the nature of the interrelationships.

A second alternative that needs to be ruled out is that the change in cognitions is unique in CT or at least is characteristic of therapies that target cognitions. Oei and Free (1995) also meta-analytically tested the relationship of non-cognitive psychological therapies and change in cognitions. It was found that cognitive therapy and other therapies did not differ significantly in terms of their effect on cognitions. Moreover, they found that drug therapies produced changes in cognitions equivalent to the two classes of psychological treatments. However, the latter conclusion has been challenged by research investigating the neural pathways of CT and antidepressant medication (DeRubeis, Siegle, & Hollon, 2008). At this point in time, the evidence is not conclusive that CT and other cognitive therapies for depression are unique in changing cognitions.

Another challenge to the specificity of cognitive treatments for depression comes from the component study conducted by Jacobson et al. (1996) discussed earlier in this chapter. This study provides compelling evidence that cognitive interventions are not needed to affect changes in cognition. Recall that there were three interventions: a) behavioral activation, b) behavioral activation plus coping skills related to automatic thoughts, and c) complete cognitive treatment, which included behavioral activation, coping skills, and identification and modification of core dysfunctional schemas. Behavioral activation contained no cognitive ingredients, whereas the latter two did contain cognitive ingredients, although only the full treatment was intended to alter core dysfunctional schemas. Nevertheless, behavioral activation altered negative thinking and dysfunctional attributional styles as well as either of the two cognitive treatments, contrary to predictions. In conjunction with the results that all three treatments were equally efficacious, the evidence from this study convincingly suggested that ingredients designed specifically to alter cognitions are not necessary in order to alter cognitions and reduce depression.

Another mediating explanation is that cognitive therapy is an efficacious treatment for depression but that change in cognitions is a result of decreased depression, not a cause (see Figure 8.2). In the first edition of this volume, we cited Ilardi and Craighead (1994), who claimed that a "majority of total symptomatic improvement [in CT] occurs *within the first three weeks of treatment* [whereas] the hypothesized mechanism of cognitive mediation, on the other hand, would probably not be expected to account for any substantial improvement observed in the earliest weeks of CBT, since the specific techniques designed to facilitate a reduction in depressive thoughts are not formally introduced until several sessions into the treatment" (pp. 140, 142). However, their conclusion was challenged by Tang and DeRubeis (1999), who presented evidence that many of the studies reviewed contained two sessions per week early in treatment and probably cognitive interventions had been introduced by the time changes in depression were achieved. As well, in two well-conducted studies, DeRubeis and colleagues (DeRubeis & Feeley, 1990; Feeley, DeRubeis, & Gelfand, 1999) found that change in depression occurs subsequent to therapists' administration of problem-focused, specific aspects of cognitive therapy. Finally, Strunk, Cooper, Ryan, DeRubeis, and Hollon (2012) found that the skills acquired in CT for depression were related to rates of relapse. Specifically, among patients who responded to CT, acquisition of cognitive coping strategies and in-session evidence of the use of cognitive skills were associated with lower rates of relapse one year later, even accounting for symptom level at the end of treatment or changes in symptoms over the course of therapy. This is informative because it indicates that specific skills learned during therapy are important for the maintenance of the benefits of psychotherapy—this may explain Bell et al.'s (2013) "sleeper" effect, which refers to the effect of an ingredient that appears to grow from end of treatment to follow-up (but see Flückiger et al., in press).

The final alternative explanation considered here is that various treatments influence a reciprocal system that, in turn, affects depression. There are several variations of the reciprocal system explanation for the efficacy of cognitive therapy. In one variation, Free and Oei (1989) hypothesized that cognitive therapy induces an adaptive cognitive style, which then affects the catecholine balance in the brain, whereas pharmacological treatments restore the catecholine balance, which in turn changes maladaptive cognitions. Ilardi and Craighead

(1994), based on their review of the timing of changes in cognitive therapy, contended that cognitive therapy (as well as other therapies) produced rapid change in depression as a result of the remoralization of the client:

> The mediational role of nonspecific processes in CBT (or any other therapeutic treatment, for that matter) might be expected to be especially prominent in the very early, as opposed to middle and later, stages of treatment. As Frank observed, "indirect support for the hypothesis [that nonspecific processes mediate clinical improvement] is that many patients improve very quickly in therapy, suggesting that their favorable response is due to the reassuring aspects of the therapeutic situation itself rather than to the specific procedure."
>
> (Ilardi & Craighead, 1994, p. 140)

Moreover, clients who are sufficiently remoralized in the early stages in therapy, according to Ilardi and Craighead, are successfully able to apply the cognitive techniques taught in CBT and, consequently, complete their recovery. Another reciprocal process could involve behavioral activation, as Jacobson et al. (1996) found that the activation component of CBT was sufficient to induce change in depression.

A final variation of the reciprocal system explanation is one in which various causal factors are fused. A fusion model, as well as the logical issues inherent in such a model, were well explicated by Hollon, DeRubeis, and Evans (1987) in a discussion of Beck's perspective on cognitions in CBT:

> Whether Beck would endorse a model based on mutual reciprocal causality between the separate components is not clear. He might argue for the correspondence between the cognitive processes and depression or between either and biological processes. In a recent monograph, Beck (1984b) suggested, "Thoughts do not cause the neurochemical changes and the neurochemical changes do not cause the thoughts. Neurochemical changes and cognitions are the *same processes* (emphasis added) examined from different perspectives" (p. 4). Although in arguing for an identity between these processes he appears to rule out causal mediation, he went on to say, "The cognitive approach, expressed in terms of the verbal and nonverbal behavior of the therapist, produces *cognitive-neurochemical* changes" (Beck, 1984b, p. 118). . . . In such a model, any change in depression, no matter how it was caused, would invariably be associated with comparable and correlated change in cognitive processes. . . . Beck's revised unitary model may well reject the notion of separation of components, obviating any causal mediation, because Beck sees those components as merely different perspectives on the same phenomenon (A. T. Beck, personal communication, March 27, 1986).
>
> (pp. 144–145 ff)

The implications of a reciprocal longitudinal model for specificity are profound, because the causal mechanism of change would be identical regardless of the treatment. That is, any efficacious treatment would ipso facto affect the unitary system composed of the various components related to depression. It would not be possible to demonstrate that a given treatment, say cognitive therapy, affects clients differently than any other treatment. Adopting a reciprocal model renders claims about specificity indeterminate, in a fundamental way.

A final study discussed here was a sophisticated examination of four mediated models for CBT for anxiety as well as depression. In a naturalistic setting, Burns and Spangler (2001), with a sample of 521 patients treated with CBT over a 12-week period, compared the evidence for four competing mediated models:

1. Changes in DAs [dysfunctional attitudes] lead to changes in depression and anxiety during treatment (the cognitive mediation hypothesis).
2. Changes in depression and/or anxiety lead to changes in DAs (the mood activation hypothesis).
3. DAs and negative emotions have reciprocal causal effect on each other (the circular causality hypothesis).
4. There are no causal links between DAs and emotions—instead, a third variable simultaneously actives DAs, depression and anxiety (the "common cause" hypothesis).

(p. 337)

In line with other studies, DAs were correlated with anxiety and depression and changes in DAs were correlated with changes in depression and anxiety over the course of therapy. Longitudinal structural equation modeling was used to compare the four hypothesized mediation models, after ensuring that the measurement model was adequate. The data did not support the first three models, but the common cause model provided a good fit: "To summarize, the data were consistent with the hypothesis that unknown variable or set of variables had simultaneous causal effects on the dysfunctional attitude, depression, and anxiety factors at both time points. . . . When controlling for the common cause, the two DA scales were not correlated with the depression and anxiety factors at either time point" (p. 356). The authors made the following conclusions:

> These findings are difficult to reconcile with Beck's (Beck, 1983; Beck et al., 1979) cognitive mediation hypothesis and with the mood activation hypothesis proposed by several investigators (Haaga et al., 1991; Persons, 1993; Teasdale, 1983). Finally, there was no support for Teasdale's hypothesis that DAs and emotions were linked by a system of circular causality . . . These findings are consistent with statements by theorists who have deemphasized the role of cognitive mediation in CBT and instead propose a simultaneous activation/model (Beck, 1984, 1996, pp. 359–360).

Recently Longmore and Worrell (2007) reviewed the evidence for cognitive mediation in CBT and concluded there was insufficient evidence to conclude that challenging thoughts were responsible for the benefits of CBT (see also Kazdin, 2007; Kazdin, 2009). Not unexpectedly, this result was itself challenged by advocates of CBT specificity (see Hofmann, 2008), which naturally resulted in a rebuttal (Worrell & Longmore, 2008). While Hofmann may or may not have had valid criticisms of Longmore and Worrell, he did not provide counter-vailing evidence to support change in cognitions as a mediator in CBT. And thus debate about the evidence for mechanisms of change for CBT goes on. At this point, the safest conclusion is that there is insufficient evidence from mediation studies to conclude that changes in cognition mediate the effects of CBT.

Evidence for Mediation in Studies Comparing Two Treatments

As discussed previously, one of the requirements of mediation is specificity, as a construct X should mediate the relationship between Treatment A and outcome, and construct Y should mediate the relationship between Treatment B and outcome. As well, longitudinal models are needed to assess the time sequence of the mediator and symptoms (Kazdin, 2007, 2009). Increasingly, studies have been designed that contain these features. Although there are insufficient numbers of studies, with replications, to make firm conclusions, a review of three such studies is instructive.

Establishment of specificity for cognitive therapy depends on finding that cognitive therapy affects a particular mediating construct differently than does a treatment that is hypothesized to operate through different mediating constructs. The NIMH Treatment of Depression Collaborative Research Program (TDCRP) compared cognitive-behavioral treatment (CBT), interpersonal psychotherapy (IPT), psychopharmacological treatment (viz., imipramine; IMI), and clinical management (CM). In this study, instruments were administered to assess the hypothesized causal mechanisms and were reported by Imber et al. (1990). As discussed in this chapter, cognitive treatments for depression are based on changing distorted cognitions. In the NIMH TDCRP, the Dysfunctional Attitude Scale (DAS) was used to measure the hypothesized mediating construct for cognitive therapy. IPT, which presumes a relation between interpersonal relations and depression, focuses on interpersonal conflict, role transitions, and social deficits. The Social Adjustment Scale (SAS) was used to assess social processes that are hypothesized to be critical to the efficacy of IPT. Imipramine is hypothesized to influence brain chemistry (neurotransmitter and receptor sensitivity) and consequently affect neurovegetative and somatic symptoms, which were measured with the Endogenous Scale from the Schedule for Affective Disorders and Schizophrenia (SADS). Specificity of therapeutic action predicts that each of the treatments would affect the mediating constructs uniquely; that is, CBT, IPT, and IMI-CM would change scores on the DAS, SAS, and SADS, respectively. Using data only from those clients who completed treatment, few of the predicted relationships were verified:

> Despite different theoretical rationales, distinctive therapeutic procedures, and presumed differences in treatment processes, none of the therapies produced clear and consistent effects at termination of acute treatment on measures related to its theoretical origins. This conclusion applies, somewhat surprisingly, not only to the two psychotherapies but also to pharmacotherapy as practiced in the TDCRP.
>
> (Imber et al., 1990, p. 357)

A limitation of this study was that the mediating constructs were assessed at the end of treatment and thus cannot rule out a reciprocal process whereby each treatment affected its hypothesized construct, which in turn affected the other constructs. Nevertheless, the TDCRP did not provide evidence to support the specificity of the three treatments.

Anholt et al. (2008) analyzed two trials that compared CT with exposure and response prevention (ERP) for the treatment of obsessive and compulsive disorder (OCD), involving 31 patients in the CT condition and 30 in the ERP condition. Obsessive and compulsive behaviors were measured weekly. The hypotheses were as follows:

> We hypothesized that the process of change in successful CT would first involve changes in obsessions, since CT primarily targets interpretation of intrusive thought, and that any decline in compulsive behavior would appear at a later stage in the treatment, once obsessions had subsided. Conversely, the process of change in ERP would presumably first appear as a decline in compulsive behavior, after which obsessions would subside as a result of the continuous refutation of dysfunctional expectations.
>
> (p. 39)

This is a hypothesis that conforms to Kazdin's (2007, 2009) specificity criterion. However, there were no differences between the two treatments in the progression of obsessive and compulsive behaviors over the course of therapy. For both treatments, contrary to the hypothesis, changes in compulsions predicted treatment effects better than changes in obsessions. The authors concluded, "One plausible explanation is that both treatments work through the same process mechanism" (p. 41), failing Kazdin's specificity criterion.

Recently, an extensive trial comparing CBT versus acceptance and commitment therapy (ACT) for mixed anxiety disorders was conducted (Arch, Eifert, et al., 2012). In this trial, 128 patients were randomly assigned to the two conditions. At termination there were no differences in outcomes on any measure, and while there were a few differences on some measures in some samples at follow-up, the general conclusion is that both treatments were effective but not different in terms of outcomes. In the trial, anxiety sensitivity and cognitive defusion were measured each session.

> Our study investigated two central questions: 1) Do CBT and ACT affect the theorized mediators for each treatment, showing greater reductions in beliefs about the harmful effects of anxiety (i.e. anxiety sensitivity) in CBT and greater increases in cognitive defusion in ACT? 2) Do changes in anxiety sensitivity and cognitive defusion mediate treatment outcomes? Specifically, do treatment specific processes mediate outcomes within the specified treatment only (anxiety sensitivity mediates CBT but not ACT outcomes, whereas cognitive defusion mediates ACT but not CBT outcomes), or, alternatively, do treatment-specific processes mediate outcomes across both treatments (anxiety sensitivity and cognitive defusion mediate outcomes across both CBT and ACT)?
>
> (Arch, Wolitzky-Taylor, Eifert, & Craske, 2012, p. 470)

The data were analyzed using sophisticated methods, namely multilevel mediation analyses. Similar to Anholt et al., 2008, a single process, in this case, cognitive defusion, was a mediator for both CBT and ACT. In the end, "The data offered little evidence for substantially distinct treatment-related mediation pathways" (Arch, Wolitzky-Taylor, et al., 2012, p. 469).

Conclusions: Mediation and Mechanisms of Change

Johansson and Høglend (2007) recently provided a critique of mediation studies in psychotherapy. In the years since Baron and Kenny presented statistical methods for conducting mediation analyses in 1986, Johansson and Høglend located 61 studies that examined mediation in psychotherapy. Their evaluation of the quality of these studies revealed numerous problems. For example, the majority of these studies were inadequate to establish the timeline of mediators and outcome. Often, mediators were not tested or tested improperly. In the end, they concluded, "Despite an increasing interest in mechanisms of change, no causal mediator has been satisfactorily demonstrated" (p. 7).

An issue for mediation is that often only the treatment-specific mediator is examined, obscuring other mediators, including those that might be common, such as the alliance. The Burns and Spangler (2001) study was one of the few to examine a competing common factor mediator (see Hoffart, Borge, Sexton, Clark, & Wampold, 2012 for another example). Perhaps the increasing sophistication of mediation studies will fulfill Kazdin's (2007, 2009) criteria for such research and reveal mechanisms of change in various treatments. However, at the present time there is insufficient evidence from mediation studies to document that any psychotherapy is mediated through its specified processes and not others.

Summary of Evidence for Specific Effects

In this chapter, we examined the evidence for specific effects by examining five areas of research: component studies, pseudo-placebos, interactions of patient characteristics and treatment, adherence and competence, and mediators of change. In each of these areas, evidence for specific effects was found to be weak or nonexistent.

Component studies examine changes in the effectiveness of removing a critical ingredient from an existing treatment (dismantling studies) or adding an ingredient that purportedly would augment the effectiveness of a treatment (additive studies). Two meta-analyses found no or small effects in these designs (Bell et al., 2013; Ahn & Wampold, 2001). Bell et al. found no significant differences between complete treatments and treatments without critical ingredients, but did find that adding a component to an existing treatment augmented the effects for targeted variables only, although the size of the effects were small.

Comparisons of a treatment to a psychological placebo creates logical and empirical difficulties due to the nature of the psychotherapy and these controls. The issues include the fact that psychotherapy trials cannot be blinded, the placebo is not indistinguishable from the treatment, the placebo and treatments effects are of the same class (i.e., are both psychological), and the incidental components in the placebo (e.g., the relationship) are active and necessary for the delivery of the purportedly active specific ingredients. Consequently, such controls are labeled as pseudo-placebos. The Medical Model and the Contextual Model make the same predictions about studies that compare treatments to pseudo-placebos and no-treatment controls but for different reasons. The Medical Model recognizes that the relationship, expectations, and remoralization will have a beneficial effect on patients and, therefore pseudo-placebos will be superior to no treatment, but a treatment with specific ingredients will outperform the pseudo-placebo. However, the Contextual Model requires that an effective treatment have a cogent rationale and treatment actions, components missing from placebo-controls. Generally, these predictions have been verified in meta-analyses: treatments intended to be therapeutic outperform pseudo-placebos, which in turn are superior to no treatment. However, when pseudo-placebos are given faithfully, permit the therapist to be caring and empathic, and are structurally equivalent to treatments, then the efficacy of the pseudo-placebos approaches that of active treatments.

An auxiliary of the Medical Model is that diagnostic schemes obscure the true nature of the psychological deficits that underlie psychological distress. Consequently, some treatments will be more effective with patients with a particular deficit, whereas other treatments will be more effective with patients with a different deficit, within a particular diagnosis. The hunt for interactions of this type has not yielded any consistent finding that a treatment by psychological deficit interaction exists. Nevertheless, there is some evidence that there is an interaction with personality variables (e.g., characterological resistance or coping style) and culture, which supports the Contextual Model.

The Medical Model predicts that adherence to a treatment protocol of an evidence-based treatment and the competence with which the therapist delivers the treatment should be related to outcome. Measurement of therapist adherence and competence is problematic because characteristics and actions of patients influence how adherent and competent the therapist appears; for example, therapists will appear less competent when working with patients who are interpersonally aggressive. Moreover, there is variability in adherence and competence across sessions within the same patient. A meta-analysis of adherence and competence revealed that ratings of these two variables and outcomes were small and generally non-significant (Webb et al., 2010).

Finally, studies have been conducted to examine whether treatments work through the purported mechanisms of change. Conducting mediation analyses in psychotherapy is difficult, and, consequently, it is not surprising that the evidence for hypothesized mechanisms of change does not clearly establish that the purported mechanism of one particular treatment is uniquely present in that treatment and not in others. As researchers begin to measure process and outcome measures frequently (e.g., every session, or even on a moment-to-moment basis within sessions) and newer growth models are applied to such data, there is the potential to establish mechanisms of change. However, such research will need to examine mechanisms that involve specific processes (e.g., changing dysfunctional cognitions) as well those related to common factors (e.g., creating expectations).

Researchers have made a concerted effort to establish the importance of specific ingredients of psychotherapy. As reviewed in this chapter, there is no compelling evidence that the specific ingredients of any particular psychotherapy or specific ingredients in general are critical to producing the benefits of psychotherapy.

Notes

1. Whether double-blinded placebo studies in medicine are truly blinded has been questioned. It appears that patients monitor themselves for the anticipated side effects to determine whether or not they have been taking the drug. Furthermore, correctly guessing that one is taking the drug affects the outcome (Fisher & Greenberg, 1997). Making this more complicated is that the treatment and psychological aspects of expectations interact, calling into question the additivity of physiochemical and psychological aspects (see Benedetti, 2011 and Chapter 7).

2. It should be noted that the authors of this study did not attempt to examine how the non-significant difference in expectancy affected the outcomes in the three groups. The authors reported that the expectancy and credibility ratings were not significant at $p > .20$. But given 55 subjects and $p = .20$, this translates into a correlation coefficient of 0.27 (Rosenthal, 1994, equation 16–23), which is large enough to account for the differences in outcomes between the active treatments and ND, particularly because the expectancy rating was so highly correlated with outcome. It is well known

that covariates with non-significant relationships with outcome can, nonetheless, have dramatic effects (Porter & Raudenbush, 1987).

3. See MacCoon et al. (2012) for a well-designed pseudo-placebo with respect to Mindfulness Based Stress Reduction (MBSR). The control condition was rigorously designed and structurally equivalent to MBSR. There were generally no differences between treatments on patient-reported outcomes. However, there was a strong patient preference for MBSR and the control was implemented in the context of a research group that generally was devoted to the study of mindfulness.

4. Liberman (1978; see Chapter 7) found an interaction between patient's level of desire for control and the internal/external attribution manipulation.

5. For example, there is existing evidence that the amount of time devoted to exposure in PE was not related to outcomes and that within-session habituation may not be necessary for successful treatment (van Minnen & Foa, 2006). There is also evidence that unattended ruptures in the therapeutic alliance predicted negative outcomes in PE (McLaughlin, Keller, Feeny, Youngstrom, & Zoellner, 2014).

6. This distinction may further breakdown in an intervention like Motivational Interviewing where therapist empathy is a core specific ingredient of the treatment approach (Moyers & Miller, 2013).

7. The authors did not test for the difference between these two coefficients, although this difference, called the contextual effect, is easily tested (see Snijders & Bosker, 1999).

Chapter 9

Beyond the Debate

Implications of the Research Synthesis for Theory, Policy, and Practice

Psychotherapy research has proliferated since the first edition of the *Great Psychotherapy Debate*. How do we make sense of the ever-accumulating evidence? Clearly there is important evidence imbedded in these results, but culling a cogent story line from this mass of evidence is not easy. With the number of psychotherapy trials and meta-analyses published each year increasing exponentially (see Chapter 4), there is some piece of evidence that one can find to support most any point of view. Consequently, and somewhat tragically, we are having some of the same debates today about psychotherapy that we have had in the past. For example, Eysenck's claims about the superiority of scientifically based treatments such as behavior therapy are being made in much the same fashion today—as are Rosenzweig's claim that treatments appear to be equally effective (see Wampold, 2013). Clearly, the evidence needs to be parsed in a coherent way.

Coherence demands a theory that can explain the preponderance of the evidence and anticipates new evidence as it appears. A single anomaly, or even multiple anomalies, should not lead to the abandonment of a research program; rather, the theory is adjusted, by the use of auxiliaries, to accommodate such anomalies. However, the hard core of the theory must survive severe tests. The theory should be able to predict what will be observed under what conditions. In a progressive research programme, challenges to conclusions should result in innovative research to examine the threats, and the theory should anticipate the results of such studies. A degenerative research programme will require many auxiliaries, many of which are generated *ad hoc* to explain anomalies and some of which are not themselves able to survive scrutiny.

In this volume, we examined two psychotherapy research programs, the Medical Model and the Contextual Model. The hard core of the Medical Model stipulates that the specific ingredients of treatments are responsible for the benefits of psychotherapy. Specifically, a) psychological dysfunction is identified, b) a treatment targets that specific dysfunction, and c) improvement occurs as a result of remediating the identified dysfunction. On the other hand, the hard core of the Contextual Model postulates that the relationship between the therapist and the client that occurs in the context of a treatment is critical to the success of therapy. This model proposes three pathways through which the benefits of psychotherapy are achieved: the real relationship, the creation of expectations through explanation and agreement about the tasks and goals of psychotherapy, and the facilitation of psychologically beneficial processes of some kind. As we have seen, the two models make very different predications about what will be observed in the same situation.

In this chapter, we discuss the implications of the evidence for theory, policy, and practice.

Implications for Theory

The Contextual Model is a Progressive Research Programme

Over the years, research syntheses of psychotherapy literature have attempted to partition the variability in outcomes to various sources, including Lambert's well-known pie chart (Lambert, 1992) and a concentric circle presentation presented in the first edition of this volume (Wampold, 2001b). Such attempts are flawed for several reasons. First, partitioning variability in outcomes to various sources assumes that the sources are independent, which they are not. For example, Lambert compared variability due to common factors with variability due to expectancy, but as we have seen, expectations is a core common factor. Similarly, therapist effects exist because therapists who are more effective are doing something that makes them more effective—for example, they are better at forming alliances. Second, the effects for various components are derived from very different research designs—that is, the effects produced depend to some extent on the research context and the experimental conditions. While we have transformed effect sizes (e.g., from correlations into Cohen's d), comparisons among effects must be interpreted cautiously. Third, any partitions of variability are often cited without consideration for the various concerns raised here.

Despite the issues with the interpretation of effect sizes, a comparison of these effects provides a starting point to understand the explanatory power of the two models. In Table 9.1 we summarize the effects produced by meta-analyses of psychotherapy effectiveness as well as various psychotherapy factors. As well, these effects are displayed as a bar graph in Figure 9.1, where the width of the bar reflects the number of studies on which the effect was based. The effects produced by the factors involved in the Contextual Model are larger than the effects produced by specific effects, a difference sometimes approaching an order of magnitude or more. The largest estimate for specific ingredients was treatment differences, but as discussed this estimate is a liberal upper bound and the best point estimate of treatment differences is zero. At the very least, these effects make it evident that the "common factors" are important considerations in the outcome of psychotherapy.

Table 9.1 Effect Sizes for Psychotherapy, Contextual Model Therapeutic Factors and Specific Ingredients Determined by Meta-analyses

Factor	# Studies	# Patients	Effect Size d	% of variability in outcomes	Chapter
Psychotherapy (vs. no treatment)					
Psychotherapy	>500		0.80	13.8	4
Contextual Model Therapeutic Factors					
Alliance[a]	190	>14,000	0.57	7.5	7
Empathy[a]	59	3599	0.63	9.0	7
Goal Consensus/Collaboration[a]	15	1302	0.72	11.5	7
Positive Regard/Affirmation[a]	18	1067	0.56	7.3	7
Congruence/Genuineness[a]	16	863	0.49	5.7	7
Expectations[a]	46	8016	0.24	1.4	7
Cultural Adaptation of EBT	21	950	0.32	2.5	7
Therapists—RCTs[b]	29	}14,519	0.35	3.0	6
Therapists—Naturalistic[b]	17		0.55	7.0	6
Specific Ingredients					
Differences between Treatments[c]	295	>5900	<0.20	<1.0	5
Specific Ingredients (dismantling)[d]	30	871	0.01	0.0	8
Adherence to Protocol[e]	28	1334	0.04	<0.1	8
Rated Competence in Delivering Particular Treatment[e]	18	633	0.14	0.5	8

[a]See various chapters in Norcross (2011).
[b]Baldwin & Imel, 2013
[c]Wampold et al. (1997b); confirmed by various other meta-analyses for specific disorders.
[d]Bell et al., 2013 (targeted variables); see also Ahn & Wampold (2001).
[e]Webb, DeRubeis, & Barber (2010).

As has been discussed in this volume, the "common factors" have either been dismissed out of hand or criticized on a number of bases. For example, the alliance outcome correlation, which is among the most established findings in psychotherapy research, was criticized due to threats related to whether it was a causal factor—perhaps early symptom improvement led to improved alliance and better outcomes, perhaps it was the patient's contribution to the alliance that was important for better outcomes rather than anything the therapist did, perhaps alliance was a "specific ingredient" for some relational therapies but unimportant for those that rely on "non-relational" specific ingredients, and so forth. Each of these issues led to innovative studies to investigate the issue and each time the conjecture that the alliance is an important therapeutic factor

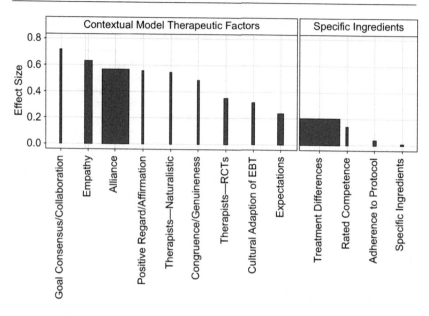

Figure 9.1 Effect sizes for therapeutic factors (width of bar reflects number of studies on which estimates are based).

has survived in the sense that the results were consistent with what would be expected if the alliance were an important therapeutic factor.

Of course, the Contextual Model employs auxiliaries, an important one of which is the allegiance of the therapist. The Contextual Model invokes the allegiance auxiliary to explain occasional studies that demonstrate treatment differences. The allegiance auxiliary states that a treatment delivered by therapists who believe that the treatment will be more effective, will be more effective than a treatment delivered by therapists who do not have that belief. As discussed in Chapter 5, researcher allegiance certainly does have an effect on outcome and most probably this is through the mechanism of therapist allegiance. Without a notable exception, the hard core of the Contextual Model is intact and when auxiliaries are used they are supported by additional research evidence.

The Contextual Model conceptualizes psychotherapy as a socially imbedded healing practice, utilizing social pathways to assist clients in alleviating various forms of psychological distress. In the Contextual Model, the influence of the relationship between the therapist and the client is central—the relationship works through direct means as well as indirect means. Even a cursory understanding of the Contextual Model conveys that the effectiveness of psychotherapy is not derived simply from having a relationship with the patient (i.e., just two people in a room talking), even if that relationship is empathic, caring, and nurturing, as important as those factors are. According to the Contextual Model, the therapist must provide an explanation of the client's problems and there must be therapeutic actions consistent with the explanation (i.e., a treatment) that involve means for overcoming or coping with the client's problems. The client needs to accept and engage in the therapeutic process—not simply be engaged with the therapist but actively working toward a goal in a coherent way. Below we will revisit the status of treatments in the Medical Model and the Contextual Model.

Medical Model Fails to Explain the Evidence

The hard core of the Medical Model emphasizes the potency of the specific ingredients. However, the evidence does not comport with predictions emanating from this hard core. Central to the Medical Model is the conjecture that some treatments should be more effective than others because the ingredients are more potent, due to their scientific nature. Since the beginning of direct comparisons between two treatments intended to be therapeutic, little evidence has been produced to show that there are differences among treatments—whatever anomalies (i.e., individual studies that show a difference) are about what would be expected by chance given that hundreds of such studies that have been conducted. Simply put, there are numerous treatments that are effective that according to a medical model should not be (e.g., Present Centered Therapy, EMDR, certain time-limited psychodynamic treatments). A logical auxiliary from the medical model would be that these treatments are actually working via accepted specific psychological processes outlined in other treatments (e.g., EMDR is simply exposure, i.e., a form of CBT). This raises the issue of another auxiliary of the Medical Model—adherence. However, if seemingly different treatments work through the same psychological mechanism (the efficacy of EMDR and CBT are due to exposure), then it is logically inferred that adherence to a particular protocol is not necessary, as exposure can be provided in a variety of ways in a variety of treatments. Ordinarily, trials specially select therapists, provide training, supervise, and monitor adherence. Regardless, trials that fail to show differences as well as those that do find significant differences are routinely criticized based on the adherence auxiliary, suggesting that it is used indiscriminately to impugn the validity of evidence. More distressing for the Medical Model, however, is that adherence does not seem to be related to outcome and thus the auxiliary itself lacks evidence. Moreover, despite the rigorous training and supervision, and other special conditions of clinical trials, in terms of outcomes, variability among therapists delivering the treatment has a larger effect than the differences between treatments.

The most direct way to identify the importance of a specific ingredient is the dismantling design in which the ingredient that purportedly addresses the psychological deficit is removed from treatment, with the expectation that the efficacy of the treatment will be attenuated. Two meta-analyses have shown that removing the critical ingredient does not attenuate the effects of treatment.

It is difficult to declare that there are zero differences between treatments in general or between two particular treatments. Nevertheless, whatever differences exist, they are clearly quite small, especially compared to other effects. The Medical Model, as a rule, venerates RCTs as the gold standard when it comes to making conclusions about research evidence, yet the evidence produced by RCTs that either compare treatments intended to be therapeutic or dismantle evidence-based treatments do not provide compelling evidence for the specific ingredients, which are central to the Medical Model. It should be noted that many, although clearly not all, advocates of the Medical Model recognize the importance of relationship factors but argue that these effects are not robust, either in terms of their magnitude or their importance, compared to specific effects.

Importance of Treatments

It is not unusual to read that some treatment is superior to a "common factor" treatment, which is a name that describes a treatment in which the therapist is trained to be empathic, warm, and accepting but is not allowed to take any action that would be interpreted as a treatment. These pseudo-placebo treatments are often given "legitimacy" by labeling them as "Rogerian Therapy," (even citing one of Rogers' books) and classifying them as a humanistic treatment but such "treatments" typically are neither treatments nor humanistic. Anyone who has studied Rogers or watched videos of his work will understand that these "common factor" treatments do not resemble what Rogers discussed and what Rogers did in therapy. Indeed, Rogers was quite strategic in his responses to patients (see Truax, 1966). In RCTs, these treatments typically are provided by therapists who are cognizant of the fact that they are indeed providing a control group therapy (e.g., Markowitz, Manber, & Rosen, 2008). Humanistic treatments have evolved since the 1950s and 1960s (Ellison & Greenberg, 2007; Greenberg, 2010), so why use a treatment popular in 1950? However, the biggest fallacy is that the Contextual Model, as well as other common factor models (see Chapter 2), *describes explicitly how some form of treatment is necessary*. In the Contextual Model, a cogent explanation of the disorder, a treatment consistent with the explanation, agreement on goals and tasks, and participation in therapeutic tasks designed to achieve the patient's goals are essential to produce the benefits of psychotherapy. It is not surprising then that treatments—treatments with cogent rationales and therapeutic actions—often outperform treatments without any structure, without any rationale for their effectiveness that can be explained to the patient, which do not help the patient make desirable changes in his or her life, and for which the therapist is often prevented from doing what he or she believes is therapeutic (see Chapter 8). Moreover, even some therapies intended to be therapeutic might indeed be less effective than other treatments if no attempt is made to orient the patient to his or her difficulties and link therapeutic actions to ways to improve, which might be the case for some humanistic treatments or psychoanalytic treatments (see e.g., Poulsen et al., 2014).

The closest a legitimate treatment might be to a "common factor" treatment is Motivational Interviewing (MI), which is a "collaborative, person-centered form of guiding to elicit and strengthen motivation for change" (Miller & Rollnick, 2009, p. 137). Although MI places emphases on common factors, particularly empathy and instilling hope (i.e., creating expectations), it provides a guide for therapists to intervene strategically to promote motivation to change, to reinforce self-efficacy and change talk, and encourage goal setting (developing discrepancy between where the client is and where they want to be). As discussed by Miller and Rollnick (2009), MI is not simply client-centered counseling:

> MI departs from traditional conceptions of client-centered counseling, however, in being consciously goal-oriented, in having intentional direction toward change. In MI, the counselor strategically listens for, elicits, and responds selectively to certain forms of speech that are collectively termed "change talk." Over the course of an MI session, the counselor seeks to increase the client's strength of expressed motivation for a target behavior change, and to diminish defenses of the status quo.
>
> (p. 135)

Moreover, MI is clearly intended to be therapeutic, is not easy to learn, and is provided by therapists who are trained in the treatment and who believe it will be effective (Miller & Rollnick, 2009).

Although the Medical Model and the Contextual Model both stipulate the necessity of a treatment, the role of treatment in the two respective theories is very different. In the Medical Model, the scientific status of the ingredients outlined in the manual is paramount—as Eysenck noted in the 1950s, treatments that contain ingredients based on scientific knowledge should be more efficacious than other treatments. We have reviewed the literature that demonstrates the lack of differences among treatments. Moreover, there are some anomalies that are very difficult to explain in the Medical Model and for which no reasonable auxiliaries have been proposed. Several treatments that are now classified as psychological treatments with strong research support began as control treatments, constructed purposefully to omit ingredients that were thought to be critical scientifically, including interpersonal therapy for depression (Weissman, 2006), behavioral activation (BA) for depression (Jacobson et al., 1996), and present-centered therapy (PCT) for PTSD (Frost, Laska, & Wampold, 2014). As discussed previously, when it was found that BA was as effective as cognitive therapy (CT) for depression, Jacobson et al. (1996) noted, "These findings run contrary to hypotheses generated by the cognitive model of depression put forth by Beck and his associates (1979), who proposed that direct efforts aimed at modifying negative schema are necessary to maximize treatment outcome and prevent relapse. If BA . . . [is] as effective as CT and also [is] as likely to modify the factors that are thought to be necessary for change to occur, then not only the theory but also the therapy may be in need of revision" (pp. 302, 303). Nonetheless, CT has not been abandoned or altered because the specific ingredients were impugned, contrary to what the Medical Model might dictate. Indeed, no treatment that has appeared on any list of evidence-based treatments has been removed due to doubts about the scientific basis of the ingredients.

Another one of these anomalies is PCT for PTSD, which was developed to "provide a credible therapeutic alternative to control for nonspecific therapeutic factors so that observed effects of prolonged exposure could be attributed to its specific effects beyond the benefits of good therapy" (Schnurr, Shea, Friedman, & Engel, 2007, p. 823), in that it was designed to omit exposure of any kind as well as any cognitive interventions. Earlier attempts to design controls for PTSD that contained neither exposure nor cognitive components, but contained no therapeutic actions other than empathic responding, were less effective than evidence-based treatments (e.g., Foa, Rothbaum, Riggs, & Murdock, 1991). However, when PCT was developed as a manualized treatment with a credible rationale that could be explained to clients and therapeutic actions that facilitated acquisition of strategies that could be used in life (viz., problem-solving skills), it became as effective as treatments with purported scientific ingredients, according to a meta-analysis of trials comparing PCT to evidence-based treatments (Frost et al., 2014). Surís, Link-Malcolm, Chard, Ahn, and North (2013) made the following conclusion, after comparing PCT to cognitive-processing therapy for PTSD:

> The current study demonstrated that CPT and PCT were both effective at reducing posttraumatic and depressive symptoms. Similar to findings from other randomized controlled clinical trials (McDonagh et al., 2005; Schnurr et al., 2007), PCT appeared to perform more like an active intervention rather than a comparison condition intended to control for the nonspecific aspects of therapy such as time and attention.
>
> (p. 7)

A troublesome anomaly for the Medical Model is Eye Movement Desensitization and Reprocessing (EMDR) for PTSD, a treatment that on the one hand has been labeled as pseudoscience and compared to Mesmerism (Herbert et al., 2000; McNally, 1999) and on the other hand is as effective as the standard evidence-based treatments and is a recommended treatment by such organizations as the National Institutes of Health and Care Excellence in the United Kingdom (Wampold et al., 2010). EMDR is listed by the Society of Clinical Psychology as a psychological treatment with "strong research support/controversial." Although there is good evidence that specific components of EMDR as outlined in the manual are not necessary (see Herbert et al., 2000; McNally, 1999), as noted previously, the same could be said for CT for depression and several other treatments. Other than the more blatant scientific implausibility of some of EMDR's specified actions, the lack of evidence for specificity appears to be similar with many other "mainline" cognitive-behavioral treatments and the reason for the "controversial" designation appears arbitrary.

The Medical Model cannot explain the efficacy of these anomalous treatments. On the other hand, the efficacy of these treatments are not anomalies in the Contextual Model—indeed, the Contextual Model predicts that a treatment that has a cogent rationale that is accepted by the patient, is provided by a therapist who believes the treatment will be effective, and induces the patient to engage in actions will be effective *regardless of the purported scientific basis* of the ingredients. Indeed, the treatment will likely result in a cascade of interrelated psychological processes, some of which might appear to be similar to what is purported to be the psychological bases of different treatments, but the content of the intervention is not necessarily a guide to what they are. The cogency of the explanation given to patients was clearly recognized by Meichenbaum (1986), a proponent of cognitive therapies, when he described the laudatory actions of a therapist:

> As part of the therapy rationale, the therapist conceptualized each client's anxiety in terms of Schacter's model of emotional arousal (Schachter, 1966). That is, the therapist stated that the client's fear reaction seemed to involve two major elements: (a) heightened physiological arousal, and (b) a set of anxiety-producing, avoidant thoughts and self-statements (e.g., disgust evoked by the phobic object, a sense of helplessness, panic thoughts of being overwhelmed by anxiety, a desire to flee). After laying this groundwork, the therapist noted that the client's fear seemed to fit Schachter's theory that an emotional state such as fear is in large part determined by the thoughts in which the client engages when physically aroused. It should be noted that the Schachter and Singer (1962) theory of emotion was used for purposes of conceptualization only. Although the theory and research upon which it is based have been criticized (Lazurus, Averill, & Opton, 1971; Plutchik & Ax, 1967*), the theory has an aura of plausibility that the clients tend to accept: The logic of the treatment plan is clear to clients in light of this conceptualization.*
>
> (Emphasis added, p. 370)

Theoretically, treatments are not analogues of medications, which contain inert ingredients and specific ingredients (see Chapter 2). Treatments by necessity contain many relational elements, which are not analogues of inert ingredients. Moreover, any treatment is an amalgamation of many different elements.

Table 9.2 Possible factors important to successful treatments of PTSD.

Cogent psychological rationale that is acceptable to patient

Systematic set of treatment actions consistent with the rationale

Development and monitoring of a safe, respectful, and trusting therapeutic relationship

Collaborative agreement about tasks and goals of therapy

Nurturing hope and creating a sense of self efficacy

Psychoeducation about PTSD

Opportunity to talk about trauma (i.e., tell stories)

Ensuring the patient's safety, especially if the patient has been victimized as in the case of domestic violence, neighborhood violence, or abuse

Helping patients learn how to avoid revictimization

Identifying patient resources, strengths, survival skills and intra and interpersonal resources and building resilience

Teaching coping skills

Examination of behavioral chain of events

Exposure (covert in session and in-vivo outside of session)

Making sense of traumatic event and patient's reaction to event

Patient attribution of change to his or her own efforts

Encouragement to generate and use social supports

Relapse prevention

Note. Reprinted from "Determining what works in the treatment of PTSD," by B.E. Wampold, Z.E. Imel, K.M. Laska, S. Benish, S.D. Miller, C. Flückiger, . . . S. Budge, 2010, *Clinical Psychology Review, 30(8)*, p. 931. Copyright 2010. Permission from Elsevier.

Wampold et al. (2010) presented a list of potentially therapeutic elements for PTSD, which is found in Table 9.2.

Most treatments for PTSD would utilize most of these elements, emphasizing some more than others, making it difficult to identify what is the "active" ingredient. Moreover, there is generally much disagreement about what are the essential elements of any "brand" of psychotherapy, as discussed by Baardseth et al. (2013):

> As discussed by Lakatos (Larvor, 1998; Lakatos, 1970; 1976), science and mathematics involve two processes. First, taxons or concepts are established, developed, and/or defined. For example, Newtonian physics posits a force called gravity; Mathematics has the class of things defined as polyhedra. Second, formal relationships among the taxons or concepts are conjectured. For gravity, Newton stated that the gravitational force is proportional to the product of the two masses and inversely proportional to the square of the distance between them. In terms of polyhedra, Euler conjectured that the characteristic of such solids, defined as the number of

vertices minus the number of edges plus the number of faces, was equal to 2. However, the manner in which the taxons or concepts are formed is critical to assessment of the truth of the formal conjectures, and the work on the formal propositions in turn creates refinements of the taxons or concepts. For Newton, the gravitational proposition was first stated in terms of point masses, which latter needed to be revised to accommodate masses with volume; similarly, for Euler's polyhedras, convex and concave polyehdra were differentiated as Euler's conjecture became a topological problem rather than a geometric solid one. Although taxons and concepts are altered in a research program, from time to time, changes need to be rational and the changes should then generate new propositions that can be investigated (Lakatos, 1970; 1976). That is, progress has been achieved based on investigations of the formal propositions, either with regard to the relation of the concepts but also on the nature of the concepts. . . . As Larvor (1998, p. 19), in his commentary on Lakatos, [stated], "Nevertheless those meanings (whatever they may be) must remain fixed from one end of the argument to the other."

(p. 402)

Unfortunately for the study of psychotherapy, what is classified as a belonging to a class of treatments, say CBT, varies from one discussion to another. For example, sometimes EMDR is classified as a CBT (e.g., Tolin, 2010) while other times it is not (Ehlers et al., 2010). Ehlers et al. (2010) made a distinction between CBT and stress management treatments (e.g., stress inoculation training). This raises the question, what are the essential features of CBT? Tolin (2010) classified a treatment as CBT if it contained *any* of the following components: relaxation training (including progressive muscle relaxation, meditation, or breathing retraining); exposure therapy (imaginal or in vivo exposure, including flooding and implosive therapy); behavior rehearsal (behavioral training in social skills, habit reversal, or problem solving); cognitive restructuring (including direct strategies to identify and alter maladaptive thought processes); or operant procedures (systematic manipulation of reinforcers or punishers for behavior, including behavioral activation). There is a strong likelihood that two treatments classified as CBT may not have any features in common! And as well, almost all treatments will have one of these features. For example, PCT, designed not to be CBT by excluding exposure and cognitive restructuring, teaches patients problem-solving skills (a behavioral intervention) for issues in the present and thus has been classified as CBT (see Bisson et al., 2007)! Consulting CBT organizations does not clarify the situation, as according to the National Association of Cognitive-Behavioral Therapists (NACBT; 2014), "Cognitive-behavioral therapy does not exist as a distinct therapeutic technique. The term cognitive-behavioral therapy (CBT) is a very general term for a classification of therapies with similarities" ("What is Cognitive-Behavioral Therapy?" para. 1), and the Association for Behavioral and Cognitive Therapies (ABCT; 2014) defines CBT as "the term used for a group of psychological treatments that are based on scientific evidence" (About Psychological Treatment section, para. 1).

The theoretical status of the Medical Model in psychotherapy is tenuous, which has implications for policy, practice, and training. As Popper noted:

> From a rational point of view we should not "rely" on any theory, for no theory has been shown to be true, or can be shown to be true. . . . But we should *prefer* as basis for action the best-tested theory.
>
> (emphasis in original, 1972, pp. 21–22)

On that basis, we might well prefer the Contextual Model. The implications of abandoning the Medical Model and tentative acceptance of the Contextual Model would seem to have radical implications for policy and practice, although not as radical as one might believe.

Policy

Research Priorities

Clinical trials continue to be the "gold standard" in more ways than one. As mentioned in Chapter 4, the number of clinical trials of psychotherapies has escalated dramatically—more and more treatments are being investigated using clinical trials. Unfortunately, what can be learned from standard psychotherapy clinical trials is limited—and moreover, clinical trials are expensive.

The limitations of clinical trials have been discussed in several instances in this volume but are summarized here. First, it is impossible to blind clinical trials. The therapist always knows which treatment is being delivered and often is aware that the treatment he or she is delivering is a "control" treatment not intended to be therapeutic. Even when two treatments intended to be therapeutic are compared, allegiance becomes an issue (see Chapter 5). In any case, therapists utilized in trials are a select sample and then typically are given extensive training, supervision, and other support. As well, patients will also know what therapy they are receiving. If they are informed honestly that one of the treatments to which they would be randomly assigned contained no therapeutic actions of known potency, they would likely infer when they were receiving the purportedly inferior treatment. Second, the use of "common factor" or as we have called them, pseudo-placebo, controls is logically flawed. In medicine, active medications and placebos are indistinguishable and, importantly, act through different systems—active medications are physiologically active while placebos are psychologically active. In psychotherapy research, the active treatment and the control group are both psychologically active. Therefore, it is difficult to add a therapeutic ingredient to a purportedly inactive psychological placebo—the relationship and other common factors in the active treatment are intrinsically different from the relationship and other common factors in the control. In addition, the delivery of specific techniques cannot be separated fully from the supposedly inactive ingredients (e.g., change in expectancy—a core "nonspecific" effect—is likely central to the benefits of cognitive therapy).

Let's examine the utility of various forms of clinical trials. The first type of comparison between a treatment intended to be therapeutic with some type of no-treatment control group (e.g., a waitlist control group) as a means to examine absolute efficacy. As described in Chapter 4, these clinical trials show demonstratively that psychotherapy works, with an effect size of about 0.80. Indeed, we know of no published report of a bona fide psychotherapy failing to separate from no-treatment, although of course this may be due to publication bias. Nevertheless, the hundreds, if not thousands, of such studies consistently find psychotherapy, of any kind, to be beneficial compared to no treatment. The second type is the comparison of two treatments intended to be therapeutic, which as seen in Chapter 5, consistently fails to find differences among treatments. The third type of clinical trial is the comparison of a treatment intended to be therapeutic to a pseudo-placebo condition, which as we have shown is insufficient to make attributions about specificity. Nevertheless, as we have seen (see Chapter 7), the pseudo-placebos are more effective than no treatment, and in many cases, approach the active treatment in terms of efficacy. Finally, trials are used to dismantle treatments that have shown to be efficacious by removing an ingredient purported to be critical for the success of the treatment. As reviewed in Chapter 8, removing the ingredient from treatments does not attenuate the benefits of the treatment. In all of these types of trials, there is a disturbing trend to give primacy to targeted variables only, ignoring the reality that patients come to treatment for a variety of concerns, including relationship problems, poor quality of life, and general feelings of distress.

Randomized clinical trials have provided much of the research reviewed in this volume and, therefore, have provided informative evidence. Moreover, clinical trials have established the efficacy of psychotherapy, thereby legitimizing psychotherapy and leading to its inclusion as a procedure within medical systems of most Western countries. Nevertheless, the wisdom of orienting scientific funding toward conducting additional trials like those discussed above has to be questioned. In the thousands of trials conducted, we have not found a particular treatment for any disorder that is reliably and clinically superior to any other treatment. When the results of a particular trial reveal some difference between treatments, the results often are impugned by the advocates of the apparently inferior treatment. No treatment that meets the definition of a psychotherapy used in this volume has ever been found to be reliably inferior or harmful. It is unclear what additional knowledge the continued use of such clinical trials will produce.

The continued use of clinical trials comes at a cost. According to Laska, Gurman, and Wampold (2014), eight studies between 1992 and 2009 funded by the NIMH that compared two treatments intended to be therapeutic produced little knowledge or actionable results. Overall, the aggregate effect of these studies was not significantly different from zero—indeed, only one of the studies produced a significant difference between treatments. That one study found that IPT was superior to CBT for depressed HIV patients (Markowitz et al., 1998), yet no clinical guideline has ever recommended that depressed HIV patients receive IPT rather than CBT. These eight studies, which seemed not to have added much clinically or scientifically (other than to further reinforce the conclusion that there are no differences between treatments), came at a cost of more than $11 million.

Of course, process research is not without its problems. While one could question what has been learned from such research, we claim the scientific return on investment has been dramatic. The research on the alliance is instructive. Heavily imbedded in theory, the research on the alliance has established it as critical therapeutic factor, and it has survived every threat raised. Instead of spending millions to compare different forms of psychotherapy, money should be spent investigating what makes various treatments work. Consider what we might learn if we had a well-funded agenda to investigate the characteristics and actions of effective therapists. Such an agenda would lead to results that would likely improve the quality of care and focus training efforts.

Quality Improvement

The Medical Model and the Contextual Model have different strategies for improving the quality of mental health services.

Medical Model Strategies

The Medical Model claims that some treatments are more effective than others, but even when there is a lack of evidence for differences, therapists should provide only treatments that have been tested in clinical trials, according to some:

> Thus, in the face of evidence that Tx A works, it is not sufficient for the practitioner who prefers Tx B to rest on the fact that no one has shown that Tx B is ineffective. Tx A remains the *ethical* choice until the success of Tx B is documented.
>
> (Chambless et al., 2006, emphasis added, p. 193)

The implication for improving the quality of care is that dissemination of evidence-based treatments into routine psychotherapy practice would improve outcomes (Baker, McFall, & Shoham, 2008; Foa, Gillihan, & Bryant, 2013; Karlin & Cross, 2014; McHugh & Barlow, 2012; Shafran et al., 2009). According to this perspective, therapists are achieving relatively poor outcomes because they are not using faithfully evidence-based treatments, and if these therapists began to use such treatments, outcomes would improve. As logical as this sounds, there are some serious problems with this strategy (see Laska et al., 2014).

The dissemination strategy assumes that therapists are achieving outcomes that are inferior to what could be achieved if only they provided an evidence-based treatment. However, as discussed in Chapter 4, therapists in practice are achieving outcomes comparable to benchmarks created in clinical trials—and doing it in fewer sessions. Moreover, when evidence-based treatments are studied in naturalistic settings, there is no convincing evidence that they are superior to treatment-as-usual, if the treatment-as-usual involves psychotherapy services, with the possible exception of the treatment of personality disorders. A second problem with dissemination efforts is that the therapists are ignored—the presumption is that if therapists are adequately trained, all therapists will achieve commendable outcomes. However, as discussed, it appears that even in specialty clinics where therapists received training in evidence-based treatments from national experts and received supervision from one of the experts, there were large differences in the outcomes achieved by the therapists (Laska, Smith, Wislocki, Minami, & Wampold, 2013).

A third problem with dissemination is that evidence-based treatments are disorder specific and a therapist would need to learn multiple treatments to serve a patients with a variety of disorders (say nothing about comorbidity), a problem noted by McHugh and Barlow (2012):

> For example, even at specialty outpatient clinical service settings, clinicians would need to receive training in multiple individual protocols to be able to treat the target patient population using ESTs. A community mental health center that serves a wider variety of clinical presentations would require training in even more protocols. Attempting to maintain fidelity to each of these individual treatments would present an enormous challenge to a clinical care system. Given the cost of didactic (e.g., workshop, written materials) and competence (e.g., supervision and feedback) training, implementing multiple treatments to a facility is often not a feasible consideration.
>
> (p. 951)

To address this issue, various transdiagnostic treatments are being developed (e.g., Barlow et al., 2011) but as yet they have not shown that they are feasible or would improve the quality of care.

The final issue for dissemination efforts is that they are expensive. Laska et al. (2014) estimated that it would cost a therapist $4,200 to learn a single evidence-based treatment, an estimate that does not include post-training consultation or retraining due to drift in therapist adherence, as recommended by dissemination advocates. For clinics or systems of care the cost could be great.

For example, the Department of Veteran Affairs spent more than $20 million to roll out evidence-based treatments between 2007 and 2010 (Ruzek, Karlin, & Zeiss, 2012). Epidemiological studies show that in the United States, around 40 percent of people who qualified for a DSM diagnosis in the past 12 months do not receive mental health services of any kind (Kessler et al., 2005; Wang et al., 2006; Wang et al., 2005). Money used to disseminate evidence-based treatments could well be spent making mental health services more *accessible*, primarily by expanding the number of providers available and ensuring that services are affordable.

Generally, clinicians are reluctant to change the manner in which they practice and the failure to use evidence-based practices is, at least to some, the root cause of poor mental health services (Baker et al., 2008; Lilienfeld, Ritschel, Lynn, Cautin, & Latzman, 2013). Indeed Baker et al. have said that clinical psychology "resembles medicine at a point in history when its practitioners were operating in a largely prescientific manner" (p. 77). However, if, as we claim, disseminating evidence-based treatment is unlikely to improve the quality of care, what is the alternative?

Contextual Model Strategies

According to the Contextual Model, a variety of different treatments will produce benefits as long the treatments are given by effective therapists. This hardly translates into a prescription that "therapists should practice as they please." Rather, the consequence of the Contextual Model for quality improvement is that each therapist is responsible for achieving commendable outcomes, regardless of the treatment they choose to use. This perspective leads to the use of "practice-based evidence," which uses data about the progress of clients in practice to improve the quality of care (Barkham, Hardy, & Mellor-Clark, 2010; Duncan, Miller, Wampold, & Hubble, 2010; Lambert, 2010; Pinsof & Wynne, 2000; Sapyta, Riemer, & Bickman, 2005).

The most researched means to use practice-based evidence is to provide therapists feedback about patient progress. Meta-analyses of clinical trials comparing feedback to no feedback have shown that providing such feedback improves outcomes, producing modest but impressive effect sizes in the neighborhood of 0.50 (Lambert & Shimokawa, 2011; Shimokawa, Lambert, & Smart, 2010). Although there are many issues involved in implementing feedback systems (Boswell, Kraus, Miller, & Lambert, in press), it provides an evidence-based alternative to the dissemination of evidence-based treatments. One of the problems with the dissemination of evidence-based treatments is that implementation of these treatments is not accompanied by outcome measurement. Thus how well the treatments work "on the ground" in any given setting is unknown. Practice-based evidence is based on actual outcomes, creating accountability based on metrics in practice settings. In one example where the Partners for Change Outcome Management System

(PCOMS; Miller, Duncan, Sorrell, & Brown, 2005) was implemented by the Center for Family Services (CFS) in Palm Beach, Florida, Bohanske and Franczak (2010) noted:

> For example, average length of stay decreased more than 40%. Cancellation and no-show rates dropped by 40% and 25%, respectively. Most impressive of all, the percentage of clients in long term treatment that experienced little to no measured improvement fell by 80%! In 1 year, CFS saved nearly $500,000, funds that were used to hire additional staff and provide more services.
>
> (p. 308)

Of course, there is no proscription from using practice-base evidence in conjunction with evidence-based practices, and many Medical Model adherents are not opposed to feedback strategies, but rarely are they mentioned as a means to improve the quality of care when evidence-based treatments are discussed.

Practice-based evidence has expanded to include data on the process of therapy. Lambert (2010) has developed clinical support tools that assess alliance, readiness for change, and social support. Other systems also have developed tools to measure the alliance and other process aspects of therapy for individuals, couples, and systems (e.g., families) (Miller et al., 2005; Pinsof et al., 2009).

The final way that practice-based evidence can be used to improve the quality of care is to monitor patient progress at the therapist level. As was clear from the review in Chapter 6, there is much variability among therapists in terms of outcomes. More importantly, it appears that the poorest therapists bring down the "average" quite dramatically. In terms of policy, any manager of an agency or a system of care should be concerned about the outcomes achieved by therapists, particularly underperforming therapists. Of course, what actions should be taken can be controversial. The very measurement of therapist performance is controversial as it impinges on professional autonomy. However, it seems to be a reasonable way to proceed given imperatives to be accountable to patients and payers, as long as underperforming therapists are given the opportunity to improve. From our perspective, therapists can achieve poor outcomes for a variety of reasons—for example, the inability to form collaborative relationships with a range of patients and the inability to respond empathically, particularly with difficult clients (see Moyers & Miller, 2013). However, some therapists may form adequate relationships with patients but fail to provide a viable and acceptable treatment structure. The former may benefit from some type of relationship enhancement work while the latter may benefit from learning particular treatments, such as evidence-based treatments.

There are some policy initiatives that make little sense from an evidentiary standpoint. Mandating that therapists only deliver a particular treatment or choose from a small set of treatments is contrary to the evidence presented in this volume. From our perspective, accountability is derived from outcomes achieved and not from insisting that only specific treatments to be delivered. We have benchmarks for some disorders and could develop them for others—as long as therapists or systems of care meet the benchmarks, why should the range of therapies (with some caveats discussed below) be restricted? Patients have preferences for different types of therapy—and indeed, a meta-analysis found that patients receiving their preferred treatment had better outcomes and had fewer premature dropouts than patients assigned to treatments they did not prefer (Swift, Callahan, & Vollmer, 2011).

This brings us to dropout. Clearly, there are many reasons for dropping out of therapy, but for whatever the reasons dropping out before the completion of treatment is problematic. Estimates of dropout vary, but a systematic review estimated that about 20 percent of psychotherapy patients drop out (Swift & Greenberg, 2012). If patients drop out because they find the treatment unacceptable, then the availability of a variety of treatments seems to be appropriate, given the evidence that no one treatment is clearly more effective than another. Let's return to Chambless et al.'s ethical imperative:

> Thus, in the face of evidence that Tx A works, it is not sufficient for the practitioner who prefers Tx B to rest on the fact that no one has shown that Tx B is ineffective. Tx A remains the *ethical* choice until the success of Tx B is documented.
>
> (emphasis added, p. 193)

This might be a perfectly reasonable way to proceed if all treatments had "equal access" to evidence. In Chapter 4 it was clear that CBT has been examined in more clinical trials than any other approach, by a rather wide margin. Part of this is due to an inclination of CBT advocates to be active in research, which perhaps confers a legitimate advantage to CBT. But there is a hegemonic aspect to this as well. The de facto requirements of clinical trials advantage treatments that are readily manualized, time limited, and focused on symptoms. Arguably, funding for CBT is more readily available, policymaking institutions are populated by CBT researchers, and top-tier journals are more inclined to publish articles that demonstrate the efficacy of CBT. Discussing the hegemony of CBT should not be interpreted as "anti-CBT." CBT, for a wide variety of disorders, is an effective treatment—for many patients, CBT is understandable, acceptable, and effective. It is the claims of superiority, the efforts to mandate CBT, and the attribution that CBT is "scientific" (vis-à-vis alternatives) that is troublesome.

A disturbing trend in RCTs and in meta-analyses of RCTs is the focus on disorder-specific symptom measures, to the exclusion of global measures of mental health, well-being, or quality of life (Crits-Christoph et al., 2008). Consider for example, McDonagh et al. (2005) who compared two treatments for PTSD, CBT, the standard evidence-based treatment, and present-centered therapy discussed earlier, with a waitlist control group. Despite superiority in targeted symptoms of PTSD, "neither treatment was superior to [waitlist] in reducing symptoms of depression, dissociation, and anger or hostility, nor in improving quality of life" (p. 520). Moreover, target symptoms are not primary for non-symptom focused treatments:

> The goals of psychodynamic therapy include, but extend beyond, allevia-tion of acute symptoms. Psychological health is not merely the absence of symptoms; it is the positive presence of inner capacities and resources that allow people to live life with a greater sense of freedom and possibility.
> (Shedler, 2010, p. 105)

The field needs to have a discussion about what is the appropriate focus of treatment. In an effort to model ourselves after medicine, we have, in many realms, focused on symptoms. But such a focus misreads trends in medicine, which are heavily involved in quality-of-life issues. If a patient's symptoms remit but the patient's quality of life, role functioning, interpersonal rela-tions, and other indicators of well-being have not improved, many would say that the therapy has not been successful. Well-being is not solely the absence of symptoms.

Good policy would expand the range of available effective treatments and ensure that patients have access to care, rather than attempting to disseminate a small set of treatments.

Practice

Entertaining the Contextual Model has implications for practice, from the per-spective of the therapist and the patient, as well as for training. Much of these conclusions mirror those made with regard to policy, albeit from a different perspective.

Therapist Perspective

Treatment Choice

As we have emphasized in this concluding chapter, there is insufficient evidence to privilege some treatments over others. The implication of this conclusion would seem to be that therapists can deliver the treatment of their choosing. However appealing this might sound, there are three important caveats.

The first caveat is that therapists must deliver a treatment that is coher-ent, explanatory, and facilitates the patient's engagement in making desir-able changes in their lives. It is not sufficient for a therapist simply to respond empathically or to deliver a set of actions that have no coherence—the latter best described as incoherent eclecticism. The essential feature of explanation and treatment is that it a) is acceptable to the patient, b) leads to expectation that the patient will have control over his or her problems, and c) engages the patient in some type of action. Therapists should understand that it is their responsibility to ensure that the patient accepts the treatment—resistance to the treatment may be due to a number of factors, some to do with the patient, some with the therapist, and some with the nature of the treatment. Therapists need to understand that patients will prefer one treatment over another or may find one more compatible with their personality, attitudes, and cultural beliefs than another. Clearly, therapists need to be aware of and take into account patients' culture, attitudes, values, economic resources, social support, and other contextual variables (see APA Presidential Task Force on Evidence-Based Practice, 2006). This suggests that therapists are flexible in how they present the treatment (see e.g., Owen & Hilsenroth, 2014), but it also implies that therapists may well need to be skilled in delivering more than one treatment. The evidence suggests that rigid adherence to a treatment protocol, particularly if it damages the relationship between therapist and patient, is detrimental.

The second caveat is that therapists are responsible for the outcomes achieved by their patients. Of course, some patients will have poorer prognoses than others, due to a number of factors outside of the control of the therapist, but overall therapists should achieve reasonable benchmarks for the types of patients being treated. This responsibility suggests that therapists measure the progress of their patients, something Paul Clement began in private practice in 1966 (Clement, 1994, 1996). Whether one uses one of the available measures or assesses patient progress toward therapeutic goals in the therapy interaction, a therapist needs to have knowledge of their effectiveness. This caveat applies to therapists delivering an evidence-based treatment as well as the therapists providing another treatment. Essentially, therapists who do not systematically monitor the effectiveness of their interventions cannot claim to be providing ethical treatment that meets current standards of care.

The third caveat is that there is a limit to the range of therapies that should be provided. Patients coming to a healer expect an explanation consistent with the healing practice and consequently the treatment provided to psychotherapy patients should have a reasonable and reasonably defensible psychological basis. There are many "crazy" therapies (Singer & Lalich, 1996) and some that may indeed be harmful, at least anecdotally (e.g., rebirthing therapies)—in our view, these therapies should be avoided. To engage in fringe therapies puts the therapist at risk but also damages the field. While interventions that do not meet the definition of psychotherapy (e.g., life coaching, religious retreats, etc.) may be useful and rely on similar psychological mechanisms, we view their application and regulation to be beyond the purview of psychotherapy research. Of course, the demarcation between acceptable treatments and those that are too deviant from a proper psychological basis is not fixed and is a decision that has to be made by the therapist.

Therapist Belief in Treatments

As reviewed in Chapter 5, there is sufficient reason to believe that therapist allegiance to the treatment delivered is important. Indeed, no client of any service wants to utilize a practitioner who does not believe in the procedures being used. If a client wants to litigate a claim against a neighbor and the lawyer does not believe that is the best course of action, the client will not have confidence that the lawyer will perform well in court and likely either will give up the desire to litigate (if the lawyer is persuasive) or change lawyers. Similarly, patients want to know that their therapist believes in the treatment being provided. This creates a bit of a dilemma for the reader, who by now has been presented convincing evidence that the particular treatment delivered is not more effective than any other treatment (with, of course, the limitations noted). How then does a therapist have the necessary belief in a treatment to deliver it with faith? Does the evidence lead to therapeutic cynicism? The way out of this dilemma is not complicated. The therapist should have the belief that the treatment being delivered by him or herself to this particular patient will be effective. The therapist should be convinced that the treatment is a good fit for him or herself and a good fit to the client, is accepted by the client, and the client is responding to the treatment. This is a useful attitude and will result in measured faith rather than blind faith (or faith that some treatment is indeed empirically privileged), which then allows for flexibility if the client finds the treatment unacceptable or is not making satisfactory progress.

Continual Improvement

Therapists have a responsibility to develop their skills over time. In the United States, psychologists, counselors, and social workers enter the field as licensed professionals with relatively little experience. Unfortunately, it appears that trainees, interns, and post-doctoral clinicians are as competent as experienced clinicians (Laska et al., 2013; Tracey, Wampold, Lichtenberg, & Goodyear, 2014; Vollmer, Spada, Caspar, & Burri, 2013). Moreover, there are many impediments to developing expertise in psychotherapy (Tracey et al., 2014), not the least of which is that we have limited knowledge about what makes an expert therapist (i.e., a therapist who achieves better-than-average outcomes— see Chapter 6). Interestingly, therapists who report having professional self-doubt have better outcomes, which suggests that a reflective attitude toward one's practice is helpful.

Patient Perspective

From the patient's perspective, finding an effective therapist is paramount. Unfortunately, little information is available to patients about the outcomes achieved by therapists, and patients typically rely on word of mouth or have to take a therapist assigned by whomever manages their care (e.g., managed care organization, government payer). Nevertheless, patients should be attentive to several factors. First, is there a treatment plan? If so, is the treatment plan acceptable?—does it make sense and does it seem that it will lead to improvement? Second, do the patient and the therapist agree on the goals of therapy and the tasks needed to achieve those goals?—that is, is there a collaborative working relationship? Third, does the patient feel understood and respected? Fourth, and most importantly, progress toward the goal should be relatively steady—is the patient making progress? Patients who feel that one or more of these factors are missing should discuss the therapy with the therapist. If after some time, and a discussion, the patient is not making progress, they should consider finding a different therapist.

Training and Supervision

Baker et al. (2008) have argued that training should be scientifically based. Of course, what this means might differ depending on whether one adopts the Medical or the Contextual Model—or perhaps not as much as one might believe at first. On the one extreme, training would focus on evidence-based treatment protocols and trainees would practice them with patients. On the other extreme, trainees would learn relationship skills, which would then be used to help clients. Hopefully, we have made it clear by now that either extreme does not follow the research evidence. Therapists need to know how to implement various treatments, so training programs need to teach a variety of treatments—and of different approaches, not simply small variations of one particular approach. Programs that only teach one approach, no matter how well taught or how well proven that the treatment is effective, will leave clinicians deficient in treating a range of patients, particularly if there is diversity in attitudes, values, cultures, and other contextual variables. As well, training that focuses on treatments and ignores relationship skills (the "how" of treatment), ignores the research evidence about what makes therapy effective. But it is also detrimental for trainees to learn relationship skills to the exclusion of learning particular approaches to psychotherapy. The optimal training programs will combine training in treatments and relationships skills—this is a scientific approach to training.

Regardless of the focus of training, training programs should be accountable for the effectiveness of their trainees. An idea that emanates from the practice-based evidence movement would be to assess the outcomes of trainees. In this way, programs could document and certify the effectiveness of trainees. There might be a day when internship applications routinely request such documentation, as controversial as that sounds presently. Of course, this practice-based evidence should be a source of feedback to trainees, trainers, and supervisors.

There are implications for supervision as well. Although the effects of supervision on the patient outcomes obtained by supervisees and on supervisee development are largely unknown, (see Bambling, King, Raue, Schweitzer, & Lambert, 2006, for a notable exception), supervision is widely practiced. Of course, supervision is required in training contexts, where unlicensed trainees are providing psychotherapeutic services. In many countries, supervision is practiced throughout professional careers. Many times we forget that in virtually every psychotherapy RCT conducted, the therapists, regardless of their expertise, are provided supervision, despite the relative paucity of research on supervision outcomes, indicating that there is an implicit importance assigned to supervision. Safe to say, supervision is widely practiced, even by those who denigrate more generally the use of untested interventions.

With regard to supervision, some troubling evidence has been presented. To help the supervisee progress, the supervisor assesses the present skill level of the supervisee and compares that to the ideal or desired skill level, keeping in mind of course the developmental level of the trainee. Using the discrepancy between present and ideal skill level assumes that the supervisor's ideal skill level will actually result in better outcomes for clients than the current level. In Chapter 8, we presented evidence that adherence and competence ratings were not correlated with outcomes. This suggests that the supervisor's assessment of the competence of the supervisee may have little to do with the supervisee's actual effectiveness and much to do with the supervisor's own implicit model of competence. This problem is compounded by the fact that the supervisor's own model of therapy will influence his or her own ideal state. A dynamic therapist, who emphasizes the expression of affect in therapy, supervising a CBT therapist who is focused on behavior and cognitions, will surely create some issues around what is the desired skill level of the therapist. In our experience, master therapists of various persuasions, viewing the same therapy session, will have very different opinions about the quality of therapy, which would have implications for supervision.

Concluding Comments

Psychotherapy, as a class of culturally situated healing practices, is documented to be an extremely effective intervention for a person experiencing psychological problems. Yet psychotherapy, often consisting of hours of unstructured, emotional dialogue, is a complex phenomenon to understand. In this volume, we have contrasted two models, the Medical Model and the Contextual Model, with the hope that reviewing the evidence with a strong theoretical scaffolding would provide understanding about the nature of psychotherapy. We make the claim that the Contextual Model offers theoreticians, researchers, clinicians, and policymakers a viable alternative to the Medical Model. According to philosophers of science, a theory cannot be proved, but sufficient evidence has been reviewed that, in Lakatosian terms, the Contextual Model is a progressive research programme—one that makes strong conjectures about what should be observed in various conditions. Pervasively, the predictions have been verified and the auxiliaries are used in a theoretically coherent and empirically justified manner. Furthermore, when criticisms have been made of the evidence, innovative methods have been applied and the Contextual Model has anticipated the results of those investigations.

Whether the Medical Model—or for that matter, the Contextual Model—will be abandoned is to be determined. The typical recommendation that is made in our field is also made here: more research is needed. We hope that this volume has furthered the explication of the Contextual and Medical Models so that testable hypotheses can be addressed in the next generation of psychotherapy research. At the very least, we hope that claims that the constructs of the Contextual Model have "marginal scientific status" (Baker et al., 2008, p. 80) will be set aside. The Contextual Model is based on scientific principles, just not those discussed in treatment manuals. Both models should have the opportunity to show their scientific worth as well as the worth of the implications for policy, practice, and training.

References

Abramowitz, J. S. (1996). Variants of exposure and response prevention in the treatment of obsessive-compulsive disorder: A meta-analysis. *Behavior Therapy, 27*, 583–600.

Abramowitz, J. S. (1997). Effectiveness of psychological and pharmacological treatments for obsessive-compulsive disorder: A quantitative review. *Journal of Consulting and Clinical Psychology, 65*, 44–52.

Adams, V. (1979, July 10). Consensus is reached: Psychotherapy works. *New York Times*, p. C1.

Addis, M. E., Hatgis, C., Krasnow, A. D., Jacob, K., Bourne, L., & Mansfield, A. (2004). Effectiveness of cognitive-behavioral treatment for panic disorder versus treatment as usual in a managed care setting. *Journal of Consulting and Clinical Psychology, 72*(4), 625–635. doi: 10.1037/0022-006x.72.4.625

Ader, R. (1997). The role of conditioning in pharmacotherapy. In A. Harrington (Ed.), *The placebo effect: An interdisciplinary exploration* (pp. 138–165). Cambridge, MA: Harvard University Press.

Ahn, H., & Wampold, B. E. (2001). Where oh where are the specific ingredients? A meta-analysis of component studies in counseling and psychotherapy. *Journal of Counseling Psychology, 48*(3), 251–257.

Albright, L., Kenny, D. A., & Malloy, T. E. (1988). Consensus in personality judgments at zero acquaintance. *Journal of Personality & Social Psychology, 55*(3), 387–395.

Amanzio, M., Pollo, A., Maggi, G., & Benedetti, F. (2001). Response variability to analgesics: A role for non-specific activation of endogenous opiods. *Pain, 90*, 205–211.

Ambady, N., & Rosenthal, R. (1993). Half a minute: Predicting teacher evaluations from thin slices of nonverbal behavior and physical attractiveness. *Journal of Personality & Social Psychology, 64*(3), 431–441.

Ambady, N., LaPlante, D., Nguen, T., Rosenthal, R., & Levinson, W. (2002). Surgeon's tone of voice: A clue to malpractice history. *Surgery, 132*, 5–9.

American Psychological Association, Office of Public Communications (1995, August). Questions and answers about memories of childhood abuse. Retrieved from www.apa.org/topics/memories.html

Anderson, A. S. (1988). Does psychotherapy make some clients worse? A reanalysis of the evidence for treatment-induced deterioration. University of Memphis, Memphis, TN.

Anderson, T., Lunnen, K. M., & Ogles, B. M. (2010). Putting models and techniques in context. In S. D. Miller, B. L. Duncan, M. A. Hubble & B. E. Wampold (Eds.), *The heart and soul of change* (2nd ed., pp. 143–163). Washington, DC: American Psychological Association.

Anderson, T., Ogles, B.M., Patterson, C.L., Lambert, M.J., & Vermeersch, D.A. (2009). Therapist effects: facilitative interpersonal skills as a predictor of therapist success. *Journal of Clinical Psychology, 65*(7), 755–768. doi: 10.1002/jclp.20583

Andrews, G., & Harvey, R. (1981). Does psychotherapy benefit neurotic patients?: A reanalysis of the Smith, Glass, and Miller data. *Archives of General Psychiatry, 38*(11), 1203–1208.

Anholt, G.E., Kempe, P., de Haan, E., van Oppen, P., Cath, D. C., Smit, J.H., & van Balkom, A.J.L.M. (2008). Cognitive versus behavior therapy: Processes of change in the treatment of obsessive-compulsive disorder. *Psychotherapy and Psychosomatics, 77*, 38–42.

APA Presidential Task Force on Evidence-Based Practice. (2006). Evidence-based practice in psychology. *American Psychologist, 61*, 271–285.

Arch, J.J., Eifert, G. H., Davies, C., Vilardaga, J.C.P., Rose, R. D., & Craske, M. G. (2012). Randomized clinical trial of cognitive behavioral therapy (CBT) versus acceptance and commitment therapy (ACT) for mixed anxiety disorders. *Journal of Consulting and Clinical Psychology* (Supplemental). doi: 10.1037/a002831010.1037/a0028310.supp

Arch, J.J., Wolitzky-Taylor, K. B., Eifert, G. H., & Craske, M. G. (2012). Longitudinal treatment mediation of traditional cognitive behavioral therapy and acceptance and commitment therapy for anxiety disorders. *Behaviour Research and Therapy, 50*(7–8), 469–478. doi: 10.1016/j.brat.2012.04.007

Arkowitz, H. (1992). Integrative theories of therapy. In D.K. Freedheim (Ed.), *History of psychotherapy: A century of change* (pp. 261–303). Washington, DC: American Psychological Association.

Arnkoff, D.B., & Glass, C.R. (1992). Cognitive therapy and psychotherapy. In D.K. Freedheim (Ed.), *History of psychotherapy: A century of change* (pp. 657–694). Washington, DC: American Psychological Association.

Arnow, B.A., Steidtmann, D., Blasey, C., Manber, R., Constantino, M.J., Klein, D.N., . . . Kocsis, J.H. (2013). The relationship between the therapeutic alliance and treatment outcome in two distinct psychotherapies for chronic depression. *Journal of Consulting and Clinical Psychology, 81*(4), 627–638. doi: 10.1037/a0031530

Asimov, I. (1983). *The roving mind.* Amherst, NY: Promethius Books.

Association for Behavioral and Cognitive Therapies (ABCT). Retrieved April 21, 2014 from www.abct.org/Information/?m=mInformation&fa=_WhatIsCBTpublic

Atkins, D. C., Steyvers, M., Imel, Z. E., & Smyth, P. (2014). Automatic evaluation of psychotherapy language with quantitative linguistic models: An initial application to Motivational Interviewing. *Implementation Science*. doi: 10.1037/a0036841

Baardseth, T. P., Goldberg, S. B., Pace, B. T., Wislocki, A. P., Frost, N. D., Siddiqui, J.R., . . . Wampold, B. E. (2013). Cognitive-behavioral therapy versus other therapies: Redux. *Clinical Psychology Review, 33*(3), 395–405. doi: 10.1016/j.cpr. 2013.01.004

Baker, T.B., McFall, R. M., & Shoham, V. (2008). Current status and future prospects of clinical psychology: Toward a scientifically principled approach to mental and behavioral health care. *Psychological Science in the Public Interest, 9*(2), 67–103. doi: 10.1111/j.1539-6053.2009.01036.x

Baldwin, S. A., Berkeljon, A., & Atkins, D. C. (2009). Rates of change in naturalistic psychotherapy: Contrasting dose-effect and good-enough level models of change. *Journal of Consulting and Clinical Psychology, 77*, 203–211.

Baldwin, S. A., & Imel, Z. E. (2013). Therapist effects: Findings and methods. In M. J. Lambert (Ed.), *Bergin and Garfield's handbook of psychotherapy and behavior change* (6th ed., pp. 258–297). New York: Wiley.

Baldwin, S. A., Murray, D. M., Shadish, W. R., Pals, S. L., Holland, J. M., Abramowtiz, J. S., . . . Watson, J. (2011). Intraclass correlation associated with therapists: Estimates and applications in planning psychotherapy research. *Cognitive Behaviour Therapy, 40*, 15–33.

Baldwin, S. A., Wampold, B. E., & Imel, Z. E. (2007). Untangling the alliance-outcome correlation: Exploring the relative importance of therapist and patient variability in the alliance. *Journal of Consulting and Clinical Psychology, 75*, 842–852.

Ball, S. A., Martino, S., Nich, C., Frankfort, T. L., Van Horn, D., Crits-Christoph, P., Woody, G. E., Obert, J. L., Farentinos, C., & Carroll, K. M. (2007). Site matters: multisite randomized trial of motivational enhancement therapy in community drug abuse clinics. *Journal of Consulting and Clinical Psychology, 75*, 556–567.

Bambling, M., King, R., Raue, P., Schweitzer, R., & Lambert, W. (2006). Clinical supervision: Its influence on client-rated working alliance and client symptom reduction in the brief treatment of major depression. *Psychotherapy Research, 16*(3), 317–331. doi: 10.1080/10503300500268524

Bandura, A. (1999). Self-efficacy: Toward a unifying theory of behavioral change. In R. F. Baumeister (Ed.), *The self in social psychology* (pp. 285–298). New York: Psychology Press.

Barber, J. P., Connolly, M. B., Crits-Christoph, P., Gladis, L., & Siqueland, L. (2009). Alliance predicts patients' outcome beyond in-treatment change in symptoms. *Personality Disorders: Theory, Research, and Treatment, S*(1), 80–89. doi: 10.1037/1949-2715.s.1.80

Barber, J. P., Gallop, R., Crits-Christoph, P., Frank, A., Thase, M. E., Weiss, R. D., & Gibbons, M. B. C. (2006). The role of therapist adherence, therapist competence, and alliance in predicting outcome of individual drug counseling: Results from the National Institute Drug Abuse Collaborative Cocaine Treatment Study. *Psychotherapy Research, 16*, 229–240.

Barber, J. P., Muran, J. C., McCarthy, K. S., & Keefe, J. R. (2013). Research on dynamic therapies. In M. J. Lambert (Ed.), *Bergin and Garfield's handbook of psychotherapy and behavior change* (6th ed., pp. 443–494). New York: Wiley.

Barcikowski, R. S. (1981). Statistical power with group mean as the unit of analysis. *Journal of Educational and Behavioral Statistics, 6*(3), 267–285.

Barker, S. L., Funk, S. C., & Houston, B. K. (1988). Psychological treatment versus nonspecific factors: A meta-analysis of conditions that engender comparable expectations for improvement. *Clinical Psychology Review, 8*, 579–594.

Barkham, M., Hardy, G. E., & Mellor-Clark, J. (2010). *Developing and delivering practice-based evidence: A guide for the psychological therapies.* Chichester, UK: Wiley Blackwell.

Barlow, D. H. (2004). Psychological treatments. *American Psychologist, 59*, 869–878.

Barlow, D. H. (2010). The dodo bird–again–and again. *The Behavior Therapist, 33*(1), 15–16.

Barlow, D. H., Farchione, T. J., Fairholme, C. P., Ellard, K. K., Boisseau, C. L., Allen, L. B., & Ehrenreich-May, J. (2011). *Unified protocol for transdiagnostic treatment of emotional disorders: Therapist guide.* New York: Oxford University Press.

Barry, J. (2004). *The great influenza: The story of the deadliest pandemic in history.* New York: Penguin.

Barth, J., Munder, T., Gerger. H., Nuesch, E., Trelle, S., et al. (2013). Comparative Efficacy of Seven Psychotherapeutic Interventions for Patients with Depression: A Network Meta-Analysis. *PLoS Medicine, 10*(5): e1001454. doi:10.1371/journal.pmed.1001454

Baskin, T. W., Tierney, S. C., Minami, T., & Wampold, B. E. (2003). Establishing specificity in psychotherapy: A meta-analysis of structural equivalence of placebo controls. *Journal of Consulting and Clinical Psychology, 71,* 973–979.

Baucom, D. H., Shoham, V., Mueser, K. T., Daiuto, A. D., & Stickle, T. R. (1998). Empirically supported couple and family interventions for marital distress and adult mental health problems. *Journal of Consulting and Clinical Psychology, 66,* 53–88.

Baumeister, R. F. (2005). *The cultural animal: Human nature, meaning, and social life.* Oxford: Oxford University Press.

Beck, A. T., & Bhar, S. S. (2009). Effectiveness of long-term psychodynamic psychotherapy: A meta-analysis: Comment. *Journal of the American Medical Association, 301*(9). doi: 10.1001/jama.2009.179

Beck, A. T., Rush, A. J., Shaw, B. F., & Emery, G. (1979). *Cognitive therapy of depression.* New York: Guilford.

Beck, A. T., Ward, C., Mendelson, M., & Erbaugh, J. (1961). An inventory for measuring depression. *Archives of General Psychiatry, 6,* 561–571.

Beecher, H. K. (1955). The powerful placebo. *Journal of the American Medical Association, 159*(17), 1602–1606.

Bell, E. C., Marcus, D. K., & Goodlad, J. K. (2013). Are the parts as good as the whole? A meta-analysis of component treatment studies. *Journal of Consulting and Clinical Psychology, 81*(4), 722–736. doi: 10.1037/a0033004

Benedetti, F. (2009). *Placebo effects: Understanding the mechanisms in health and disease.* New York: Oxford University Press.

Benedetti, F. (2011). *The patient's brain: The neuroscience behind the doctor-patient relationship.* New York: Oxford University Press.

Benish, S. G., Imel, Z. E., & Wampold, B. E. (2008). The relative efficacy of bona fide psychotherapies for treating post-traumatic stress disorder: A meta-analysis of direct comparisons. *Clinical Psychology Review, 28,* 746–758.

Benish, S. G., Quintana, S., & Wampold, B. E. (2011). Culturally adapted psychotherapy and the legitimacy of myth: A direct-comparison meta-analysis. *Journal of Counseling Psychology, 58*(3), 279–289. doi: 10.1037/a0023626

Benjamin, L. S. (1994). SASB: A bridge between personality theory and clinical psychology. *Psychological Inquiry, 5,* 273–316.

Bergin, A. E. (1963). The effects of psychotherapy: Negative results revisited. *Journal of Counseling Psychology, 10,* 244–250.

Bergin, A. E. (1971). The evaluation of therapeutic outcomes. In S. L. Garfield & A. E. Bergin (Eds.), *Handbook of psychotherapy and behavior change* (pp. 217–270). New York: Wiley.

Bergin, A. E., & Lambert, M. J. (1978). The evaluation of therapeutic outcomes. In S. L. Garfield & A. E. Bergin (Eds.), *Handbook of psychotherapy and behavior change: An empirical analysis* (2nd ed., pp. 139–190). New York: Wiley.

Berglund, M., Thelander, S., Salaspuro, M., Franck, J., Andréasson, S., & Öjehagen, A. (2003). Treatment of alcohol abuse: An evidence-based review. *Alcoholism: Clinical and Experimental Research, 27,* 1645–1656.

Berman, J. S., Miller, C., & Massman, P. J. (1985). Cognitive therapy versus systematic desensitization: Is one treatment superior? *Psychological Bulletin, 97,* 451–461.

Beutler, L. E. (1998). Identifying empirically supported treatments: What if we didn't? *Journal of Consulting and Clinical Psychology, 66,* 113–120.

Beutler, L. E., & Baker, M. (1998). The movement toward empirical validation. In K. S. Dobson & K. D. Craig (Eds.), *Empirically supported therapies: Best practice in professional psychology* (pp. 43–65). Thousand Oaks, CA: Sage.

Beutler, L. E., & Castonguay, L. G. (Eds.). (2006). *Principles of therapeutic change that work.* New York: Oxford.

Beutler, L. E., & Clarkin, J. (1990). *Differential treatment selection: Toward targeted therapeutic interventions.* New York: Brunner/Mazel.

Beutler, L. E., Frank, M., Schieber, S. C., Calvert, L., & Gaines, J. (1984). Comparative effects of group psychotherapies in a short-term inpatient setting: An experience with deterioration effects. *Psychiatry, 44,* 67–76.

Beutler, L. E., & Harwood, T. M. (2000). *Perscriptive psychotherapy: A practical guide to systematic treatment selection.* New York: Oxford University Press.

Beutler, L. E., Harwood, T. M., Alimohamed, S., & Malik, M. (2002). Functional impairment and coping style. In J. C. Norcross (Ed.), *Psychotherapy relationships that work: Therapist contributions and responsiveness to patients* (pp. 145–170). New York: Oxford University.

Beutler, L. E., Harwood, T. M., Kimpara, S., Verdirame, D., & Blau, K. (2011). Coping style. *Journal of Clinical Psychology, 67*(2), 176–183. doi: 10.1002/jclp.20752

Beutler, L. E., Harwood, T. M., Michelson, A., Song, X., & Holman, J. (2011). Resistance/reactance level. *Journal of Clinical Psychology, 67*(2), 133–142. doi: 10.1002/jclp.20753

Beutler, L. E., Malik, M., Alimohamed, S., Harwood, T. M., Talebi, H., Noble, S., & Wong, E. (2004). Therapist variables. In M. J. Lambert (Ed.), *Bergin and Garfield's handbook of psychotherapy and behavior change* (5th ed., pp. 227–306). New York: Wiley.

Bhar, S. S., & Beck, A. T. (2009). Treatment integrity of studies that compare short-term psychodynamic psychotherapy with cognitive-behavior therapy. *Clinical Psychology: Science and Practice, 16*(3), 370–378. doi: 10.1111/j.1468-2850.2009.01176.x

Bisson, J. I., Ehlers, A., Matthews, R., Pilling, S., Richards, D., & Turner, S. (2007). Psychological treatments for chronic post-traumatic stress disorder: Systematic review and meta-analysis. *The British Journal of Psychiatry, 190*(2), 97–104. doi:10.1192/bjp.bp.106.021402

Bisson, J., & Andrew, M. (2009). Psychological Treatment of Post-traumatic Stress Disorder (PTSD) (Review). The Cochrane Library, *2,* www.thecochranelibrary.com

Blatt, S. J., Sanislow III, C. A., Zuroff, D. C., & Pilkonis, P. A. (1996). Characteristics of effective therapists: further analyses of data from the National Institute of Mental Health Treatment of Depression Collaborative Research Program. *Journal of Consulting and Clinical psychology, 64*(6), 1276.

Bleiberg, K. L., & Markowitz, J. C. (2005). A pilot study of interpersonal psychotherapy for posttraumatic stress disorder. *The American Journal of Psychiatry, 162*(1), 181–183. doi: 10.1176/appi.ajp.162.1.181

Boffey, P. M. (1982, June 28). Alcoholism study under new attack. *New York Times,* pp. 12.

Bohanske, R. T., & Franczak, M. (2010). Transforming public behavioral health care: A case example of consumer-directed services, recovery, and the common factors. In B. L. Duncan, S. D. Miller, B. E. Wampold & M. A. Hubble (Eds.), *The heart and soul of change: Delivering what works in therapy* (2nd ed., pp. 299–322). Washington, DC: American Psychological Association.

Bohart, A. C., & Tallman, K. (1999). *How Clients Make Therapy Work: The Process of Active Self-Healing.* Washington, DC: American Psychological Association.

Bohart, A. C., & Wade, A. G. (2013). The client in psychotherapy. In M. J. Lambert (Ed.), *Bergin and Garfield's handbook of pyschotherapy and behavior change* (6th ed., pp. 219–257). Hoboken, NJ: Wiley.

Bordin, E. S. (1979). The generalizability of the psychoanalytic concept of the working alliance. *Psychotherapy: Theory, Research & Practice, 16*(3), 252–260. doi: 10.1037/h0085885

Borkovec, T. D. (1990). Control groups and comparison groups in psychotherapy outcome research. *National Institute on Drug Abuse Research Monograph, 104,* 50–65.

Borkovec, T. D., & Castonguay, L. G. (1998). What is the scientific meaning of empirically supported therapy? *Journal of Consulting and Clinical Psychology, 66,* 136–142.

Borkovec, T. D., & Costello, E. (1993). Efficacy of applied relaxation and cognitive-behavioral therapy in the treatment of generalized anxiety disorder. *Journal of Consulting and Clinical Psychology, 61,* 611–619.

Boswell, J. F., Gallagher, M. W., Sauer-Zavala, S. E., Bullis, J., Gorman, J. M., Shear, M. K., . . . Barlow, D. H. (2013). Patient characteristics and variability in adherence and competence in cognitive-behavioral therapy for panic disorder. *Journal of Consulting and Clinical Psychology, 81*(3), 443–454. doi: 10.1037/a0031437

Boswell, J. F., Kraus, D. R., Miller, S. D., & Lambert, M. J. (in press). Implementing routine outcome monitoring in clinical practice: Benefits, challenges, and solutions. *Psychotherapy Research.*

Bowers, T. G., & Clum, G. A. (1988). Relative contributions of specific and nonspecific treatment effects: Meta-analysis of placebo-controlled behavior therapy research. *Psychological Bulletin, 103,* 315–323.

Bowlby, J. (1969). *Attachment and loss. Vol. 1: Attachment.* New York: Basic Books.

Bowlby, J. (1973). *Attachment and loss, Vol. 2: Separation-anxiety and anger.* New York: Basic Books.

Bowlby, J. (1980). *Attachment and loss, Vol. 3: Loss-sadness and depression.* New York: Basic Books.

Boyer, P., & Barrett, H. C. (2005). Domain specificity and intuitive ontologies. In D. M. Buss (Ed.), *The handbook of evolutionary psychology* (pp. 96–118). Hoboken, NJ: Wiley.

Bradley, R., Greene, J., Russ, E., Dutra, L., & Westen, D. (2005). A multidimensional meta-analysis of psychotherapy for PTSD. *American Journal of Psychiatry, 162,* 214–227.

Braun, S. R., Gregor, B., Tran, U. S. (2013). Comparing bona fide psychotherapies of depression in adults with two meta-analytical approaches. *PLoS ONE, 8*(6):e68135. doi: 10.1371/journal.pone.0068135

Brody, N. (1980). *Placebos and the philosophy of medicine: Clinical, conceptual, and ethical issues.* Chicago: The University of Chicago Press.

Budge, S. L., Baardseth, T. P., Wampold, B. E., & Flückiger, C. (2010). Researcher allegiance and supportive therapy: Pernicious affects on results of randomized clinical trials. *European Journal of Counselling and Psychotherapy, 12,* 23–39.

Budge, S. L., Moore, J. T., Del Re, A. C., Wampold, B. E., Baardseth, T. P., & Nienhuis, J. B. (2013). The effectiveness of evidence-based treatments for personality disorders when comparing treatment-as-usual and bona fide treatments. *Clinical Psychology Review, 33,* 1057–1066. doi: 10.1016/j.cpr.2013.08.003

Buranelli, V. (1975). *The wizard from Vienna: Franz Anton Mesmer.* New York: Coward, McCann & Geoghegan.

Burns, D. D., & Spangler, D. L. (2001). Do changes in dysfunctional attitudes mediate changes in depression and anxiety in cognitive behavioral therapy? *Behavior Therapy, 32*(2), 337–369. doi: 10.1016/s0005-7894(01)80008-3

Butler, A. C., Chapman, J. E., Forman, E. M., & Beck, A. T. (2006). The empirical status of cognitive-behavioral therapy: A review of meta-analyses. *Clinical Psychology Review, 26*, 17–31. doi: 10.1016/j.cpr.2005.07.003

Butler, G., Fennell, M., Robson, P., & Gelder, M. (1991). Comparison of behavior therapy and cognitive behavior therapy in the treatment of generalized anxiety disorder. *Journal of Consulting and Clinical Psychology, 59*(1), 167–175.

Cacioppo, J. T., Fowler, J. H., & Christakis, N. A. (2009). Alone in the crowd: The structure and spread of loneliness in a large social network. *Journal of Personality and Social Psychology, 97*(6), 977–991. doi: 10.1037/a0016076

Cacioppo, S., & Cacioppo, J. T. (2012). Decoding the invisible forces of social connections. *Frontiers in Integrative Neuroscience, 6.* doi: 10.3389/fnint.2012.00051

Calhoun, K. S., Moras, K., Pilkonis, P. A., & Rehm, L. (1998). Empirically supported treatments: Implications for training. *Journal of Consulting and Clinical Psychology, 66*, 151–161.

Campbell, D. T., & Kenny, D. A. (1999) *A primer on regression artifacts.* New York: Guilford.

Caplan, E. (1998). *Mind games: American culture and the birth of psychotherapy.* Berkeley: University of California Press.

Carbajal, R., Chauvet, X., Couderc, S., & Oliver-Martin, M. (1999). Randomised trial of analgesic effects of sucrose, glucose, and pacifiers in term neonates. *British Medical Journal, 319*, 1393–1397.

Carroll, K. M., Rounsaville, B. J., & Nich, C. (1994). Blind man's bluff: Effectiveness and significance of psychotherapy and pharmacoptherapy blinding procedures in a clinical trial. *Journal of Consulting and Clinical Psychology, 62*, 276–280.

Castonguay, L. G. (1993). "Common factors" and "nonspecific variables": Clarification of the two concepts and recommendations for research. *Journal of Psychotherapy Integration, 3*, 267–286.

Castonguay, L. G., & Beutler, L. E. (Eds.). (2006). *Principles of therapeutic change that work.* New York: Oxford University Press.

Castonguay, L. G., Goldfried, M. R., Wiser, S., Raue, P. J., & Hayes, A. M. (1996). Predicting the effect of cognitive therapy for depression: A study of unique and common factors. *Journal of Consulting and Clinical Psychology, 64*, 497–504.

Chambless, D. L., Baker, M. J., Baucom, D. H., Beutler, L. E., Calhoun, K. S., Daiuto, A., et al. (1998). Update on empirically validated therapies, II. *The Clinical Psychologist, 51*, 3–16.

Chambless, D. L., & Crits-Christoph, P. (2006). What should be validated? The treatment method. In J. C. Norcross, L. E. Beutler & R. F. Levant (Eds.), *Evidence-based practices in mental health: Debate and dialogue on the fundamental questions* (pp. 191–200). Washington, DC: American Psychological Association.

Chambless, D. L., & Gillis, M. M. (1993). Cognitive therapy of anxiey disorders. *Journal of Consulting and Clinical Psychology, 61*, 248–260.

Chambless, D. L., & Hollon, S. D. (1998). Defining empirically supported therapies. *Journal of Consulting and Clinical Psychology, 66*, 7–18.

Chambless, D. L., Sanderson, W. C., Shoham, V., Johnson, S. B., Pope, K. S., Crits-Christoph, P., et al. (1996). An update on empirically validated therapies. *The Clinical Psychologist, 49*(2), 5–18.

Christakis, N. A., & Fowler, J. H. (2007). The spread of obesity in a large social network over 32 years. *The New England Journal of Medicine, 357*(4), 370–379. doi: 10.1056/NEJMsa066082

Clark, D. M. (2013). Psychodynamic therapy or cognitive therapy for social anxiety disorder. *American Journal of Psychiatry, 170*(11), 1365.

Clark, D. M., Ehlers, A., Hackmann, A., McManus, F., Fennell, M., Grey, N., . . . & Wild, J. (2006). Cognitive therapy versus exposure and applied relaxation in social phobia: a randomized controlled trial. *Journal of Consulting and Clinical Psychology, 74*(3), 568–578.

Clark, D. M., Ehlers, A., McManus, F., Hackmann, A., Fennell, M., Campbell, H., . . . & Louis, B. (2003). Cognitive therapy versus fluoxetine in generalized social phobia: a randomized placebo-controlled trial. *Journal of Consulting and Clinical Psychology, 71*(6), 1058–1067.

Clark, D. M., Fairburn, C. G., & Wessely, S. (2008). Psychological treatment outcomes in routine NHS services: A commentary on Stiles et al. (2007). *Psychological Medicine, 38*, 629–634. doi: 10.1017/S0033291707001869

Clark, D. M., Salkovskis, P. M., Hackmann, A., Middleton, H., Anastasiades, P., & Gelder, M. (1994). A comparison of cognitive therapy, applied relaxation, and imipramine in the treatment of panic disorder. *British Journal of Psychiatry, 164*, 759–769.

Clarkin, J. F., & Levy, K. N. (2004). The infuence of client variables on psychotherapy. In M. J. Lambert (Ed.), *Bergin and Garfield's handbook of psychotherapy and behavior change* (5th ed., pp. 194–226). Hoboken, NJ: Wiley.

Clement, P. W. (1994). Quantitative evaluation of 26 years of private practice. *Professional Psychology: Research and Practice, 25*(2), 173–176. doi: 10.1037/0735-7028.25.2.173

Clement, P. W. (1996). Evaluation in private practice. *Clinical Psychology: Science and Practice, 3*(2), 146–159. doi: 10.1111/j.1468-2850.1996.tb00064.x

Clum, G. A., Clum, G. A., & Surls, R. (1993). A meta-analysis of treatments for panic disorder. *Journal of Consulting and Clinical Psychology, 61*, 317–326.

Cohen, J. (1988). *Statistical power analysis for the behavioral sciences* (2nd ed.). Hillsdale, NJ: Erlbaum.

Cohen, A. S., Barlow, D. H., & Blanchard, E. B. (1985). Psychophysiology of relaxation-associated panic attacks. *Journal of Abnormal Psychology, 94*, 96–101.

Cohen, S., & Syme, S. L. (1985). *Social support and health.* San Diego, CA: Academic Press.

Compas, B. E., Haaga, D. A. F., Keefe, F. J., Leitenberg, H., & Williams, D. A. (1998). Sampling of empirically supported psychological treatments from health psychology: Smoking, chronic pain, cancer, and bulimia nervosa. *Journal of Consulting and Clinical Psychology, 66*, 89–112.

Connell, J., Grant, S., & Mullin, T. (2006). Client initiated termination of therapy at NHS primary care counselling services. *Counselling & Psychotherapy Research, 6*(1), 60–67. doi: 10.1080/14733140600581507

Constantino, M. J., Arnkoff, D. B., Glass, C. R., Ametrano, R. M., & Smith, J. Z. (2011). Expectations. *Journal of Clinical Psychology, 67*(2), 184–192. doi: 10.1002/jclp.20754

Constantino, M. J., Glass, C. R., Arnkoff, D. B., Ametrano, R. M., & Smith, J. Z. (2011). Expectations. In J. C. Norcross (Ed.), *Psychotherapy relationships that work: Evidence-based responsiveness (2nd ed.).* (pp. 354–376). New York: Oxford University Press.

Cook, T. D., & Campbell, D. T. (1979). *Quasi-experimentation: Design and analysis for field settings.* Chicago: Rand McNally.

Cooper, H., & Hedges, L. V. (Eds.). (1994). *The handbook of research synthesis.* New York: Russell Sage Foundation.

Cooper, H., Hedges, L. V., & Valentine, J. C. (Eds.). (2009). *The handbook of research synthesis and meta-analysis* (2nd ed.). New York: Russell Sage Foundation.

Craske, M. G., Meadows, E. A., & Barlow, D. H. (1994). *Therapist guide for the mastery of your anxiety and panic II and agoraphobia supplement.* Albany, NY: Graywind Publications Incorporated.

Cremer, S., & Sixt, M. (2009). Analogies in the evolution of individual and social immunity. *Philosophical Transactions of the Royal Society B: Biological Sciences, 364*(1513), 129–142.

Critelli, J. W., & Neumann, K. F. (1984). The placebo: Conceptual analysis of a construct in transition. *American Psychologist, 39*, 32–39.

Crits-Christoph, P. (1997). Limitations of the dodo bird verdict and the role of clinical trials in psychotherapy research: Comment on Wampold et al. (1997). *Psychological Bulletin, 122*, 216–220.

Crits-Christoph, P., Baranackie, K., Kurcias, J. S., Carroll, K., Luborsky, L., McLellan, T., . . . Zitrin, C. (1991). Meta-analysis of therapist effects in psychotherapy outcome studies. *Psychotherapy Research, 1*, 81–91.

Crits-Christoph, P., Gallop, R., Temes, C. M., Woody, G., Ball, S. A., Martino, S., & Carroll, K. M. (2009). The alliance in motivational enhancement therapy and counseling as usual for substance use problems. *Journal of Consulting and Clinical Psychology, 77*(6), 1125–1135. doi: 10.1037/a0017045

Crits-Christoph, P., Gibbons, M.B.C., Hamilton, J., Ring-Kurtz, S., & Gallop, R. (2011). The dependability of alliance assessments: The alliance–outcome correlation is larger than you might think. *Journal of Consulting and Clinical Psychology, 79*(3), 267–278. doi: 10.1037/a0023668

Crits-Christoph, P., Gibbons, M. B., & Hearon, B. (2006). Does the alliance cause good outcome? Recommendations for future research on the alliance. *Psychotherapy: Theory, Research, Practice, Training, 43*(3), 280–285.

Crits-Christoph, P., Gibbons, M.B.C., Ring-Kurtz, S., Gallop, R., Stirman, S., Present, J., . . . Goldstein, L. (2008). Changes in positive quality of life over the course of psychotherapy. *Psychotherapy: Theory, Research, Practice, Training, 45*(4), 419–430. doi: 10.1037/a0014340

Crits-Christoph, P., & Mintz, J. (1991). Implications of therapist effects for the design and analysis of comparative studies of psychotherapies. *Journal of Consulting and Clinical Psychology, 59*(1), 20–26.

Cronbach, L. J., & Snow, R. E. (1977). *Aptitudes and instructional methods: A handbook for research on interactions.* Oxford: Irvington.

Cuijpers, P. (1997). Bibliotherapy in unipolar depression: A meta-analysis. *Journal of Behavior Therapy and Experimental Psychiatry, 28*(2), 139–147. doi: 10.1016/s0005-7916(97)00005-0

Cuijpers, P., Driessen, E., Hollon, S. D., van Oppen, P., Barth, J., & Andersson, G. (2012). The efficacy of non-directive supportive therapy for adult depression: A meta-analysis. *Clinical Psychology Review, 32*, 280–291. doi: 10.1016/j.cpr.2012.01.003

Cuijpers, P., van Straten, A., Andersson, G., & van Oppen, P. (2008a). Psychotherapy for depression in adults: A meta-analysis of comparative outcome studies. *Journal of Consulting and Clinical Psychology, 76*(6), 909–922. doi:10.1037/a0013075

Cuijpers, P., van Straten, A., Warmerdam, L., & Andersson, G. (2008b). Psychological treatment of depression: A meta-analytic database of randomized studies. *BMC Psychiatry, 8*(1), 36. doi:10.1186/1471-244X-8-36

Curran, P. J., & Bauer, D. J. (2011). The disaggregation of within-person and between person effects in longitudinal models of change. *Annual Review of Psychology, 62*, 5833–5619. doi: 10.1146/annurev.psych.093008.100356

Currier, J. M., Neimeyer, R. A., & Berman, J. S. (2008). The effectiveness of psychotherapeutic interventions for bereaved persons: A comprehensive quantitative review.
Psychological Bulletin, 134, 648–661.

Cushman, P. (1992). Psychotherapy to 1992: A history situated interpretation. In D. K.
Freedheim (Ed.), *History of psychotherapy: A century of change* (pp. 21–64). Washington,
DC: American Psychological Association.

Dance, K. A., & Neufeld, R. W. J. (1988). Aptitude-treatment interaction research in the
clinic setting: A review of attempts to dispel the "patient uniformity" myth. *Psychological Bulletin, 104,* 192–213.

Danziger, K. (1990). *Constructing the subject: Historical origins of psychological research.* Cambridge, UK: Cambridge University Press.

Davidson, P. R., & Parker, K. C. H. (2001). Eye movement desensitization and reprocessing (EMDR): A meta-analysis. *Journal of Consulting and Clinical Psychology, 69,*
305–316.

Davies, D. L. (1962). Normal drinking in recovered addicts. *Quarterly Journal of Studies on
Alcohol, 23,* 94–104.

Davison, G. C. (1998). Being bolder with the Boulder Model: The challenge of education and training in empirically supported treatments. *Journal of Consulting and Clinical
Psychology, 66,* 163–167.

De Bolle, M., Johnson, J. G., & De Fruyt, F. (2010). Patient and clinician perceptions
of therapeutic alliance as predictors of improvement in depression. *Psychotherapy and
Psychosomatics, 79*(6), 378–385. doi: 10.1159/000320895

de Waal, F. B. M. (2008). Putting the altruism back into altruism: The evolution of empathy. *Annual Review of Psychology, 59,* 279–300. doi: 10.1146/annurev.psych.59.103006.
093625

Del Re, A. C., Flückiger, C., Horvath, A. O., Symonds, D., & Wampold, B. E. (2012).
Therapist effects in the therapeutic alliance–outcome relationship: A restricted-
maximum likelihood meta-analysis. *Clinical Psychology Review, 32*(7), 642–649. doi:
10.1016/j.cpr.2012.07.002

Del Re, A. C., Spielmans, G. I., Flückiger, C., & Wampold, B. E. (2013). Efficacy of new
generation antidepressants: Differences seem illusory. *PLoS ONE, 8*(6): e63509. doi:
10.1371/journal.pone.0063509

DeRubeis, R. J., Brotman, M. A., & Gibbons, C. J. (2005). A Conceptual and Methodological Analysis of the Nonspecifics Argument. *Clinical Psychology: Science and Practice,
12*(2), 174–183.

DeRubeis, R. J., & Crits-Christoph, P. (1998). Empirically supported individual and
group psychological treatments for mental disorders. *Journal of Consulting and Clinical
Psychology, 66,* 37–52.

DeRubeis, R. J., & Feeley, M. (1990). Determinants of change in cognitive therapy for
depression. *Cognitive Therapy and Research, 14,* 469–482.

DeRubeis, R. J., Siegle, G. J., & Hollon, S. D. (2008). Cognitive therapy versus medication for depressions: Treatment outcomes and neural mechanisms. *Nature Reviews
Neuroscience, 9*(10), 788–796. doi: 10.1038/nrn2345

Desrosières, A. (1998). *The politics of large numbers: A history of statistical reasoning* (C. Naish,
Trans.). Cambridge, MA: Harvard University Press.

Devilly, G. J., & Foa, E. B. (2001). The investigation of exposure and cognitive therapy:
Comment on Tarrier et al. (1999). *Journal of Consulting and Clinical Psychology, 69*(1),
114–116. doi: 10.1037/0022-006x.69.1.114

Dinger, U., Strack, M., Leichsenring, F., Wilmers, F., & Schauenburg, H. (2008). Therapist effects on outcome and alliance in inpatient psychotherapy. *Journal of Clinical Psychology, 64*(3), 344–354. doi: 10.1002/jclp.20443

Dishion, T. J., McCord, J., & Poulin, F. O. (1999). When interventions harm: Peer groups and problem behavior. *American Psychologist, 54*, 755–764.

Dobson, K. S. (1989). A meta-analysis of the efficacy of cognitive therapy for depression. *Journal of Consulting and Clinical Psychology, 57*, 414–419.

Dollard, J., & Miller, N. E. (1950). *Personality and psychotherapy: An analysis in terms of learning, thinking, and culture.* New York: McGraw Hill.

Duncan, B. L., Miller, S. D., & Sparks, J. A. (2004). *The heroic client: a revolutionary way to improve effectiveness through client-directed, outcome-informed therapy* (Rev. ed.). San Francisco: Jossey-Bass.

Duncan, B. L., Miller, S. D., Wampold, B. E., & Hubble, M. A. (2010). *The heart and soul of change: Delivering what works in therapy (2nd ed.).* Washington, DC: American Psychological Association.

Dush, D. M., Hirt, M. L., & Schroeder, H. (1983). Self-statement modification with adults: A meta-analysis. *Psychological Bulletin, 94*, 408–422.

Ehlers, A., Bisson, J., Clark, D. M., Creamer, M., Pilling, S., Richards, D., . . . Yule, W. (2010). Do all psychological treatments really work the same in post-traumatic stress disorder? *Clinical Psychology Review, 30*(2), 269–276. doi: 10.1016/j.cpr.2009.12.001

Elkin, I. (1994). The NIMH Treatment of Depression Collaborative Research Program: Where we began and where we are. In A. E. Bergin & S. L. Garfield (Eds.), *Handbook of psychotherapy and behavior change* (4th ed., pp. 114–139). New York: Wiley.

Elkin, I., Gibbons, R. D., Shea, M. T., & Shaw, B. F. (1996). Science is not a trial (but it can sometimes be a tribulation). *Journal of Consulting and Clinical Psychology, 64*, 92–103.

Elkin, I., Parloff, M. B., Hadley, S. W., & Autry, J. H. (1985). NIMH treatment of depression collaborative research program: Background and research plan. *Archives of General Psychiatry, 42*(3), 305–316.

Elkin, I., Shea, T., Watkins, J. T., Imber, S. D., Sotsky, S. M., Collins, J. F., . . . Parloff, M. B. (1989). National Institute of Mental Health Treatment of Depression Collaborative Research Program. *Archives of General Psychiatry, 46*, 971–982.

Ellickson, P. L., Bell, R. M., & McGuigan, K. (1993). Preventing adolescent drug use: Long-term results of a junior high program. *American Journal of Public Health, 83*, 856–861.

Elliott, R., Bohart, A. C., Watson, J. C., & Greenberg, L. S. (2011). Empathy. *Psychotherapy, 48*(1), 43–49. doi: 10.1037/a0022187

Elliott, R., Greenberg, L. S., Watson, J., Timulak, L., & Freire, E. (2013). Research on humanistic-experiential psychotherapies. In M. J. Lambert (Ed.), *Bergin and Garfield's handbook of psychotherapy and behavior change* (6th ed., pp. 495–538). New York: Wiley.

Ellis, A. (1957). Outcome of emplying three techniques of psychotehrapy. *Journal of Clinical Psychology, 13*, 344–350.

Ellison, J. A., & Greenberg, L. S. (2007). *Emotion-focused experiential therapy.* New York: Springer Science.

Ellsworth, J. R., Lambert, M. J., & Johnson, J. (2006). A comparison of the Outcome Questionnaire-45 and Outcome Questionnaire-30 in classification and prediction of treatment outcome. *Clinical Psychology & Psychotherapy, 13*(6), 380–391.

Emmelkamp, P.M.G. (2004). Behavior therapy with adults. In M. Lambert (Ed.), *Bergin and Garfield's handbook of psychotherapy and behavior change* (5th ed., pp. 393–446). Oxford: Wiley & Sons.

Emmelkamp, P.M.G. (2013). Behavior therapy with adults. In M.J. Lambert (Ed.), *Bergin and Garfield's handbook of psychotherapy and behavior change* (6th ed., pp. 343–392). New York: Wiley.

Eysenck, H.J. (1952). The effects of psychotherapy: An evaluation. *Journal of Consulting Psychology, 16,* 319–324.

Eysenck, H.J. (1961). The effects of psychotherapy. In H.J. Eysenck (Ed.), *Handbook of abnormal psychology* (pp. 697–725). New York: Basic Books.

Eysenck, H.J. (1966). *The effects of psychotherapy.* New York: International Science Press.

Eysenck, H.J. (1978). An exercise in meta-silliness. *American Psychologist, 33,* 517.

Eysenck, H.J. (1984). Meta-analysis: An abuse of research integration. *The Journal of Special Education, 18*(1), 41–59.

Falkenström, F., Granström, F., & Holmqvist, R. (2013). Therapeutic alliance predicts symptomatic improvement session by session. *Journal of Counseling Psychology, 60*(3), 317–328. doi: 10.1037/a0032258

Falkenström, F., Granström, F., & Holmqvist, R. (2014). Working alliance predicts psychotherapy outcome even while controlling for prior symptom improvement. *Psychotherapy Research, 24*(2), 146–159. doi:10.1080/10503307.2013.847985

Falkenström, F., Markowitz, J.C., Jonker, H., Philips, B., & Holmqvist, R. (2013). Can psychotherapists function as their own controls? Meta-analysis of the crossed therapist design in comparative psychotherapy trials. *Journal of Clinical Psychiatry, 74*(5), 482–491. doi: 10.4088/JCP.12r07848

Farber, B.A., & Doolin, E.M. (2011). Positive regard and affirmation. In J.C. Norcross (Ed.), *Psychotherapy relationships that work: Evidence-based responsiveness* (2nd ed., pp. 168–186). New York: Oxford University Press.

Feeley, M., DeRubeis, R.J., & Gelfand, L.A. (1999). The temporal relation of adherence and alliance to symptom change in cognitive therapy for depression. *Journal of Consulting and Clinical Psychology, 67,* 578–582.

Fisher, R.A. (1935). *The design of experiments.* Edinburgh: Oliver and Boyd.

Fisher, S., & Greenberg, R.P. (1997). The curse of the placebo: Fanciful pursuit of a pure biological therapy. In S. Fisher & R.P. Greenberg (Eds.), *From placebo to panacea: Putting psychiatric drugs to the test* (pp. 3–56). New York: Wiley.

Fishman, D.B., & Franks, C.M. (1992). Evolution and differentiation within behavior therapy: A theoretical and epistemological review. In D.K. Freedheim (Ed.), *History of psychotherapy: A century of change* (pp. 159–196). Washington, DC: American Psychological Association.

Flückiger, C., Del Re, A.C., Horvath, A.O., Symonds, D., Ackert, M., & Wampold, B.E. (2013). Substance use disorders and racial/ethnic minorities matter: A meta-analytic examination of the relation between alliance and outcome. *Journal of Counseling Psychology, 60*(4), 610–616. doi: 10.1037/a0033161

Flückiger, C., Del Re, A.C., & Wampold, B.E. (in press). The Sleeper Effect: Artifact or Phenomenon—A brief comment on *Are the Parts as Good as the Whole? A Meta-Analysis of Component Treatment Studies (Bell, Marcus & Goodlad, 2013). Journal of Consulting and Clinical Psychology.*

Flückiger, C., Del Re, A.C., Wampold, B.E., Symonds, D., & Horvath, A.O. (2012). How central is the alliance in psychotherapy? A multilevel longitudinal meta-analysis. *Journal of Counseling Psychology, 59*(1), 10–17. doi: 10.1037/a0025749

Flückiger, C., Holtforth, M. G., Znoj, H. J., Caspar, F., & Wampold, B. E. (2013). Is the relation between early post-session reports and treatment outcome an epiphenomenon of intake distress and early response? A multi-predictor analysis in outpatient psychotherapy. *Psychotherapy Research, 23*(1), 1–13. doi: 10.1080/10503307.2012.693773

Foa, E. B., Gillihan, S. J., & Bryant, R. A. (2013). Challenges and successes in dissemination of evidence-based treatments for posttraumatic stress: Lessons learned from prolonged exposure therapy for PTSD. *Psychological Science in the Public Interest, 14*(2), 65–111. doi: 10.1177/1529100612468841

Foa, E. B., Hembree, E. A., & Rothbaum, B. O. (2007). *Prolonged exposure therapy for PTSD: Emotional processing of traumatic experiences: Therapist guide*. New York: Oxford University Press.

Foa, E. B., & Kozak, M. J. (1986). Emotional processing of fear: Exposure to corrective information. *Psychological Bulletin, 99*(1), 20–35. doi: 10.1037/0033-2909.99.1.20

Foa, E. B., Rothbaum, B. O., Riggs, D. S., & Murdock, T. B. (1991). Treatment of post-traumatic stress disorder in rape victims: A comparison between cognitive-behavioral procedures and counseling. *Journal of Consulting and Clinical Psychology, 59*, 715–723.

Follette, W. C., & Houts, A. C. (1996). Models of scientific progress and the role of theory in taxonomy development: A case study of the DSM. *Journal of Consulting and Clinical Psychology, 64*, 1120–1132.

Fortner, B. V. (1999). The effectiveness of grief counseling and therapy: A quantitative review. University of Memphis, Memphis, TN.

Fowler, J. H., & Christakis, N. A. (2009). Dynamic spread of happiness in a large social network: Longitudinal analysis over 20 years in the Framingham Heart Study. *British Medical Journal, 338*(7685), 1–13. doi: 10.1136/bmj.b1

Fowler, J. H., & Christakis, N. A. (2010). Cooperative behavior cascades in human social networks. *Proceedings of the National Academy of Sciences of the United States of America, 107*(12), 5334–5338. doi: 10.1073/pnas.0913149107

Frank, J. D. (1961). *Persuasion and healing: A comparative study of psychotherapy*. Baltimore: Johns Hopkins University Press.

Frank, J. D. (1973). *Persuasion and healing: A comparative study of psychotherapy* (Rev. Ed. ed.). Baltimore: Johns Hopkins University Press.

Frank, J. D. (1992). Historical developments in research centers: The Johns Hopkins Psychotherapy Research Project. In D. K. Freedheim (Ed.), *History of psychotherapy: A century of change* (pp. 392–396). Washington, DC: American Psychological Association.

Frank, J. D., & Frank, J. B. (1991). *Persuasion and healing: A comparative study of psychotherapy* (3rd ed.). Baltimore: Johns Hopkins University Press.

Free, M. L., & Oei, T. P. (1989). Biological and psychological processes in the treatment and maintenance of depression. *Clinical Psychology Review, 9*, 653–688.

French, T. M. (1933). Interrelations between psychoanalysis and the experimental work of Pavlov. *The American Journal of Psychiatry, 12*, 1165–1203.

Friedlander, M. L., Escudero, V., Heatherington, L., & Diamond, G. M. (2011). Alliance in couple and family therapy. *Psychotherapy, 48*(1), 25–33. doi: 10.1037/a0022060

Frost, N. D., Laska, K. M., & Wampold, B. E. (2014). The evidence for present-centered therapy as a treatment for posttraumatic stress disorder: Present-centered therapy. *Journal of Traumatic Stress, 27*(1), 1–8. doi:10.1002/jts.21881

Gabbard, G. O., Beck, J. S., & Holmes, J. (2005). *Oxford textbook of psychotherapy*. New York: Oxford University Press.

Gaffan, E. A., Tsaousis, I., Kemp-Wheeler, S. M. (1995). Researcher allegiance and meta-analysis: the case of cognitive therapy for depression. *Journal of Consulting and Clinical Psychology, 63*(6), 966–980.

Gallo, D. A., & Finger, S. (2000). The power of a musical instrument: Franklin, the Mozarts, Mesmer, and the glass harmonica. *History of Psychology, 3*, 326–343.

Gardner, R. (1998). The brain and communication are basic for human clinical sciences. *British Journal of Medical Psychology, 71*, 493–508.

Garfield, S. L. (1992). Eclectic pyschotherapy: A common factors approach. In J. C. Norcross & M. R. Goldfried (Eds.), *Handbook of psychotherapy integration* (pp. 169–201). New York: Basic Books.

Garfield, S. L. (1994). Research on client variables in psychotherapy. In A. E. Bergin & S. L. Garfield (Eds.), *Handbook of psychotherapy and behavior change* (4th ed., pp. 191–228). New York: Wiley.

Garfield, S. L. (1995). *Psychotherapy: An eclectic-integrative approach*. New York: Wiley & Sons.

Garfield, S. L. (1998). Some comments on empirically supported treatments. *Journal of Consulting and Clinical Psychology, 66*, 121–125.

Gaston, L., Marmar, C. R., Gallagher, D., & Thompson, L. W. (1991). Alliance prediction of outcome beyond in-treatment symptomatic change as psychotherapy processes. *Psychotherapy Research, 1*(2), 104–112. doi: 10.1080/10503309112331335531

Gauld, A. (1992). *A history of hypnotism*. Cambridge: Cambridge University Press.

Gehan, E., & Lemak, N. A. (1994). *Statistics in medical research: Developments in clinical trials*. New York: Plenum Medical Book.

Gelso, C. (2014). A tripartite model of the therapeutic relationship: Theory, research, and practice. *Psychotherapy Research, 24*(2), 117–131. doi:10.1080/10503307.2013.845920

Gelso, C. J. (2009). The real relationship in a postmodern world: Theoretical and empirical explorations. *Psychotherapy Research, 19*(3), 253–264. doi: 10.1080/10503300802389242

Gelso, C. J., & Carter, J. A. (1994). Components of the psychotherapy relationship: Their interaction and unfolding during treatment. *Journal of Counseling Psychology, 41*(3), 296–306. doi: 10.1037/0022-0167.41.3.296

Gelso, C. J., & Hayes, J. A. (2007). *Countertransference and the therapist's inner experience: Perils and possibilities*. Mahwah, NJ: Lawrence Erlbaum Associates Publishers.

Gilbert, P. (2010). *Compassion focused therapy: Distinctive features*. New York: Routledge/ Taylor & Francis Group.

Gilboa-Schechtman, E., Foa, E. B., Shafran, N., Aderka, I. M., Powers, M. B., Rachamim, L., . . . & Apter, A. (2010). Prolonged exposure versus dynamic therapy for adolescent PTSD: a pilot randomized controlled trial. *Journal of the American Academy of Child & Adolescent Psychiatry, 49*(10), 1034–1042.

Glass, G. V. (1976). Primary, secondary, and meta-analysis of research. *Educational Researcher, 5*, 3–8.

Gleick, J. (2003). *Isaac Newton*. New York: Pantheon Books.

Gleser, L. J., & Olkin, I. (2009). Stochastically dependent effect sizes. In H. Cooper, L. V. Hedges & J. C. Valentine (Eds.), *The handbook of research synthesis and meta-analysis* (2nd ed., pp. 357–376). New York: Russell Sage Foundation.

Gloaguen, V., Cottraux, J., Cucherat, M., Blackburn, I. (1998). A meta-analysis of the effects of cognitive therapy in depressed patients. *Journal of Affective Disorders, 49*, 59–72.

Goldfried, M. R. (1980). Toward the delineation of therapeutic change principles. *American Psychologist, 35*, 991–999.

Goldfried, M. R., & Wolfe, B. E. (1996). Psychotherapy practice and research: Repairing a strained alliance. *Journal of Consulting and Clinical Psychology, 51*, 1007–1016.

Goldstein, E., & Farmer, K. (Eds.) (1994). *Confabulations: Creating false memories, destroying families.* Boca Raton, FL: SIRS Books.

Gould, S. J. (1989). The chain of reason vs. the chain of thumbs. *Natural History, 7*, 12–21.

Gould, S. J. (1991). *Bully for Brontosaurus.* New York: Norton.

Greenberg, L. S. (2007). A guide to conducting a task analysis of psychotherapeutic change. *Psychotherapy Research, 17*, 15–30.

Greenberg, L. S. (2010). *Emotion-focused therapy.* Washington, DC: American Psychological Association.

Grencavage, L. M., & Norcross, J. C. (1990). Where are the commonalities among the therapeutic common factors? *Professional Psychology: Research and Practice, 21*, 372–378.

Greenberg, L. S. and Watson, J. C. (2005). *Emotion-Focused Therapy for Depression.* Washington, DC: American Psychological Association Press.

Greenberg, L. S., & Webster, M. C. (1982). Resolving decisional conflict by Gestalt two-chair dialogue: Relating process to outcome. *Journal of Counseling Psychology, 29*, 468–477.

Greenberg, R. P., Constantino, M. J., & Bruce, N. (2006). Are patient expectations still relevant for psychotherapy process and outcome? *Clinical Psychology Review, 26*, 657–678.

Grissom, R. J. (1996). The magical number .7 + - .2: Meta-meta-analysis of the probability of superior outcome in comparisons involving therapy, placebo, and control. *Journal of Consulting and Clinical Psychology, 64*, 973–982.

Grünbaum, A. (1981). The placebo concept. *Behaviour Research and Therapy, 19*, 157–167.

Guess, H. A., Kleinman, A., Kusek, J. W., & Engel, L. W. (2002). *The science of placebo: Toward an interdisciplinary research agenda.* London: BMJ Books.

Harrington, A. (1997). *The placebo effect: An interdiscipinary exploration.* Cambridge, MA: Harvard University Press.

Hatcher, R. L., & Barends, A. W. (1996). Patients' view of the alliance in psychotherapy: Exploratory factor analysis of three alliance measures. *Journal of Consulting and Clinical Psychology, 64*(6), 1326–1336. doi: 10.1037/0022-006x.64.6.1326

Hatcher, R. L., & Barends, A. W. (2006). How a Return to Theory Could Help Alliance Research. *Psychotherapy: Theory, Research, Practice, Training, 43*(3), 292–299.

Hays, W. L. (1988). *Statistics.* New York: Holt, Rinehart and Winston.

Hedges, L. V. (1981). Distribution theory for Glass's estimator of effect size and related estimators. *Journal of Educational Statistics, 6*(2), 107–128. doi: 10.2307/1164588

Hedges, L. V., & Olkin, I. (1985). *Statistical methods for meta-analysis.* San Diego: Academic Press.

Heide, F. J., & Borkovec, T. D. (1984). Relaxation-induced anxiety: Mechanisms and theoretical implications. *Behaviour Research and Therapy, 22*, 1–12.

Henry, W. P., Schacht, T. E., Strupp, H. H., Butler, S. F., & Binder, J. (1993). Effects of training in time-limited dynamic psychotherapy: Mediators of therapists' responses to training. *Journal of Consulting and Clinical Psychology, 61*, 441–447.

Henry, W. P., Strupp, H. H., Butler, S. F., Schacht, T. E., & Binder, J. (1993). Effects of training in time-limited psychotherapy: Changes in therapist behavior. *Journal of Consulting and Clinical Psychology, 61*, 434–440.

Hentschel, E., Brandstätter, G., Dragosics, B., Hirschl, A. M., Nemec, H., Schütze, K., . . . Wurzer, H. (1993). Effect of ranitidine and amoxicillin plus metronidazole on the eradication of Helicobacter pylori and the recurrence of duodenal ulcer. *The New England Journal of Medicine, 328*(5), 308–312.

Heppner, P.P., & Claiborn, C.D. (1989). Social influence research in counseling: A review and critique. *Journal of Counseling Psychology, 36*, 365–387.

Heppner, P.P., Kivlighan, D.M., & Wampold, B.E. (2008). *Research design in counseling* (3rd ed.). Belmont, CA: Thomson Brooks/Cole.

Herbert, J.D., Lilienfeld, S.O., Lohr, J.M., Montgomery, R.W., O'Donohue, W.T., Rosen, G.M., & Tolin, D.F. (2000). Science and pseudoscience in the development of eye movement desensitization and reprocessing: Implications for clinical psychology. *Clinical Psychology Review, 20*(8), 945–971.

Hill, C.E. (1986). An overview of the Hill counselor and client verbal response modes category systems. In L.S. Greenberg & W.M. Pinsof (Eds.), *The psychotherapeutic process: A research handbook* (pp. 131–159). New York: Guilford.

Hill, C.E., O'Grady, K.E., & Elkin, I. (1992). Applying the Collaborative Study Psychotherapy Rating Scale to rate therapist adherence in cognitive-behavior therapy, interpersonal therapy, and clinical management. *Journal of Consulting and Clinical Psychology, 60*, 73–79.

Hoffart, A., Borge, F.M., Sexton, H., Clark, D.M., & Wampold, B.E. (2012). Psychotherapy for social phobia: How do alliance and cognitive process interact to produce outcome? *Psychotherapy Research, 22*(1), 82–94. doi: 10.1080/10503307.2011.626806

Hoffart, A., Øktedalen, T., Langkaas, T.F., & Wampold, B.E. (2013). Alliance and outcome in varying imagery procedures for PTSD: A study of within-person processes. *Journal of Counseling Psychology, 60*(4), 471–482. doi: 10.1037/a0033604

Hofmann, S.G. (2008). Common misconceptions about cognitive mediation of treatment change: A commentary to Longmore and Worrell (2007*). Clinical Psychology Review, 28*(1), 67–70. doi: 10.1016/j.cpr.2007.03.003

Hofmann, S.G., & Lohr, J.M. (2010). To kill a dodo bird. *The Behavior Therapist, 33*(1), 14–15.

Holland, P.W. (1986). Statistics and causal inference. *Journal of the American Statistical Association, 81*(396), 945–960. doi: 10.2307/2289064

Holland, P.W. (1993). Which comes first, cause or effect? In G. Keren, C. Lewis, G. Keren & C. Lewis (Eds.), *A handbook for data analysis in the behavioral sciences: Methodological issues.* (pp. 273–282). Hillsdale, NJ: Lawrence Erlbaum Associates, Inc.

Hollon, S.D., & Beck, A.T. (2013). Cognitive and cognitive-behavioral therapies. In M.J. Lambert (Ed.), *Bergin and Garfield's handbook of psychotherapy and behavior change* (6th ed., pp. 393–442). New York: Wiley.

Hollon, S.D., DeRubeis, R.J., & Evans, M.D. (1987). Causal mediation of change in treatment for depression: Discriminating between nonspecificity and noncausality. *Psychological Bulletin, 102*, 139–149.

Holt-Lunstad, J., Smith, T.B., & Layton, J.B. (2010). Social relationships and mortality risk: a meta-analytic review. *Plos Medicine, 7*(7), e1000316.

Honyashiki, M., Furukawa, T.A., Noma, H., Tanaka, S., Chen, P., Ono, M., . . . Caldwell, D.M. (2014). Specificity of CBT for depression: A contribution from multiple treatments meta-analyses. *Cognitive Therapy and Research 38*, 249–260, doi: 10.1007/s10608-014-9599-7

Horvath, A.O. (2006). The alliance in context: Accomplishments, challenges, and future directions. *Psychotherapy: Theory, Research, Practice, Training, 43*(3), 258–263. doi: 10.1037/0033-3204.43.3.258

Horvath, A.O., & Bedi, R.P. (2002). The alliance. In J.C. Norcross (Ed.), *Psychotherapy relationships that work: Therapist contributions and responsiveness to patients* (pp. 37–70). New York: Oxford University.

Horvath, A. O., Del Re, A. C., Flückiger, C., Symonds, D. (2011a). Alliance in individual psychotherapy. In J. C. Norcross (Ed.), *Psychotherapy relationships that work: Evidence-based responsiveness* (2nd ed., pp. 25–69). New York: Oxford.

Horvath, A. O., Del Re, A. C., Flückiger, C., & Symonds, D. (2011b). Alliance in individual psychotherapy. *Psychotherapy, 48*(1), 9–16. doi: 10.1037/a0022186

Horvath, A. O., & Greenberg, L. S. (1989). Development and validation of the Working Alliance Inventory. *Journal of Counseling Psychology, 36*(2), 223–233. doi: 10.1037/0022-0167.36.2.223

Horvath, A. O., & Symonds, B. D. (1991). Relation between working alliance and outcome in psychotherapy: A meta-analysis. *Journal of Counseling Psychology, 38*, 139–149.

Horvath, P. (1988). Placebos and common factors in two decades of psychotherapy research. *Psychological Bulletin, 104*, 214–225.

Howard, K. I., Krause, M. S., & Orlinsky, D. E. (1986). The attrition dilemma: Toward a new strategy for psychotherapy research. *Journal of Consulting and Clinical Psychology, 54*, 106–110.

Howard, K. I., Krause, M. S., Saunders, S. M., & Kopta, S. M. (1997). Trials and tribulations in the meta-analysis of treatment differences: Comment on Wampold et al. (1997). *Psychological Bulletin, 122*, 221–225.

Hoyt, W. T., & Del Re, A. C. (2013). *Comparison of methods for aggregating dependent effect sizes in meta-analysis.* Manuscript submitted for publication.

Hoyt, W. T., & Larson, D. G. (2008). A realistic approach to drawing conclusions from the scientific literature: Response to Bonanno and Lilienfeld. *Professional Psychology Research and Practice, 39*(3), 378–379.

Hróbjartsson, A., & Gøtzsche, P. C. (2001). Is the placebo powerless? An analysis of clinical trials comparing placebo with no treatment. *The New England Journal of Medicine, 344*(21), 1594–1602.

Hróbjartsson, A., & Gøtzsche, P. C. (2004). Is the placebo powerless? Update of a systematic review with 52 new randomized trials comparing placebo with no treatment. *Journal of Internal Medicine, 256*(2), 91–100. doi: 10.1111/j.1365-2796.2004.01355.x

Hróbjartsson, A., & Gøtzsche, P. C. (2006). Unsubstantiated claims of large effects of placebo on pain: Serious errors in meta-analysis of placebo analgesia mechanism stuidies. *Journal of Clinical Epidemiology, 59*, 336–338.

Hróbjartsson, A., & Gøtzsche, P. C. (2007a). Powerful spin in the conclusion of Wampold et al.'s re analysis of placebo versus no-treatment trials despite similar results as in original review. *Journal of Clinical Psychology, 63*(4), 373–377. doi: 10.1002/jclp.20357

Hróbjartsson, A., & Gøtzsche, P. C. (2007b). Wampold et al.'s reiterate spin in the conclusion of a re-analysis of placebo versus no-treatment trials despite similar results as in original review. *Journal of Clinical Psychology, 63*(4), 405–408. doi: 10.1002/jclp.20356

Hubble, M. A., Duncan, B. L., & Miller, S. D. (Eds.). (1999). *The heart & soul of change: What works in therapy.* Washington, DC: American Psychological Association.

Huey, S. J., Jr, Tilley, J. L., Jones, E. O., & Smith, C. (in press). The contribution of cultural competence to evdince-based care for ethnically diverse populations. *Annual Review of Clinical Psychology.*

Hunsley, J., & Westmacott, R. (2007). Interpreting the magnitude of the placebo effect: Mountain or molehill? *Journal of Clinical Psychology, 63*(4), 391–399. doi: 10.1002/jclp.20352

Hunt, M. (1997). *How science takes stock: The story of meta-analysis*. New York: Russell Sage Foundation.

Hunt, M., & Corman, R. (November 11, 1962). Analysis of Psychoanalysis. *New York Times*, p. 248.

Ilardi, S. S., & Craighead, W. E. (1994). The role of nonspecific factors in cognitive-behavior therapy for depression. *Clinical Psychology, 1*, 138–156.

Imber, S. D., Pilkonis, P. A., Sotsky, S. M., Elkin, I., Watkins, J. T., Collins, J. F., . . . Glass, D. R. (1990). Mode-specific effects among three treatments for depression. *Journal of Consulting and Clinical Psychology, 58*, 352–359.

Imel, Z. E., Baer, J. S., Martino, S., Ball, S. A., & Carroll, K. M. (2011). Mutual influence in therapist competence and adherence to motivational enhancement therapy. *Drug and Alcohol Dependence, 115*(3), 229–236. doi: 10.1016/j.drugalcdep.2010.11.010

Imel, Z. E., Barco, J. S., Brown, H., Baucom, B. R., Baer, J. S., Kircher, J., & Atkins, D. C. (2014). Synchrony in vocally encoded arousal as an indicator of therapist empathy in motivational interviewing. *Journal of Counseling Psychology, 61*(1), 146–153.

Imel, Z.E., Sheng, E., Baldwin, S.A., & Atkins, D.C. (in press). Removing very low-performing therapists: A simulation of performance-based retention in psychotherapy. *Psychotherapy*.

Imel, Z. E., Steyvers, M., Atkins, D.C. (in press). Computational Psychotherapy Research: Scaling up the evaluation of patient provider interactions. *Psychotherapy*.

Imel, Z. E., Wampold, B. E., Miller, S. D., & Fleming, R. R. (2008). Distinctions without a difference: Direct comparisons of psychotherapies for alcohol use disorders. *Psychology of Addictive Behaviors, 22*(4), 533–543. doi: 10.1037/a0013171

Jacobson, N. S. (1991). To be or not to be behavioral when working with couples: What does it mean? *Journal of Family Psychology, 4*, 436–445.

Jacobson, N. S., Dobson, K. S., Truax, P. A., Addis, M. E., Koerner, K., Gollan, J. K., . . . Price, S. E. (1996). A component analysis of cognitive-behavioral treatment for depression. *Journal of Consulting and Clinical Psychology, 64*, 295–304.

Jacobson, N. S., & Hollon, S. D. (1996a). Cognitive-behavior therapy versus pharmacotherapy: Now that the jury's returned its verdict, it's time to present the rest of the evidence. *Journal of Consulting and Clinical Psychology, 64*, 74–80.

Jacobson, N. S., & Hollon, S. D. (1996b). Prospects for future comparisons between drugs and psychotherapy: Lessons from the CBT-versus-pharmacotherapy exchange. *Journal of Consulting and Clinical Psychology, 64*, 104–108.

Johansson, P., & Høglend, P. (2007). Identifying mechanisms of change in psychotherapy: Mediators of treatment outcome. *Clinical Psychology & Psychotherapy, 14*(1), 1–9. doi: 10.1002/cpp.514

Kaptchuk, T. J., Kelley, J. M., Conboy, L. A., Davis, R. B., Kerr, C. E., Jacobson, E. E., . . . Lembo, A. J. (2008). Components of placebo effect: Randomised controlled trial in patients with irritable bowel syndrome. *BMJ: British Medical Journal, 336*(7651), 999–1003. doi: 10.1136/bmj.39524.439618.25

Karlin, B. E., & Cross, G. (2014). From the laboratory to the therapy room: National dissemination and implementation of evidence-based psychotherapies in the U.S. Department of Veterans Affairs Health Care System. *American Psychologist, 69*(1), 19–33. doi: 10.1037/a0033888

Kazdin, A. E. (1994) Methodology, design, and evaluation in pyschotherapy research. In A.E. Bergin & S.L. Garfield (Eds.), *Handbook of psychotherapy and behavior change* (4th ed., pp. 19–71). New York: Wiley.

Kazdin, A. E. (2000). *Psychotherapy for children and adolescents: Directions for research and practice*. New York: Oxford University Press.

Kazdin, A. E. (2002*). Research design in clinical psychology* (4th ed.). Needham Heights, MA: Allyn & Bacon.

Kazdin, A. E. (2007). Mediators and mechanisms of change in psychotherapy research. *Annual Review of Clinical Psychology, 3*, 1–27. doi: 10.1146/annurev.clinpsy.3.022806.091432

Kazdin, A. E. (2009). Understanding how and why psychotherapy leads to change. *Psychotherapy Research, 19*(4–5), 418–428. doi: 10.1080/10503300802448899

Kazdin, A. E. & Bass, D. (1989). Power to detect differences between alternative treatments in comparative psychotherapy outcome research. *Journal of Consulting and Clinical Psychology, 57*, 138–147.

Kazdin, A. E., Esveldt-Dawson, K., French, N. H., & Unis, A. S. (1987). Effects of parent management training and problem-solving skills training combined in the treatment of antisocial child behavior. *Journal of the American Academy of Child & Adolescent Psychiatry, 26*(3), 416–424. doi: 10.1097/00004583-198705000-00024

Kazdin, A. E., & Weisz, J. R. (1998). Identifying and developing empirically supported child and adolescent treatments. *Journal of Consulting and Clinical Psychology, 66*, 19–36.

Kelley, J. M., Lembo, A. J., Ablon, J. S., Villanueva, J. J., Conboy, L. A., Levy, R., . . . Kaptchuk, T. J. (2009). Patient and practitioner influences on the placebo effect in irritable bowel syndrome. *Psychosomatic Medicine, 71*(7), 789–797. doi: 10.1097/PSY.0b013e3181acee12

Kendall, P. C. (1998). Empirically supported psychological therapies. *Journal of Consulting and Clinical Psychology, 66*, 3–6.

Kenny, D. A., & Judd, C. M. (1986). Consequences of violating the independence assumption in analysis of variance. *Psychological Bulletin, 99*(3), 422–431.

Kessler, R. C., Demler, O., Frank, R. G., Olfson, M., Pincus, H. A., Walters, E. E., . . . Zaslavsky, A. M. (2005). Prevalence and Treatment of Mental Disorders, 1990 to 2003. *New England Journal of Medicine, 352*, 2515–2523.

Kiesler, D. J. (1966). Some myths of psychotherapy research and the search for a paradigm. *Psychological Bulletin, 65*(2), 110–136. doi: 10.1037/h0022911

Kiesler, D. J. (1994). Standardization of intervention: The tie that binds psychotherapy research and practice. In P. F. Talley, H. H. Strupp & S. F. Butler (Eds.), *Psychotherapy research and practice: Bridging the gap* (pp. 143–153). New York: Basic Books.

Kiesler, D. J. (1996). *Contemporary interpersonal theory and research: Personality, psychopathology, and psychotherapy*. Oxford: John Wiley and Sons.

Kim, D. M., Wampold, B. E., & Bolt, D. M. (2006). Therapist effects in psychotherapy: A random effects modeling of the NIMH TDCRP data. *Psychotherapy Research, 16*, 161–172.

Kirk, R. E. (1995). *Experimental design: Procedures for the behavioral sciences* (3rd ed.). Pacific Grove, CA: Brooks/Cole

Kirsch, I. (1985). Response expectancy as a determinant of experience and behavior. *American Psychologist, 40*, 1189–1202.

Kirsch, I. (1999). *How expectancies shape experience*. Washington, DC: American Psychological Association.

Kirsch, I. (2000). Are drug and placebo effects in depression additive? *Biological Psychiatry, 47*(8), 733–735. doi: 10.1016/s0006-3223(00)00832-5

Kirsch, I. (2002). Yes, there *is* a placebo effect, but is there a powerful antidepressant drug effect? *Prevention & Treatment, 5*(1), 22.

Kirsch, I. (2005). Placebo Psychotherapy: Synonym or Oxymoron? *Journal of Clinical Psychology, 61*(7), 791–803.

Kirsch, I. (2009). Antidepressants and the placebo response. *Epidemiology and Psychiatric Sciences, 18*(4), 318–322.

Kirsch, I. (2010). *The emperor's new drugs: Exploding the antidepressant myth.* New York: Basic Books.

Kirsch, I., Deacon, B. J., Huedo-Medina, T. B., Scoboria, A., Moore, T. J., & Johnson, B. T. (2008). Initial severity and antidepressant benefits: A meta-analysis of data submitted to the food and drug administration. *Plos Medicine, 5*(2), 260–268. doi: 10.1371/journal.pmed.0050045

Kirsch, I., & Low, C. B. (2013). Suggestion in the treatment of depression. *American Journal of Clinical Hypnosis, 55*(3), 221–229. doi: 10.1080/00029157.2012.738613

Kirsch, I., Moore, T. J., Scoboria, A., & Nicholls, S. S. (2002). The emperor's new drugs: An analysis of antidepressant medication data submitted to the U.S. Food and Drug Administration. *Prevention & Treatment, 5,* article 23.

Kirsch, I., & Sapirstein, G. (1998). Listening to Prozac but hearing placebo: A meta-analysis of antidepressant medication. *Prevention & Treatment, 1*(2), 2a. doi:10.1037/1522-3736.1.1.12a

Kirsch, I., Scoboria, A., & Moore, T. J. (2002). Antidepressants and placebos: Secrets, revelations, and unanswered questions. *Prevention & Treatment, 5*(1), 33. doi:10.1037/1522-3736.5.1.533r

Kivlighan, D. M., Jr., & Shaughnessy, P. (2000). Patterns of working alliance development: A typology of client's working alliance ratings. *Journal of Counseling Psychology, 47*(3), 362–371. doi: 10.1037/0022-0167.47.3.362

Klein, D. F. (1996). Preventing hung juries about therapy studies. *Journal of Consulting and Clinical Psychoogy, 64,* 81–87.

Klein, D. N., Schwartz, J. E., Santiago, N. J., Vivian, D., Vocisano, C., Castonguay, L. G., . . . Keller, M. B. (2003). Therapeutic alliance in depression treatment: Controlling for prior change and patient characteristics. *Journal of Consulting and Clinical Psychology, 71*(6), 997–1006.

Klerman, G. L., Weissman, M. M., Rounsaville, B. J., & Chevron, E. S. (1984). *Interpersonal psychotherapy of depression.* New York: Basic Books.

Kohlenberg, R. J. & Tsai, M. (2007). *Functional Analytic Psychotherapy: A guide for creating intense and curative therapeutic relationships* (2nd ed.). New York: Springer.

Kolden, G. G., Klein, M. H., Wang, C.-C., & Austin, S. B. (2011). Congruence/genuineness. In J. C. Norcross (Ed.), *Psychotherapy relationships that work: Evidence-based responsiveness* (2nd ed., pp. 187–202). New York: Oxford University Press.

Kong, J., Kaptchuk, T. J., Polich, G., Kirsch, I., Vangel, M., Zyloney, C., . . . Gollub, R. (2009). Expectancy and treatment interactions: A dissociation between acupuncture analgesia and expectancy evoked placebo analgesia. *NeuroImage, 45*(3), 940–949. doi: 10.1016/j.neuroimage.2008.12.025

Konrad, M., Vyleta, M. L., Theis, F. J., Stock, M., Tragust, S., Klatt, M., . . . Cremer, S. (2012). Social transfer of pathogenic fungus promotes active immunisation in ant colonies. *PLoS Biology, 10*(4). doi: 10.1371/journal.pbio.1001300

Kraemer, H. C., & Kupfer, D. J. (2006). Size of treatment effects and their importance to clinical research and practice. *Biological Psychiatry, 2006,* 990–996.

Kuhn, T. S. (1962). *The structures of scientific revolutions.* Chicago: University of Chicago.

Kuhn, T. S. (1970). Logic of discovery or psychology of research. In I. Lakatos & A. Musgrave (Eds.), *Criticism and the growth of knowledge* (pp. 1–23). Cambridge: Cambridge University Press.

Lakatos, I. (1970). Falsification and the methodology of scientific research programmes. In I. Lakatos & A. Musgrave (Eds.), *Criticism and the growth of knowledge* (pp. 91–196). Cambridge: Cambridge University Press.

Lakatos, I. (1976). *Proofs and refutations: The logic of mathematical discovery.* Cambridge: Cambridge University Press.

Lakatos, I., & Musgrave, A. (Eds.). (1970). *Criticism and the growth of knowledge.* Cambridge: Cambridge University Press.

Lambert, M.J. (1992). Psychotherapy outcome research: Implications for integrative and eclectic therapists. In J.C. Norcross & M.R. Goldfried (Eds.), *Handbook of psychotherapy integration* (pp. 94–129). New York: Basic Books.

Lambert, M.J. (2010). *Prevention of treatment failure: The use of measuring, monitoring, and feedback in clinical practice.* Washington, DC: American Psychological Association.

Lambert, M.J. (Ed.). (2013). *Bergin and Garfield's handbook of psychotherapy and behavior change.* Hoboken, NJ: Wiley.

Lambert, M.J., & Bergin, A.E. (1994). The effectiveness of psychotherapy. In A.E. Bergin & S.L. Garfield (Eds.), *Handbook of psychotherapy and behavior change* (4th ed., pp. 143–189). New York: Wiley.

Lambert, M.J., Bergin, A.E., & Collins, J.L. (1997). Therapist-induced deterioration in psychotherapy. In A.S. Gurman & A.M. Razin (Eds.), *The therapist's contributions to effective treatment: An empirical assessment.* New York: Pergamon.

Lambert, M.J., Gregersen, A.T., & Burlingame, G.M. (2004). The Outcome Questionnaire-45. In M.E. Murish (Ed.), *Use of psychological testing for treatment planning and outcome assessment* (3rd ed., Vol. 3, pp. 191–234). Mahway, NJ: Erlbaum.

Lambert, M.J., & Ogles, B.M. (2004). The efficacy and effectiveness of psychotherapy. In M.J. Lambert (Ed.), *Bergin and Garfield's handbook of psychotherapy and behavior change* (5th ed., pp. 139–193). New York: Wiley.

Lambert, M.J., & Shimokawa, K. (2011). Collecting client feedback. In J.C. Norcross (Ed.), *Psychotherapy relationships that work: Evidence-based responsiveness* (2nd ed., pp. 203–223). New York: Oxford University Press.

Landman, J.T., & Dawes, R.M. (1982). Psychotherapy outcome: Smith and Glass' conclusions stand up under scrutiny. *American Psychologist, 37*(5), 504–516. doi: 10.1037/0003-066X.37.5.504

Langman, P.F. (1997). White culture, Jewish culture, and the origins of psychotherapy. *Psychotherapy, 34,* 207–218.

Larson, D.G., & Hoyt, W.T. (2007). What has become of grief counseling? An evaluation of the empirical foundations of the new pessimism. *Professional Psychology: Research and Practice, 38,* 347–355.

Larvor, B. (1998). *Lakatos: An introduction.* London: Routledge.

Laska, K.M., Gurman, A.S., & Wampold, B.E. (2014). Expanding the lens of evidence-based practice in psychotherapy: A common factors perspective. *Psychotherapy, 51,* 467–481.

Laska, K.M., Smith, T.L., Wislocki, A.P., Minami, T., & Wampold, B.E. (2013). Uniformity of evidence-based treatments in practice? Therapist effects in the delivery of cognitive processing therapy for PTSD. *Journal of Counseling Psychology, 60*(1), 31–41. doi: 10.1037/a0031294

Latour, B. (1999). *Pandora's hope: Essays on the reality of science studies.* Cambridge, MA: Harvard University Press.

Lau, A. S. (2006). Making the case for selective and directed cultural adaptations of evidence-based treatments: Examples from parent training. *Clinical Psychology: Science and Practice, 13*, 295–310.

Lazarus, A. A. (1981). *The practice of multimodal therapy*. New York: McGraw-Hill.

Leary, T. (1955). Psychiatry. *Journal for the Study of Interpersonal Processes, 18*, 147–161.

Leichsenring, F., Rabung, S., & Leibing, E. (2004). The efficacy of short-term psychodynamic psychotherapy in specific psychiatric disorders: a meta-analysis. *Archives of General Psychiatry, 61*,1208–1216.

Leichsenring, F., Salzer, S., Beutel, M. E., Herpertz, S., Hiller, W., Hoyer, J., . . . Leibing, E. (2013). Psychodynamic therapy and cognitive-behavioral therapy in social anxiety disorder: A multicenter randomized controlled trial. *The American Journal of Psychiatry, 170*(7), 759–767.

Leichsenring, F., Salzer, S., & Leibing, E. (2013). Response to Clark. *American Journal of Psychiatry, 170*(11), 1365–1366.

Leykin, Y., & DeRubeis, R. J. (2009). Allegiance in psychotherapy outcome research: Separating association from bias. *Clinical Psychology: Science and Practice, 16*, 54–65.

Liberman, B. L. (1978). The role of mastery in psychotherapy: Maintenance of improvement and prescriptive change. In J. D. Frank, R. Hoehn-Saric, S. D. Imber, B. L. Liberman & A. R. Stone (Eds.), *Effective ingredients of successful psychotherapy* (pp. 35–72). Baltimore: Johns Hopkins University Press.

Lieberman, M. D. (2013). *Social: Why our brains are wired to connect*. New York: Crown Publishing Group.

Lilienfeld, S. O. (2007). Psychological treatments that cause harm. *Perspectives on Psychological Science, 2*, 53–70.

Lilienfeld, S. O., Ritschel, L. A., Lynn, S. J., Cautin, R. L., & Latzman, R. D. (2013). Why many clinical psychologists are resistant to evidence-based practice: Root causes and constructive remedies. *Clinical Psychology Review, 33*(7), 883–900. doi: 10.1016/j.cpr.2012.09.008

Lillard, A. (1998). Ethnopsychologies: Cultural variations in theories of mind. *Psychological Bulletin, 123*(1), 3–32. doi: 10.1037/0033-2909.123.1.3

Lipsey, M. W., & Wilson, D. B. (1993). The efficacy of psychological, educational, and behavioral treatment: confirmation from meta-analysis. *American Psychologist, 48*(12), 1181–1209.

Loftus, E. F., & Davis, D. (2006). Recovered memories. *Annual Review of Clinical Psychology, 2*, 469–498.

Longmore, R. J., & Worrell, M. (2007). Do we need to challenge thoughts in cognitive behavior therapy? *Clinical Psychology Review, 27*(2), 173–187. doi: 10.1016/j.cpr.2006.08.001

Luborsky, L. (1954). A note on Eysenck's article "The effects of psychotherapy: an evaluation."*British Journal of Psychology, 45*, 129–131.

Luborsky, L., Crits-Christoph, P., McLellan, A. T., Woody, G., Piper, W., Liberman, B., . . . & Pilkonis, P. (1986). Do therapists vary much in their success? Findings from four outcome studies. *American Journal of Orthopsychiatry, 56*(4), 501–512.

Luborsky, L., & DeRubeis, R. J. (1984). The use of psychotherapy treatment manuals: A small revolution in psychotherapy research style. *Clinical Psychology Review, 4*, 5–14.

Luborsky, L., Diguer, L., Seligman, D. A., Rosenthal, R., Krause, E. D., Johnson, S., . . . Schweizer, E. (1999). The researcher's own therapy allegiances: A "wild card" in comparisons of treatment efficacy. *Clinical Psychology: Science and Practice, 6*(1), 95–106.

Luborsky, L., McLellan, A. T., Diguer, L., Woody, G., & Seligman, D. A. (1997). The Psychotherapist Matters: Comparison of Outcomes Across Twenty-Two Therapists and Seven Patient Samples. *Clinical Psychology: Science and Practice, 4*(1), 53–65.

Luborsky, L., Singer, B., & Luborsky, L. (1975). Comparative studies of psychotherapies: Is it true that "everyone has won and all must have prizes?" *Archives of General Psychiatry, 32*(8), 995–1008.

Luo, Y., Hawkley, L. C., Waite, L. J., & Cacioppo, J. T. (2012). Loneliness, health, and mortality in old age: A national longitudinal study. *Social Science & Medicine, 74*(6), 907–914. doi: 10.1016/j.socscimed.2011.11.028

MacCoon, D. G., Imel, Z. E., Rosenkranz, M. A., Sheftel, J. G., Weng, H. Y., Sullivan, J. C., . . . Lutz, A. (2012). The validation of an active control intervention for Mindfulness Based Stress Reduction (MBSR). *Behaviour Research and Therapy, 50*(1), 3–12. doi: 10.1016/j.brat.2011.10.011

MacKenzie, D. L., Wilson, D. B., & Kider, S. B. (2001). Effects of correctional boot camps on offending. *Annals of the American Academy of Political and Social Science, 578*, 126–143.

Madsen, M. V., Gøtzsche, P. C., & Hróbjartsson, A. (2009). Acupuncture treatment for pain: Systematic review of randomised clinical trials with acupuncture, placebo acupuncture, and no acupuncture groups. *British Medical Journal, 338*(7690). doi: 10.1136/bmj.a3115

Markowitz, J. C., Klerman, G. L., Clougherty, K. F., Spielman, L. A., Jacobsberg, L. B., Fishman, B., . . . Perry, S. W. (1995). Individual psychotherapies for depressed HIV-positive patients. *American Journal of Psychiatry, 152*, 1504–1509.

Markowitz, J. C., Kocsis, J. H., Fishman, B., Spielman, L. A., Jacobsberg, L. B., Frances, A. J., . . . Perry, S. W. (1998). Treatment of depressive symptoms in human immunodeficiency virus-positive patients. *Archives of General Psychiatry, 55*(5), 452–457. doi: 10.1001/archpsyc.55.5.452

Markowitz, J. C., Manber, R., & Rosen, P. (2008). Therapists' response to training in brief supportive psychotherapy. *American Journal of Psychotherapy, 62*(1), 67–81.

Markowitz, J. C., Milrod, B., Bleiberg, K., & Marshall, R. D. (2009). Interpersonal factors in understanding and treating posttraumatic stress disorder. *Journal of Psychiatric Practice, 15*(2), 133–140. doi: 10.1097/01.pra.0000348366.34419.28

Marlatt, G. A. (1983). The controlled-drinking controversy: A commentary. *American Psychologist, 38*, 1097–1110.

Marlatt, G. A. (1985). Abstinence and controlled drinking: Alternative treatment goals for alcoholism and problem drinking? *Bulletin of the Society of Psychologists in Addictive Behaviors, 4*, 123–150.

Marlatt, G. A., & Gordon, J. (1985). *Relapse prevention: Maintenance strategies in the treatment of addictive behaviors.* New York: Guilford.

Martin, D. J., Garske, J. P., & Davis, M. K. (2000). Relation of the therapeutic alliance with outcome and other variables: A meta-analytic review. *Journal of Consulting and Clinical Psychology, 68*, 438–450.

Mattick, R. P., Andrews, G., Hadzi-Pavlovic, D., & Christensen, H. (1990). Treatment of panic and agoraphobia: An integrative review. *The Journal of Nervous and Mental Disease, 178*(9), 567–576.

Mavissakalian, M., & Michelson, L. (1986). Agoraphobia: Relative and combined effectiveness of therapist-assisted in vivo exposure and imipramine. *Journal of Clinical Psychiatry, 47*, 117–122.

Mays, V. M., & Albee, G. W. (1992). Psychotherapy and ethnic minorities. In D. K. Freedheim (Ed.), *History of psychotherapy: A century of change* (pp. 552–570). Washington, DC: American Psychological Association.

McCall, W. A. (1923). *How to experiment in education.* New York: Macmillan.

McCullough, L., & Magill, M. (2009). Affect-focused short-term dynamic therapy. In R. A. Levy & J. S. Ablon (Eds.), *Handbook of evidence-based psychodynamic psychotherapy: Bridging the gap between science and practice.* (pp. 249–277). Totowa, NJ: Humana Press.

McDonagh, A., Friedman, M., McHugo, G., Ford, J., Sengupta, A., Mueser, K., . . . Descamps, M. (2005). Randomized trial of cognitive-behavioral therapy for chronic posttraumatic stress disorder in adult female survivors of childhood sexual abuse. *Journal of Consulting and Clinical Psychology, 73*, 515–524.

McHugh, R. K., & Barlow, D. H. (2012). Dissemination and implementation of evidence-based psychological interventions: Current status and future directions. In R. K. McHugh & D. H. Barlow (Eds.), *Dissemination and implementation of evidence-based psychological interventions* (pp. 247–263). New York: Oxford University Press.

McKay, K. M., Imel, Z. E., & Wampold, B. E. (2006). Psychiatrist effects in the psychopharmacological treatment of depression. *Journal of Affective Disorders, 92*(2), 287–290.

McLaughlin, A. A., Keller, S. M., Feeny, N. C., Youngstrom, E. A., & Zoellner, L. A. (2014). Patterns of therapeutic alliance: Rupture–repair episodes in prolonged exposure for posttraumatic stress disorder. *Journal of Consulting and Clinical Psychology, 82*(1), 112.

McNally, R. J. (1999). EMDR and Mesmerism: A comparative historical analysis. *Journal of Anxiety Disorders, 13*, 225–236.

McNally, R. J., Bryant, R. A., & Ehlers, A. (2003). Does early psychological intervention promote recovery from posttraumatic stress? *Psychological Science in the Public Interest, 4*, 45–79.

McNamara, K., & Horan, J. J. (1986). Experimental construct validity in the evaluation of cognitive and behavioral treatments for depression. *Journal of Counseling Psychology, 33*: 23–30. doi:10.1037//0022-0167.33.1.23

Meehl, P. E. (1967). Theory-testing in psychology and physics: A methodological paradox. *Philosophy of Science, 34*, 103–115.

Meehl, P. E. (1978). Theoretical risks and tabular asterisks: Sir Karl, Sir Ronald, and the slow progress of soft psychology. *Journal of Consulting and Clinical Psychology, 46*(4), 806–834. doi: 10.1037/0022-006x.46.4.806

Meichenbaum, D. (1986). Cognitive-behavior modification. In F. H. Kanfer & A. P. Goldstein (Eds.), *Helping people change: A textbook of methods* (3rd ed., pp. 346–380). New York: Pergamon Press.

Meltzoff, J., and Kornreich, M. (1970). *Research in psychotherapy.* Chicago: Adline

Mercer, J. (2002). Attachment therapy: A treatment without empirical support. *The Scientific Review of Mental Health Practice, 1,* 105–112.

Merrill, K. A., Tolbert, V. E., & Wade, W. A. (2003). Effectiveness of cognitive therapy for depression in a community mental health center: A benchmarking study. *Journal of Consulting and Clinical Psychology, 71*(2), 404–409. doi: 10.1037/0022-006x.71.2.404

Mesmer, F. A. (1980). *Mesmerism: A translation of the original scientific and medical writings of E. A. Mesmer* (G. Bloch, Trans.). Los Altos, CA: William Kaufman. (Original work published 1766)

Milgrom, J., Negri, L. M., Gemmill, A. W., McNeil, M., Martin, P. R. (2005). A randomized controlled trial of psychological interventions for postnatal depression. *British Journal of Clinical Psychology, 44*: 529–542. doi:10.1348/014466505x34200

Miller, D. (1994). *Critical rationalism: A restatement and defense.* Chicago: Open Court.

Miller, G. A. (1996). How we think about cognition, emotion, and biology in psychopathology. *Psychophysiology, 33,* 615–628.

Miller, S. D., Duncan, B. L., Sorrell, R., & Brown, G. S. (2005). The Partners for Change Outcome Management System. *Journal of Clinical Psychology, 61*(2), 199–208. doi: 10.1002/jclp.20111

Miller, W. R., Andrews, N. R., Wilbourne, P., & Bennett, M. E. (1998). A wealth of alternatives: Effective treatments for alcohol problems. In W. R. Miller, & N. Heather (Eds.), *Treating addictive behaviors* (2nd ed., pp. 203–216). New York: Plenum Press.

Miller, W. R., & Rollnick, S. (2002). *Motivational interviewing* (2nd ed.). New York: Guilford.

Miller, W. R., & Rollnick, S. (2009). Ten things that motivational interviewing is not. *Behavioural and Cognitive Psychotherapy, 37*(2), 129–140. doi: 10.1017/s1352465809005128

Miller, W. R., & Rollnick, S. (2012). *Motivational interviewing* (3rd ed.). New York: Guilford Press.

Miller, W. R., & Rose, G. S. (2009). Toward a theory of motivational interviewing. *American Psychologist, 64,* 527–537.

Mills, K. C., Sobell, M. B., & Schaefer, H. H. (1971). Training social drinking as an alternative to abstinence for alcoholics. *Behavior Therapy, 2,* 18–27.

Minami, T., & Wampold, B. E. (2008). Adult psychotherapy in the real world. In W. B. Walsh (Ed.), *Biennial Review of Counseling Psychology* (Vol. I, pp. 27–45). New York: Taylor and Francis.

Minami, T., Davies, D. R., Tierney, S. C., Bettmann, J. E., McAward, S. M., Averill, L. A., . . . Wampold, B. E. (2009). Preliminary evidence on the effectiveness of psychological treatments delivered at a university counseling center. *Journal of Counseling Psychology, 56*(2), 309–320. doi: 10.1037/a0015398

Minami, T., Serlin, R. C., Wampold, B. E., Kircher, J., & Brown, G. S. (2008). Using clinical trials to benchmark effects produced in clinical practice. *Quality and Quantity, 42,* 513–525.

Minami, T., Wampold, B. E., Serlin, R. C., Hamilton, E., Brown, G. S., & Kircher, J. (2008). Benchmarking the effectiveness of psychotherapy treatment for adult depression in a managed care environment: A preliminary study. *Journal of Consulting and Clinical Psychology, 76,* 116–124.

Minami, T., Wampold, B. E., Serlin, R. C., Kircher, J. C., & Brown, G. S. J. (2007). Benchmarks for psychotherapy efficacy in adult major depression. *Journal of Consulting and Clinical Psychology, 75*(2), 232–243.

Mohr, D. C. (1995). Negative outcome in psychotherapy: A critical review. *Clinical Psychology: Science and Practice, 2,* 1–27.

Mohr, D. C., Beutler, L. E., Engle, D., Shoham-Salomon, V., Bergan, J., Kaszniak, A. W., et al. (1990). Identification of patients at risk for nonresponse and negative outcome in psychotherapy. *Journal of Consulting and Clinical Psychology, 58,* 622–628.

Mohr, D. C., Spring, B., Freedland, K. E., Beckner, V., Arean, P., Hollon, S. D., . . . & Kaplan, R. (2009). The selection and design of control conditions for randomized controlled trials of psychological interventions. *Psychotherapy and Psychosomatics, 78*(5), 275–284.

Molden, D. C., & Dweck, C. S. (2006). Finding "Meaning" in Psychology: A Lay Theories Approach to Self-Regulation, Social Perception, and Social Development. *American Psychologist, 61*(3), 192–203. doi: 10.1037/0003-066x.61.3.192

Montgomery, G. H., & Kirsch, I. (1997). Classical conditioning and the placebo effect. *Pain, 72,* 107–113.

Moos, R. H. (2005). Iatrogenic effects of psychosocial interventions for substance use disorders: Prevalence, predictors, prevention. *Addiction, 100,* 595–604.

Morris, D. B. (1997). Placebo, pain, and belief: A biocultural model. In A. Harrington (Ed.), *The placebo effect: An interdisciplinary exploration* (pp. 187–207). Cambridge, MA: Harvard University Press.

Morris, D. B. (1998). *Illness and culture in the postmodern age.* Berkeley: University of California Press.

Moses, E. B., & Barlow, D. H. (2006). A new unified treatment approach for emotional disorders based on emotion science. *Current Directions in Psychological Science, 15,* 146–150.

Moyers, T. B., & Miller, W. R. (2013). Is low therapist empathy toxic? *Psychology of Addictive Behaviors, 27*(3), 878–884. doi: 10.1037/a0030274

Moyers, T. B., Miller, W. R., & Hendrickson, S. M. L. (2005). How does motivational interviewing work? Therapist interpersonal skill predicts client involvement within motivational interviewing sessions. *Journal of Consulting and Clinical Psychology, 73*(4), 590–598. doi: 10.1037/0022-006x.73.4.590

Munder, T., Brütsch, O., Leonhart, R., Gerger, H., & Barth, J. (2013). Researcher allegiance in psychotherapy outcome research: An overview of reviews. *Clinical Psychology Review, 33*(4), 501–511. doi: 10.1016/j.cpr.2013.02.002

Munder, T., Gerger, H., Trelle, S., & Barth, J. (2011). Testing the allegiance bias hypothesis: A meta-analysis. *Psychotherapy Research, 21,* 670–684.

Munder, T., Flückiger, C., Gerger, H., Wampold, B. E. & Barth, J. (2012). Is the allegiance effect an epiphenomenon of true efficacy differences between treatments? A meta-analysis. *Journal of Counseling Psychology, 59,* 632–637.

Nash, E., Hoehn-Sacric, R., Battle, C., Stone, A., Imber, S. D., & Frank, J. (1965). Systematic preparation of patients for short-term psychotherapy: 2. Relation to characteristics of patient, therapist, and the psychotherapeutic process. *Journal of Nervous and Mental Disorders, 140,* 374–383.

National Association of Cognitive-Behavioral Therapists (NACBT) (2014). Retrieved April 21, 2014, from www.nacbt.org/whatiscbt.aspx

National Collaborating Centre for Mental Health (2005). Post-traumatic stress disorder: The management of PTSD in adults and children in primary and secondary care. London, Royal College of Psychiatrists and Leicester, The British Psychological Society.

Neimeyer, R. A. (2000). Searching for the meaning of meaning: Grief therapy and the process of reconstruction. *Death Studies, 24,* 541–558.

Niedenthal, P. M., & Brauer, M. (2012). Social functionality of human emotion. *Annual Review of Psychology, 63,* 259–285. doi: 10.1146/annurev.psych.121208.131605

Nissen-Lie, H. A., Monsen, J. T., & Rønnestad, M. H. (2010). Therapist predictors of early patient-rated working alliance: A multilevel approach. *Psychotherapy Research, 20*(6), 627–646. doi: 10.1080/10503307.2010.497633

Nitschke, J. B., Dixon, G. E., Sarinopoulos, I., Short, S. J., Cohen, J. D., Smith, E. E., . . . Davidson, R. J. (2006). Altering expectancy dampens neural response to aversive taste in primary taste cortex. *Nature Neuroscience, 9*(3), 435–442.

Norcross, J. C. (2011). *Psychotherapy relationships that work: Evidence-based responsiveness.* New York: Oxford University Press.

Norcross, J. C., & Goldfried, M. R. (1992). *Handbook of psychotherapy integration.* New York: Basic Books.

Norcross, J. C., & Goldfried, M. R. (2005). *Handbook of psychotherapy integration* (2nd ed.). New York: Oxford University Press.

Norcross, J. C., & Karpiak, C. P. (2012). Clinical psychologists in the 2010s: 50 years of the APA division of clinical psychology. *Clinical Psychology: Science and Practice, 19*(1), 1–12. doi: 10.1111/j.1468-2850.2012.01269.x

Norcross, J. C., Karpiak, C. P., & Santoro, S. O. (2005). Clinical psychologists across the years: The division of clinical psychology from 1960 to 2003. *Journal of Clinical Psychology, 61*(12), 1467–1483. doi: 10.1002/jclp.20135

Norcross, J. C., & Newman, C. F. (1992). Psychotherapy integration: Setting the context. In J. C. Norcross & M. R. Goldfried (Eds.), *Handbook of psychotherapy integration* (pp. 3–45). New York: Basic Books.

Nowinski J, Baker S, & Carroll, K. (1992). *Twelve step facilitation therapy manual: A clinical research guide for therapists treating individuals with alcohol abuse and dependence.* Rockville, MD: NIAA.

Oei, T. P. S., & Free, M. L. (1995). Do cognitive behaviour therapies validate cognitive models of mood disorders? A review of the empirical evidence. *International Journal of Psychology, 30*, 145–179.

Okiishi, J., Lambert, M. J., Nielsen, S. L., & Ogles, B. M. (2003). Waiting for supershrink: An empirical analysis of therapist effects. *Clinical Psychology & Psychotherapy, 10*(6), 361–373.

Orlinsky, D. E., & Howard, K. I. (1986). Process and outcome in psychotherapy. In S. L. Garfield & A. E. Bergin (Eds.), *Handbook of psychotherapy and behavior change* (3rd ed., pp. 311–381). New York: Wiley.

Öst, L. G. (1987). Applied relaxation: Description of a coping technique and review of controlled studies. *Behaviour Research and Therapy*, 25, 397–409.

Ougrin, D. (2011). Efficacy of exposure versus cognitive therapy in anxiety disorders: systematic review and meta-analysis. *BMC psychiatry, 11*(1), 200.

Owen, J., & Hilsenroth, M. J. (2014). Treatment adherence: The importance of therapist flexibility in relation to therapy outcomes. *Journal of Counseling Psychology, 61,* 280-288.

Papakostas, Y. G., & Daras, M. D. (2001). Placebos, placebo effect, and the response to the healing situation: The evolution of a concept. *Epilepsia, 42*(12), 1614–1625.

Parloff, M. B. (1986). Frank's "Common elements" in psychotherapy: Nonspecific factors and placebos. *American Journal of Orthopsychiatry, 56*, 521–529.

Pattie, F. A. (1994). *Mesmer and animal magnetism: A chapter in the history of medicine.* Hamilton, NY: Edmonston.

Paul, G. L. (1969). Behavior modification research: Design and tactics. In C. M. Franks (Ed.), *Behavior therapy: Appraisal and status* (pp. 29–62). New York: McGraw-Hill.

Pendery, M. L., Maltzman, I. M., & West, L. J. (1982). Controlled drinking by alcoholics? New findings and a reevaluation of a major affirmative study. *Science, 217*, 169–175.

Perepletchikova, F. (2009). Treatment integrity and differential treatment effects. *Clinical Psychology: Science and Practice, 16*(3), 379–382. doi: 10.1111/j.1468-2850.2009.01177.x

Persons, J. B., & Silberschatz, G. (1998). Are results of randomized controlled trials useful to psychotherapists? *Journal of Consulting and Clinical Psychology, 66*, 126–135.

Petrosino, A., Turpin-Petrosino, C., & Buehler, J. (2003). Scared Straight and other juvenile awareness programs for preventing juvenile delinquency: A systematic review of the randomized experimental evidence. *Annals of the American Academy of Political and Social Science, 589*, 41–62.

Phillips, E. L. (1957). *Psychotherapy: A modern theory and practice.* London: Staples.

Pilkonis, P. A., Imber, S. D., Lewis, P., & Rubinsky, P. (1984). A comparative outcome study of individual, group, and conjoint psychotherapy. *Archives of General Psychiatry, 41*, 431–437.

Piper, W. E., Debbane, E. G., Bienvenu, J. P., & Garant, J. (1984). A comparative study of four forms of psychotherapy. *Journal of Consulting and Clinical Psychology, 52*(2), 268–279.

Pinsof, W. M., & Wynne, L. C. (2000). Toward progress research: Closing the gap between family therapy practice and research. *Journal of Marital and Family Therapy, 26*(1), 1–8. doi: 10.1111/j.1752-0606.2000.tb00270.x

Pinsof, W. M., Zinbarg, R. E., Lebow, J. L., Knobloch-Fedders, L. M., Durbin, E., Chambers, A., . . . Friedman, G. (2009). Laying the foundation for progress research in family, couple, and individual therapy: The development and psychometric features of the initial Systemic Therapy Inventory of Change. *Psychotherapy Research, 19*(2), 143–156. doi: 10.1080/10503300802669973

Piper, W. E., Debbane, E. G., Bienvenu, J. P., & Garant, J. (1984). A comparative study of four forms of psychotherapy. *Journal of Consulting and Clinical Psychology, 52*(2), 268–279.

Plassmann, H., O'Doherty, J., Shiv, B., & Rangel, A. (2008). Marketing actions can modulate neural representations of experienced pleasantness. *Proceedings of the National Academy of Sciences, 105*(3), 1050–1054.

Pollo, A., Amanzio, M., Arslanian, A., Casadio, C., Maggi, G., & Benedetti, F. (2001). Response expectancies in placebo analgesia and their clinical relevance. *Pain, 93*(1), 77–84. doi: 10.1016/s0304-3959(01)00296-2

Popper, K. R. (1963). *Conjectures and refutations.* London: Routledge.

Popper, K. R. (1962). On the sources of knowledge and of ignorance. *Conjectures and refutations: The growth of scientific knowledge.* New York: Basic Books.

Popper, K. R. (1972). *Objective knowledge: An evolutionary approach.* Oxford: Oxford University Press.

Porter, A. C., & Raudenbush, S. W. (1987). Analysis of covariance: Its model and use in psychological research. *Journal of Counseling Psychology, 34*, 383–392.

Poulsen, S., Lunn, S., Daniel, S.I.F., Folke, S., Mathiesen, B. B., Katznelson, H., & Fairburn, C. G. (2014). A randomized controlled trial of psychoanalytic psychotherapy or cognitive-behavioral therapy for bulimia nervosa. *The American Journal of Psychiatry, 171*(1), 109–116. doi: 10.1176/appi.ajp.2013.12121511

Powers, M. B., Halpern, J. M., Ferenschak, M. P., Gillihan, S. J., & Foa, E. B. (2010). A meta-analytic review of prolonged exposure for posttraumatic stress disorder. *Clinical Psychology Review, 30*, 635–641.

Powers, M. B., Smits, J.A.J., Whitley, D., Bystritsky, A., & Telch, M. J. (2008). The effect of attributional processes concerning medication taking on return of fear. *Journal of Consulting and Clinical Psychology, 76*(3), 478–490.

Preston, S. D., & de Waal, F.B.M. (2002). Empathy: Its ultimate and proximate bases. *Behavioral and Brain Sciences, 25,* 1–20.

Price, D. P., Finniss, D. G., & Benedetti, F. (2008). A comprehensive review of the placebo effect: Recent advances and current thought. *Annual Review of Psychology, 59,* 565–590.

Prochaska, J. O., & Norcross, J. C. (2002). Stages of change. In J. C. Norcross (Ed.), *Psychotherapy relationships that work: Therapist contributions and responsiveness to patients* (pp. 303–313). New York: Oxford University.

Project MATCH Research Group. (1997). Matching alcoholism treatments to client heterogeneity: Project MATCH Posttreatment drinking outcomes. *Journal of Studies on Alcohol, 58,* 7–29.

Project MATCH Research Group. (1998). Therapist effects in three treatments for alcohol problems. *Psychotherapy Research, 8*(4), 455–474.

Propst, L. R., Ostrom, R., Watkins, P., Dean, T., & Mashburn, D. (1992). Comparative efficacy of religious and nonreligious cognitive-behavioral therapy for the treatment of clinical depression in religious individuals. *Journal of Consulting and Clinical Psychology, 60,* 94–103.

Puschner, B., Wolf, M., & Kraft, S. (2008). Helping alliance and outcome in psychotherapy: What predicts what in routine outpatient treatment? *Psychotherapy Research, 18*(2), 167–178. doi: 10.1080/10503300701367984

Rachman, S. (1971). *The effects of psychotherapy* (Vol. 15). Oxford: Pergamon.

Rachman, S. (1977). Double standards and single standards. *Bulletin of the British Psychological Society, 30*(AUG), 295–295.

Rachman, S., & Wilson, G. T. (1980). *The effects of psychological therapy.* Oxford: Pergamon Press.

Ramseyer, F., & Tschacher, W. (2011). Nonverbal synchrony in psychotherapy: Coordinated body movement reflects relationship quality and outcome. *Journal of Consulting and Clinical Psychology, 79,* 284–295.

Raudenbush, S. W. (2009). Analyzing effect sizes: Random-effects models. In H. Cooper, L. V. Hedges & J. C. Valentine (Eds.), *The handbook of research synthesis and meta-analysis* (2nd ed., pp. 295–316). New York: Russell Sage Foundation.

Rhule, D. M. (2005). Take care to do no harm: Harmful interventions for youth problem behavior. *Professional Psychology: Research and Practice, 36,* 618–625.

Rice, L. N., & Greenberg, L. S. (1992). Humanistic approaches to psychotherapy. In D. K. Freedheim (Ed.), *History of psychotherapy: A century of change* (pp. 197–224). Washington, DC: American Psychological Association.

Robinson, L. A., Berman, J. S., & Neimeyer, R. A. (1990). Psychotherapy for the treatment of depression: A comprehensive review of controlled outcome research. *Psychological Bulletin, 108,* 30–49.

Rogers, C. R. (1951a). *Client-centered therapy.* Boston: Houghton Mifflin.

Rogers, C. R. (1951b). A research program in client-centered therapy. *Research publications—Association for Research in Nervous and Mental Disorders, 31,* 106–113.

Rosa-Alcázar, A.I., Sánchez-Meca, J., Gómez-Conesa, A., & Marín-Martínez, F. (2008). Psychological treatment of obsessive–compulsive disorder: A meta-analysis. *Clinical Psychology Review, 28,* 1310–1325.

Rose, S., Bisson, J., & Wessely, S. (2001). Psychological debriefing for preventing post traumatic stress disorder (PTSD). (Cochrane Library, Issue 3.) Oxford: Update Software.

Rosen, G. M. (1999). Treatment fidelity and research on Eye Movement Desensitization and Reprocessing (EMDR). *Journal of Anxiety Disorders, 13,* 173–184.

Rosenbaum, D. P., & Hanson, G. S. (1998). Assessing the effects of school-based drug education: A six-year multilevel analysis of Project D.A.R.E. *Journal of Research in Crime and Delinquency, 35*(4), 381–412.

Rosenquist, J. N., Fowler, J. H., & Christakis, N. A. (2011). Social network determinants of depression. *Molecular Psychiatry, 16*(3), 273–281. doi: 10.1038/mp.2010.13

Rosenthal, D., & Frank, J. D. (1956). Psychotherapy and the placebo effect. *Psychological Bulletin, 53,* 294–302.

Rosenthal, R. (1994). Parametric measures of effect size. In H. Cooper & L. V. Hedges (Eds.), *The handbook of research synthesis* (pp. 231–260). New York: Russell Sage Foundation.

Rosenzweig, S. (1936). Some implicit common factors in diverse methods of psychotherapy: "At last the Dodo said, 'Everybody has won and all must have prizes'." *American Journal of Orthopsychiatry, 6,* 412–415.

Rosenzweig, S. (1954). A transvaluation of psychotherapy: a reply to Hans Eysenck. *The Journal of Abnormal and Social Psychology, 49,* 298–304.

Roth, W. T., Wilhelm, F. H., & Petit, D. (2005). Are current theories of panic falsifiable? *Psychological Bulletin, 131,* 171–192.

Rubin, D. B. (1986). Statistics and causal inference—which ifs have causal answers. *Journal of the American Statistical Association, 81*(396), 961–962. doi: 10.2307/2289065

Ruzek, J. I., Karlin, B. E., & Zeiss, A. (2012). Implementation of evidence-based psychological treatments in the Veterans Health Administration. In R. K. McHugh & D. H. Barlow (Eds.), *Dissemination and implementation of evidence-based psychological interventions* (pp. 78–96). New York: Oxford University Press.

Sackett, D. L., Straus, S. E., Richardson, W. S., Rosenberg, W., & Haynes, R. B. (2000). *Evidence-based medicine: How to practice and teach EBM* (2nd ed.). London: Churchill Livingstone.

Safran, J. D., & Muran, J. C. (2000). *Negotiating the therapeutic alliance.* New York: Guilford.

Safran, J. D., Muran, J. C., & Eubanks-Carter, C. (2011). Repairing alliance ruptures. *Psychotherapy, 48*(1), 80–87. doi: 10.1037/a0022140

Sagan, C. In P. G Blacketor (2009). *Everyday useful quotes.* Xlibris.

Sánchez-Meca, J., Rosa-Alcázar, A. I., Marín-Martínez, F., & Gómez-Conesa, A. (2010). Psychological treatment of panic disorder with or without agoraphobia: a meta-analysis. *Clinical Psychology Review, 30*(1), 37–50.

Sapyta, J., Riemer, M., & Bickman, L. (2005). Feedback to Clinicians: Theory, Research, and Practice. *Journal of Clinical Psychology, 61*(2), 145–153. doi: 10.1002/jclp.20107

Saxon, D., & Barkham, M. (2012). Patterns of therapist variability: Therapist effects and the contribution of patient severity and risk. *Journal of Consulting and Clinical Psychology, 80*(4), 535–546. doi: 10.1037/a0028898

Schneider Institute for Health Policy, Brandeis University for the Robert Wood Johnson Foundation. (2001). *Substance abuse: The nation's number one health problem: Key indicators for policy update.* Princeton, NJ: The Robert Wood Johnson.

Schnurr, P. P., Friedman, M. J., Engel, C. C., Foa, E. B., Shea, M. T., Chow, B. K., et al. (2007). Cognitive behavioral therapy for posttraumatic stress disorder in women: A randomized controlled trial. *JAMA: Journal of the American Medical Association, 297,* 820–830.

Schnurr, P. P., Shea, M. T., Friedman, M. J., & Engel, C. C. (2007). 'Posttraumatic stress disorder and cognitive behavioral therapy': In reply. *Journal of the American Medical Association, 297*(24). doi: 10.1001/jama.297.24.2695

Seidler, G. H., & Wagner, F. E. (2006). Comparing the efficacy of EMDR and trauma-focused cognitive-behavioral therapy in the treatment of PTSD: a meta-analytic study. *Psychological Medicine, 36*(11), 1515–1522.

Seligman, M. E. (1995). The effectiveness of psychotherapy: The Consumer Reports study. *American Psychologist, 50*(12), 965–974.

Serlin, R. C., & Lapsley, D. K. (1985). Rationality in psychological research: The good-enough principle. *American Psychologist, 40*(1), 73–83. doi: 10.1037/0003-066x. 40.1.73

Serlin, R. C., & Lapsley, D. K. (1993). Rational appraisal of psychological research and the good-enough principle. In G. Keren, C. Lewis, G. Keren & C. Lewis (Eds.), *A handbook for data analysis in the behavioral sciences: Methodological issues* (pp. 199–228). Hillsdale, NJ: Lawrence Erlbaum Associates, Inc.

Serlin, R. C., Wampold, B. E., & Levin, J. R. (2003). Should providers of treatment be regarded as a random factor? If it ain't broke, don't "Fix" it: A comment on Siemer and Joorman (2003). *Psychological Methods, 8,* 524–534.

Shadish, W. R., & Haddock, C. K. (2009). Combining estimates of effect size. In H. Cooper, L. V. Hedges & J. C. Valentine (Eds.), *The handbook of research synthesis and meta-analysis* (2nd ed., pp. 257–277). New York: Russell Sage Foundation.

Shadish, W. R., Matt, G. E., Navarro, A. M., & Phillips, G. (2000). The effects of psychological therapies in clinically representative conditions: A meta-analysis. *Psychological Bulletin, 126,* 512–529.

Shadish, W. R., Matt, G. E., Navarro, A. M., Siegle, G., Crits-Christoph, P., Hazelrigg, M. D., . . . Weiss, B. (1997). Evidence that therapy works in clinically representative conditions. *Journal of Consulting and Clinical Psychology, 65,* 355–365.

Shadish, W. R., Montgomery, L. M., Wilson, P., Wilson, M. R., Bright, I., & Okwumabua, T. (1993). Effects of family and marital psychotherapies: A meta-analysis. *Journal of Consulting and Clinical Psychology, 61*(6), 992.

Shadish, W. R., & Sweeney, R. B. (1991). Mediators and moderators in meta-analysis: There's a reason we don't let dodo birds tell us which psychotherapies should have prizes. *Journal of Consulting and Clinical Psychology, 59*(6), 883–893

Shafran, R., Clark, D. M., Fairburn, C. G., Arntz, A., Barlow, D. H., Ehlers, A., . . . Wilson, G. T. (2009). Mind the gap: Improving the dissemination of CBT. *Behaviour Research and Therapy, 47*(11), 902–909. doi: 10.1016/j.brat.2009.07.003

Shapiro, D. A., Barkham, M., Rees, A., Hardy, G. E., Reynolds, S., & Startup, M. (1994). Effects of treatment duration and severity of depression on the effectiveness of cognitive-behavioral and psychodynamic-interpersonal psychotherapy. *Journal of Consulting and Clinical Psychology, 62,* 522–534.

Shapiro, A. K., & Morris, L. A. (1978). The placebo effect in medical and psychological therapies. In S. L. Garfield & A. E. Bergin (Eds.), *Handbook of psychotherapy and behavior change* (2nd ed., pp. 369–410). New York: Wiley.

Shapiro, A. K., & Shapiro, E. S. (1997a). The placebo: Is it much ado about nothing? In A. Harrington (Ed.), *The placebo effect: An interdisciplinary exploration.* Cambridge, MA: Harvard University Press.

Shapiro, A. K., & Shapiro, E. S. (1997b). *The powerful placebo: From ancient priest to modern medicine*. Baltimore: The Johns Hopkins University Press.

Shapiro, D. A., & Shapiro, D. (1982). Meta-analysis of comparative therapy outcome studies: A replication and refinement. *Psychological Bulletin, 92*, 581–604.

Shaw, B. F., Elkin, I., Yamaguchi, J., Olmsted, M., Vallis, T. M., Dobson, K. S., . . . Imber, S. D. (1999). Therapist competence ratings in relation to clinical outcome in cognitive therapy of depression. *Journal of Consulting and Clinical Psychology, 67*, 837–846.

Shedler, J. (2010). The efficacy of psychodynamic psychotherapy. *American Psychologist, 65*(2), 98–109. doi: 10.1037/a0018378

Shepherd, M. (1993). The placebo: From specificity to the non-specific and back. *Psychological Medicine, 23*(3), 569–578.

Sherman, J. J. (1998). Effects of psychotherapeutic treatments for PTSD: A meta-analysis of controlled clinical trial. *Journal of Traumatic Stress, 11*, 413–435.

Shimokawa, K., Lambert, M. J., & Smart, D. W. (2010). Enhancing treatment outcome of patients at risk of treatment failure: Meta-analytic and mega-analytic review of a psychotherapy quality assurance system. *Journal of Consulting and Clinical Psychology, 78*(3), 298–311. doi: 10.1037/a0019247

Shirk, S. R., Karver, M. S., & Brown, R. (2011). The alliance in child and adolescent psychotherapy. *Psychotherapy, 48*(1), 17–24. doi: 10.1037/a0022181

Siev, J., & Chambless, D. L. (2007). Specificity of treatment effects: Cognitive therapy and relaxation for generalized anxiety and panic disorders. *Journal of Consulting and Clinical Psychology, 75*, 513–522.

Siev, J., Huppert, J. D., & Chambless, D. L. (2009). The dodo bird, treatment technique, and disseminating empirically supported treatments. *The Behavior Therapist, 32*, 69–76.

Simon, G., Imel, Z. E., & Steinfield, B. J. (2012). Is dropout after a first psychotherapy visit always a bad outcome? *Psychiatric Services, 63*, 705–7.

Simon G.E. & Ludman, E. J. (2010). Predictors of early dropout from psychotherapy for depression in community practice. *Psychiatric Services, 61*, 684–689.

Simpson, S. H., Eurich, D. T., Majumdar, S. R., Padwal, R. S., Tsuyuki, S. T., Varney, J., & Johnson, J. A. (2006). A meta-analysis of the association between adherence to drug therapy and mortality. *British Medical Journal, 3–4.* doi:10.1136/bmj.38875.675486.55.

Singer, M. T., & Lalich, J. (1996). *"Crazy" therapies: What are they? Do they work?* New York: Jossey-Bass.

Sloane, R. B., Staples, F. R., Cristol, A. H., Yorkston, N. J., & Whipple, K. (1975). *Psychotherapy versus behavior therapy*. Cambridge, MA: Harvard University Press.

Smith, B., & Sechrest, L. (1991). Treatment of Aptitude × Treatment Interactions. *Journal of Consulting and Clinical Psychology, 59*(2), 233–244. doi: 10.1037/0022-006x.59.2.233

Smith, M. L., & Glass, G. V (1977). Meta-analysis of psychotherapy outcome studies. *American Psychologist, 32*, 752–760.

Smith, M. L., Glass, G. V, & Miller, T. I. (1980). *The benefits of psychotherapy*. Baltimore: The Johns Hopkins University Press.

Snijders, T., & Bosker, R. (1999). *Multilevel analysis: An introduction to basic and advanced multilevel modeling*. London: Sage.

Snyder, D. K., & Wills, R. M. (1989). Behavioral versus insight-oriented marital therapy: Effects on individual and interpersonal functioning. *Journal of Consulting and Clinical Psychology, 57*, 39–46.

Snyder, D. K., & Wills, R. M. (1991). Facilitating change in marital therapy and research. *Journal of Family Psychology, 4*, 426–435.

Snyder, D. K., Wills, R. M., & Grady-Fletcher, A. (1991). Long term effectiveness of behavioral versus insight oriented marital therapy: A 4-year follow-up study. *Journal of Consulting and Clinical Psychology, 59*, 138–141.

Sobell, L. C., Sobell, M. B., & Christelman, W. C. (1972). The myth of "one drink." *Behaviour Research and Therapy, 10*, 119–123.

Sobell, M. B. & Sobell, L. C. (1973). Alcoholics treated by individualized behavior therapy: One year treatment outcomes. *Behavior Research and Therapy, 11*, 599–618.

Sobell, M. B., & Sobell, L. C. (1976). Second year treatment outcome of alcoholics treated by individualized behavior therapy: Results. *Behaviour Research and Therapy, 14*, 195–215.

Sobell, M. B., & Sobell, L. C. (1984a). The aftermath of heresy: A response to Pendery et al.'s (1982) critique of 'Individualized behavior therapy for alcoholics'. *Behaviour Research and Therapy, 22*, 413–440.

Sobell, M. B., & Sobell, L. C. (1984b). Under the microscope yet again: A commentary on walker and roach's critique of the dickens committee's enquiry into our research. *British Journal of Addiction, 79*, 157–168.

Society of Clinical Psychology. (2007). Website on Research Supported Psychological Treatments, www.div12.org/PsychologicalTreatments/index.html

Spiegel, A. (2004). Cognitive behavior therapy: Thinking positive [Radio series episode]. "All Things Considered." Washington, DC: National Public Radio. Retrieved from www.npr.org/templates/story/story.php?storyId=1920052

Spielmans, G. I., Gatlin, E. T., & McFall, J. P. (2010). The efficacy of evidence-based psychotherapies versus usual care for youths: Controlling confounds in a meta-reanalysis. *Psychotherapy Research, 20*(2), 234–246. doi: 10.1080/10503300903311293

Spielmans, G. I., & Kirsch, I. (in press). Drug approval and drug effectiveness. *Annual Review of Clinical Psychology.* doi: 10.1146/annurev-clinpsy-050212-185533

Spielmans, G. I., Pasek, L. F., & McFall, J. P. (2007). What are the active ingredients in cognitive and behavioral psychotherapy for anxious and depressed children? A meta-analytic review. *Clinical Psychology Review, 27*(5), 642–654. doi:10.1016/j.cpr.2006.06.001

Stangier, U., Schramm, E., Heidenreich, T., Berger, M., & Clark, D. M. (2011). Cognitive therapy vs interpersonal psychotherapy in social anxiety disorder: a randomized controlled trial. *Archives of General Psychiatry, 68*(7), 692–700.

Stevens, S. E., Hynan, M. T., & Allen, M. (2000). A meta-analysis of common factor and specific treatment effects across domains of the phase model of psychotherapy. *Clinical Psychology: Science and Practice, 7*, 273–290.

Stiles, W. B., Shapiro, D. A., & Elliott, R. (1986). Are all psychotherapies equivalent? *American Psychologist, 41*, 165–180.

Strunk, D. R., Brotman, M. A., & DeRubeis, R. J. (2010). The process of change in cognitive therapy for depression: Predictors of early inter-session symptom gains. *Behaviour Research and Therapy, 48*(7), 599–606. doi: 10.1016/j.brat.2010.03.011

Strunk, D. R., Cooper, A. A., Ryan, E. T., DeRubeis, R. J., & Hollon, S. D. (2012). The process of change in cognitive therapy for depression when combined with antidepressant medication: Predictors of early intersession symptom gains. *Journal of Consulting and Clinical Psychology, 80*(5), 730–738. doi: 10.1037/a0029281

Strupp, H. H., & Howard, K. I. (1992). A brief history of psychotherapy research. In D. K. Freedheim (Ed.), *History of psychotherapy: A century of change* (pp. 309–334). Washington, DC: American Psychological Association.

Sullivan, H. S. (1953). *The interpersonal theory of psychiatry.* New York: Routledge.

Surgeon General. (1999). *Mental Health: A Report of the Surgeon General—Executive Summary.* Rockville, MD: U.S. Department of Health and Human Services, Substance

Abuse and Mental Health Services Administration, Center for Mental Health Services, National Institutes of Health, National Institute of Mental Health.

Surís, A., Link-Malcolm, J., Chard, K., Ahn, C., & North, C. (2013). A randomized clinical trial of cognitive processing therapy for veterans with PTSD related to military sexual trauma. *Journal of Traumatic Stress, 26*(1), 28–37. doi: 10.1002/jts.21765

Sutton, A.J. (2009). Publication bias. In H. Cooper, L.V. Hedges & J.C. Valentine (Eds.), *The hanbook of research synthesis and meta-analysis* (2nd ed., pp. 435–454). New York: Russell Sage Foundation.

Swift, J.K., Callahan, J.L., & Vollmer, B.M. (2011). Preferences. *Journal of Clinical Psychology, 67*(2), 155–165. doi: 10.1002/jclp.20759

Swift, J.K., & Greenberg, R.P. (2012). Premature discontinuation in adult psychotherapy: A meta-analysis. *Journal of Consulting and Clinical Psychology, 80*(4), 547–559. doi: 10.1037/a0028226

Tang, T.Z., & DeRubeis, R.J. (1999). Reconsidering rapid early response in cognitive behavioral therapy for depression. *Clinical Psychology: Science and Practice, 6*(3), 283–288. doi: 10.1093/clipsy/6.3.283

Tarrier, N., Pilgrim, H., Sommerfield, C., Faragher, B., Reynolds, M., Graham, E., & Barrowclough, C. (1999). A randomized trial of cognitive therapy and imaginal exposure in the treatment of chronic posttraumatic stress disorder. *Journal of Consulting and Clinical Psychology, 67*, 13–18.

Tasca, G.A., & Lampard, A.M. (2012). Reciprocal influence of alliance to the group and outcome in day treatment for eating disorders. *Journal of Counseling Psychology, 59*(4), 507–517. doi: 10.1037/a0029947

Task Force on Promotion and Dissemination of Psychological Procedures. (1995). Training in and dissemination of empirically-validated psychological treatment: Report and recommendations. *The Clinical Psychologist, 48*, 2–23.

Taylor, E. (1999). *Shadow culture: Psychology and spirituality in America*. Washington, DC: Counterpoint.

Taylor, S. (1996). Meta-analysis of cognitive-behavioral treatments for social phobia. *Journal of Behaviour Therapy and Experimental Psychiatry, 27*, 1–9.

Taylor, S., Thordarson, D.S., Maxfield, L., Fedoroff, I.C., Lovell, K., & Ogrodniczuk, J. (2003). Comparative efficacy, speed, and adverse effects of three PTSD treatments: Exposure therapy, EMDR, and relaxation training. *Journal of Consulting and Clinical Psychology, 71*(2), 330–338. doi:10.1037/0022-006X.71.2.330

Thomas, R.M. (2001). *Folk psychologies across cultures*. Thousand Oaks, CA: Sage.

Tolin, D.F. (2010). Is cognitive–behavioral therapy more effective than other therapies?: A meta-analytic review. *Clinical Psychology Review, 30*(6), 710–720. doi: 10.1016/j.cpr.2010.05.003

Tracey, T.J.G., Wampold, B.E., Lichtenberg, J.W., & Goodyear, R.K. (2014). Expertise in Psychotherapy: An Elusive Goal? *American Psychologist*. doi: 10.1037/a0035099

Truax, C.B. (1966). Reinforcement and nonreinforcement in Rogerian psychotherapy. *Journal of Abnormal Psychology, 71*(1), 1–9. doi: 10.1037/h0022912

Tryon, G.S., & Winograd, G. (2011). Goal consensus and collaboration. In J.C. Norcross (Ed.), *Psychotherapy relationships that work: Evidence-based responsiveness* (2nd ed., pp. 153–167). New York: Oxford University Press.

UKATT Research Team. (2007). UK alcohol treatment trial: client-treatment matching effects. *Addiction, 103*, 228–238.

Ulvenes, P. G., Berggraf, L., Hoffart, A., Stiles, T. C., Svartberg, M., McCullough, L., & Wampold, B. E. (2012). Different processes for different therapies: Therapist actions, therapeutic bond, and outcome. *Psychotherapy, 49*(3), 291–302. doi: 10.1037/a0027895

van Balkom, A. J., van Oppen, P., Vermeulen, A. W., van Dyck, R., Nauta, M. C., & Vorst, H. (1994). A meta-analysis on the treatment of obsessive compulsive disorder: a comparison of antidepressants, behavior, and cognitive therapy. *Clinical Psychology Review, 14*(5), 359–381.

van Emmerik, A. A. P., Kamphuis, J. H., Hulsbosch, A. M., & Emmelkamp, P. M. G. (2002). Single session debriefing after psychological trauma: A meta-analysis. *The Lancet, 360*, 766–771.

van Minnen, A., & Foa, E. B. (2006). The Effect of Imaginal Exposure Length on Outcome of Treatment for PTSD. *Journal of Traumatic Stress, 19*(4), 427–438. doi: 10.1002/jts.20146

VandenBos, G. R., Cummings, N. A., & DeLeon, P. H. (1992). A century of psychotherapy: Economic and environmental influences. In D. K. Freedheim (Ed.), *History of psychotherapy: A century of change* (pp. 65–102). Washington, DC: American Psychological Association.

Vase, L., Riley III, J. L., & Price, D. P. (2002). A comparison of placebo effects in clinical analgesic trials versus studies of placebo analgesia. *Pain, 99*, 443–452.

Vollmer, S., Spada, H., Caspar, F., & Burri, S. (2013). Expertise in clinical psychology. The effects of university training and practical experience on expertise in clinical psychology. *Frontiers in Psychology, 4*, article 141.

Vos, S. P. F., Huibers, M. J. H., Diels, L., & Arntz, A. (2012). A randomized clinical trial of cognitive behavioral therapy and interpersonal psychotherapy for panic disorder with agoraphobia. *Psychological Medicine, 42*(12), 2661–2672. doi:10.1017/S0033291712000876

Wachtel, P. L. (1977). *Psychoanalysis and behavior therapy: Toward an integration.* New York: Basic Books.

Wade, W. A., Treat, T. A., & Stuart, G. L. (1998). Transporting an empircally supported treatment for panic disorder to a service clinic setting: A benchmarking strategy. *Journal of Consulting and Clinical Psychology, 66*, 231–239.

Walach, H. (2003). Placebo and placebo effects—a concise review. *Focus on Alternative and Complementary Therapies, 8*, 178–187.

Walsh, J. E. (1947). Concerning the effect of intraclass correlation on certain significance tests. *The Annals of Mathematical Statistics, 18*(1), 88–96.

Walsh, R. (2011). Lifestyle and mental health. *American Psychologist, 66*(7), 579–592. doi: 10.1037/a0021769

Waltz, J., Addis, M. E., Koerner, K., & Jacobson, N. S. (1993). Testing the integrity of a psychotherapy protocol: Assessment of adherence and competence. *Journal of Consulting and Clinical Psychology, 61*, 620–630.

Wampold, B. E. (1997). Methodological problems in identifying efficacious psychotherapies. *Psychotherapy Research, 7*, 21–43.

Wampold, B. E. (2001a). Contextualizing psychotherapy as a healing practice: Culture, history, and methods. *Applied and Preventive Psychology, 10*, 69–86.

Wampold, B. E. (2001b). *The great psychotherapy debate: Model, methods, and findings.* Mahwah, NJ: Lawrence Erlbaum Associates.

Wampold, B. E. (2007). Psychotherapy: *The* humanistic (and effective) treatment. *American Psychologist, 62*, 857–873.

Wampold, B. E. (2013). The good, the bad, and the ugly: A 50-year perspective on the outcome problem. *Psychotherapy, 50*(1), 16–24. doi: 10.1037/a0030570

Wampold, B. E., & Bhati, K. S. (2004). Attending to the omissions: A historical examination of the evidenced-based practice movement. *Professional Psychology: Research and Practice, 35*, 563–570.

Wampold, B. E., & Brown, G. S. (2005). Estimating therapist variability: A naturalistic study of outcomes in managed care. *Journal of Consulting and Clinical Psychology, 73*, 914–923.

Wampold, B. E., & Budge, S. L. (2012). The 2011 Leona Tyler Award Address: The Relationship—and Its Relationship to the Common and Specific Factors of Psychotherapy. *The Counseling Psychologist, 40*(4), 601–623. doi: 10.1177/0011000011432709

Wampold, B. E., Budge, S. L., Laska, K. M., Del Re, A. C., Baardseth, T. P., Flückiger, C., . . . Gunn, W. (2011). Evidence-based treatments for depression and anxiety versus treatment-as-usual: A meta-analysis of direct comparisons. *Clinical Psychology Review, 31*(8), 1304–1312. doi: 10.1016/j.cpr.2011.07.012

Wampold, B. E., & Drew, C. J. (1990). *Theory and application of statistics*. New York: McGraw-Hill College.

Wampold, B. E., Goodheart, C. D., & Levant, R. F. (2007). Evidence-based practice in psychology: Clarification and elaboration. *American Psychologist, 62*, 616–618.

Wampold, B. E. & Imel, Z. E. (2006). Psychotherapy stories: A textbook case of privilege. Review of the *Oxford Textbook of Psychotherapy*. *Contemporary Psychology: APA Review of Books, 51*(20).

Wampold, B. E., Imel, Z. E., Bhati, K. S., & Johnson Jennings, M. D. (2006). Insight as a common factor. In L. G. Castonguay & C. E. Hill (Eds.), *Insight in psychotherapy*, 119–139. Washington, DC: American Psychological Association.

Wampold, B. E., Imel, Z. E., Laska, K. M., Benish, S., Miller, S. D., Flückiger, C., . . . Budge, S. (2010). Determining what works in the treatment of PTSD. *Clinical Psychology Review, 30*(8), 923–933. doi: 10.1016/j.cpr.2010.06.005

Wampold, B. E., Imel, Z. E., & Miller, S. D. (2009). Barriers to the dissemination of empirically supported treatments: Matching messages to the evidence. *The Behavior Therapist, 32*(7), 144–155.

Wampold, B. E., Imel, Z. E., & Minami, T. (2007a). The placebo effect: 'Relatively large' and 'robust' enough to survive another assault. *Journal of Clinical Psychology, 63*(4), 401–403. doi: 10.1002/jclp.20350

Wampold, B. E., Imel, Z. E., & Minami, T. (2007b). The story of placebo effects in medicine: Evidence in context. *Journal of Clinical Psychology, 63*, 379–390.

Wampold, B. E., Minami, T., Baskin, T. W., & Callen Tierney, S. (2002). A meta-(re)analysis of the effects of cognitive therapy versus 'other therapies' for depression. *Journal of Affective Disorders, 68*(2), 159–165.

Wampold, B. E., Minami, T., Tierney, S. C., Baskin, T. W., & Bhati, K. S. (2005). The placebo is powerful: Estimating placebo effects in medicine and psychotherapy from clinical trials. *Journal of Clinical Psychology, 61*, 835–854.

Wampold, B. E., Mondin, G. W., Moody, M., & Ahn, H. (1997a). The flat earth as a metaphor for the evidence for uniform efficacy of bona fide psychotherapies: Reply to Crits-Christoph (1997) and Howard et al. (1997). *Psychological Bulletin, 122*, 226–230.

Wampold, B. E., Mondin, G. W., Moody, M., Stich, F., Benson, K., & Ahn, H. (1997b). A meta-analysis of outcome studies comparing bona fide psychotherapies: Empirically, "All must have prizes." *Psychological Bulletin, 122*, 203–215.

Wampold, B. E., & Serlin, R. C. (2000). The consequences of ignoring a nested factor on measures of effect size in analysis of variance. *Psychological Methods, 5*, 425–433.

Wampold, B. E., & Serlin, R. C. (2014). Meta-analytic methods to test relative efficacy. *Quality and Quantity, 48*, 755–765. doi: 10.1007/s11135-012-9800-6

Wang, P. S., Demler, O., Olfson, M., Pincus, H. A., Wells, K. B., & Kessler, R. C. (2006). Changing profiles of service sectors used for mental health care in the United States. *American Journal of Psychiatry, 163*, 1187–1198.

Wang, P. S., Lane, M., Olfson, M., Pincus, H. A., Wells, K. B., & Kessler, R. C. (2005). Twelve-month use of mental health services in the United States: Results from the National Comorbidity Survey Replication. *Archives of General Psychiatry, 62*, 629–640.

Watson, J. B., & Rayner, R. (1920). Conditioned emotional reactions. *Experimental psychology, 3*, 1–14.

Watson, J. C., Gordon, L. B., Stermac, L., Kalogerakos, F., & Steckley, P. (2003). Comparing the effectiveness of process-experiential with cognitive-behavioral psychotherapy in the treatment of depression. *Journal of Consulting and Clinical Psychology*, 71, 773–781.

Webb, C. A., DeRubeis, R. J., Amsterdam, J. D., Shelton, R. C., Hollon, S. D., & Dimidjian, S. (2011). Two aspects of the therapeutic alliance: Differential relations with depressive symptom change. *Journal of Consulting and Clinical Psychology, 79*(3), 279–283. doi: 10.1037/a0023252

Webb, C. A., DeRubeis, R. J., & Barber, J. P. (2010). Therapist adherence/competence and treatment outcome: A meta-analytic review. *Journal of Consulting and Clinical Psychology, 78*(2), 200–211. doi: 10.1037/a0018912

Weersing, V. R., & Weisz, J. R. (2002). Community clinic treatment of depressed youth: Benchmarking usual care against CBT clinical trials. *Journal of Consulting and Clinical Psychology, 70*(2), 299–310.

Weiss, B., Caron, A., Ball, S., Tapp, J., Johnson, M., & Weisz, J. R. (2005). Iatrogenic effects of group treatment for antisocial youths. *Journal of Consulting and Clinical Psychology, 73*, 1036–1044.

Weissman, M. M. (2006). A Brief History of Interpersonal Psychotherapy. *Psychiatric Annals, 36*(8), 553–557.

Weisz, J. R., Jensen-Doss, A., & Hawley, K. M. (2006). Evidence-based youth psychotherapies versus usual clinical care: A meta-analysis of direct comparisons. *American Psychologist, 61*(7), 671–689. doi: 10.1037/0003-066x.61.7.671

Werch, C. E., & Owen, D. M. (2002). Iatrogenic effects of alcohol and drug prevention programs. *Journal of Studies on Alcohol, 63*, 581–590.

West, S. L, & O'Neal, K. K. (2004). Project D.A.R.E. outcome effectiveness revisited. *American Journal of Public Health, 94*, 1027–1029.

Westen, D. (1998). The scientific legacy of Sigmund Freud: Toward a psychodynamically informed psychological science. *Psychological Bulletin, 124*, 333–371.

Westen, D., & Bradley, R. (2005). Empirically Supported Complexity. Rethinking Evidence-Based Practice in Psychotherapy. *Current Directions in Psychological Science, 14*(5), 266–271.

Westen, D., Novotny, C. M., & Thompson-Brenner, H. (2004). The empirical status of empirically supported psychotherapies: assumptions, findings, and reporting in controlled clinical trials. *Psychological Bulletin, 130*, 631–663.

Westen, D., Novotny, C. M., & Thompson-Brenner, H. (2005). EBP =/ EST: Reply to Crits-Christoph et al. (2005) and Weisz et al. (2005). *Psychological Bulletin, 131*(3), 427–433.

White, W. L. (1998). *Slaying the dragon: The history of addiction treatment and recovery in America.* Bloomington, IL: Chestnut Health Systems.

Wilkins, W. (1983). Failure of placebo groups to control for nonspecific events in therapy outcome research. *Psychotherapy: Theory, Research and Practice, 20,* 31–37.

Wilkins, W. (1984). Psychotherapy: The powerful placebo. *Journal of Consulting and Clinical Psychology, 52,* 570–573.

Williams, A.C.d.C. (2002). Facial expression of pain: An evolutionary account. *Behavioral and Brain Sciences, 25*(4), 439–488. doi: 10.1017/s0140525x02000080

Willis, J., & Todorov, A. (2006). First Impressions: Making Up Your Mind After a 100-Ms Exposure to a Face. *Psychological Science, 17*(7), 592–598. doi: 10.1111/j.1467-9280.2006.01750.x

Wilson, E. O. (1978). *On human nature.* Cambridge, MA: Harvard University Press.

Wilson, E. O. (2012). *The social conquest of earth.* New York: Liveright Publishing

Wilson, G. T. (1982). How Useful is Meta-analysis in Evaluating the Effects of Different Psychological Therapies? *Behavioural Psychotherapy, 10,* 221–231.

Wilson, G. T. (1996). Manual-based treatments: The clinical application of research findings. *Behaviour Research and Therapy, 34,* 295–314.

Wilson, G. T., & Rachman, S. J. (1983). Meta-analysis and the evaluation of psychotherapy outcome: Limitations and liabilities. *Journal of Consulting and Clinical Psychology, 51*(1), 54.

Wolpe, J. (1952a). Experimental neuroses as learned behavior. *British Journal of Psychology, 43,* 243–268.

Wolpe, J. (1952b). Objective psychotherapy of the neuroses. *South African Medical Journal, 26,* 825–829.

Wolpe, J. (1954). Reciprocal inhibition as the main basis of psychotherapeutic effects. *American Medical Association Archives of Neurological Psychiatry, 72,* 205–226.

Wolpe, J. (1958). *Psychotherapy by reciprocal inhibition.* Palo Alto, CA: Stanford University.

Woody, G. E., Luborsky, L., McLellan, A. T., Obrien, C. P., Beck, A. T., Blaine, J., . . . Hole, A. (1983). Psychotherapy for opiate addicts—does it help? *Archives of General Psychiatry, 40*(6), 639–645.

Worrell, M., & Longmore, R. J. (2008). Challenging Hofmann's negative thoughts: A rebuttal. *Clinical Psychology Review, 28*(1), 71–74. doi: 10.1016/j.cpr.2007.03.004

Zuroff, D. C., & Blatt, S. J. (2006). The therapeutic relationship in brief treatment of depression: Contributions to clinical improvement and enhanced adaptive capacities. *Journal of Consulting and Clinical Psychology, 74,* 130–140.

Zuroff, D. C., Kelly, A. C., Leybman, M. J., Blatt, S. J., & Wampold, B. E. (2010). Between-therapist and within-therapist differences in the quality of the therapeutic relationship: Effects on maladjustment and self-critical perfectionism. *Journal of Clinical Psychology, 66,* 681–697. doi: 10.1002/jclp.20683

Index